T0177468

Flexibility within Fidelity

Flexibility within Fidelity

Breathing Life into a Psychological Treatment Manual

EDITED BY PHILIP C. KENDALL

OXFORD

UNIVERSITY PRESS

Oxford University Press is a department of the University of Oxford. It furthers
the University's objective of excellence in research, scholarship, and education
by publishing worldwide. Oxford is a registered trade mark of Oxford University
Press in the UK and certain other countries.

Published in the United States of America by Oxford University Press
198 Madison Avenue, New York, NY 10016, United States of America.

© Oxford University Press 2022

All rights reserved. No part of this publication may be reproduced, stored in
a retrieval system, or transmitted, in any form or by any means, without the
prior permission in writing of Oxford University Press, or as expressly permitted
by law, by license, or under terms agreed with the appropriate reproduction
rights organization. Inquiries concerning reproduction outside the scope of the
above should be sent to the Rights Department, Oxford University Press, at the
address above.

You must not circulate this work in any other form
and you must impose this same condition on any acquirer.

Library of Congress Cataloging-in-Publication Data
Names: Kendall, Philip C., editor.
Title: Flexibility within fidelity: Breathing life into a psychological treatment manual /
[edited by Philip C. Kendall].
Description: New York, NY : Oxford University Press, [2022] |
Includes bibliographical references and index.
Identifiers: LCCN 2021012194 (print) | LCCN 2021012195 (ebook) |
ISBN 9780197552155 (paperback) | ISBN 9780197552179 (epub) |
ISBN 9780197552186
Subjects: LCSH: Psychotherapy. | Adaptability (Psychology) |
Medicine, Empirical.
Classification: LCC RC480.F557 2021 (print) | LCC RC480 (ebook) |
DDC 616.89/14—dc23
LC record available at https://lccn.loc.gov/2021012194
LC ebook record available at https://lccn.loc.gov/2021012195

DOI: 10.1093/med-psych/9780197552155.001.0001

9 8 7 6 5 4 3 2 1

Printed by Marquis, Canada

CONTENTS

CONTRIBUTORS

Jennifer R. Alexander, PhD
Postdoctoral Associate
Department of Psychiatry and
  Behavioral Sciences
University of Minnesota

Jafar Bakhshaie, MD, PhD
Clinical and Research Fellow
Integrated Brain Health Clinical and
  Research Program, Department of
  Psychiatry
Massachusetts General Hospital/
  Harvard Medical School

Christiana Bratiotis, PhD
Associate Professor
School of Social Work
The University of British
  Columbia

Haley M. Brickman, PhD
Postdoctoral Scientist
Big Lots Behavioral Health Services
  and Division of Child and Family
  Psychiatry
Nationwide Children's Hospital

Rachel M. Butler, MA
Doctoral Candidate
Department of Psychology
Temple University

Margaret E. Crane, MA
Clinical Psychology PhD Student
Department of Psychology
Temple University

Michelle G. Craske, PhD
Professor
Department of Psychology
University of California

Laura Nelson Darling, MA
Doctoral Student
Department of Psychological and
  Brain Sciences
Boston University

James D. Doorley, PhD
Clinical and Research Fellow
Integrated Brain Health Clinical and
  Research Program, Department of
  Psychiatry
Massachusetts General Hospital/
  Harvard Medical School

Iony D. Ezawa, PhD
Department of Psychology
The Ohio State University

Martin E. Franklin, PhD
Director of Clinical Services
Rogers Behavioral Health in
  Philadelphia

Mary A. Fristad, PhD
Director, Academic Affairs and
  Research Development
Division of Child and Family
  Psychiatry/Big Lots Behavioral
  Health Services
Nationwide Children's
  Hospital

Elizabeth A. Gosch, PhD, ABPP
Professor
Department of Clinical
  Psychology
Philadelphia College of Osteopathic
  Medicine

Victoria A. Grunberg, PhD
Clinical and Research Fellow
Integrated Brain Health Clinical and
  Research Program, Department of
  Psychiatry
Massachusetts General Hospital/
  Harvard Medical School

Richard G. Heimberg, PhD
Thaddeus L. Bolton Professor
Department of Psychology
Temple University

Shannon Jones, MSW
Program Manager
Center for Youth Development and
  Intervention
University of Alabama

Sarah G. Turk Karan, BA
Research Assistant
Department of Psychology
Brandeis University

Philip C. Kendall, PhD, ABPP
Distinguished University Professor
  and Laura H. Carnell Professor of
  Psychology
Department of Psychology
Temple University

Ethan G. Lester, PhD
Assistant Director of Clinical
  Innovation
Integrated Brain Health Clinical and
  Research Program, Department of
  Psychiatry
Massachusetts General Hospital/
  Harvard Medical School

Ovsanna Leyfer, PhD
Research Assistant Professor
Department of Psychological and
  Brain Sciences
Boston University

Scott Litwack, PhD
Staff Psychologist and Assistant
  Professor
Mental Health and Department of
  Psychiatry
VA Boston Healthcare System and
  Boston University School of
  Medicine

John E. Lochman, PhD
Saxon Professor Emeritus of
  Psychology
Department of Psychology
The University of Alabama

Ryan A. Mace, PhD
Clinical and Research Fellow
Integrated Brain Health Clinical and
  Research Program, Department of
  Psychiatry
Massachusetts General Hospital/
  Harvard Medical School

Abby Adler Mandel, PhD
Assistant Professor
Department of Psychology
The Catholic University of America

Lindsay Myerberg, MA
Department of Psychology
Temple University

Lesley A. Norris, MA
Graduate Student
Department of Clinical
  Psychology
Temple University

Emily B. O'Day, MA
Clinical Psychology Doctoral
  Student
Department of Psychology
Temple University

John D. Otis, PhD
Research Associate Professor
Department of Psychological and
  Brain Sciences
Boston University

Suzanne Otte, MS, MBA, MSW, LCSW
Lecturer
School of Social Work
Boston University

Donna B. Pincus, PhD
Professor
Department of Psychological and
  Brain Sciences
Boston University

Nicole P. Powell, PhD, MPH
Research Psychologist
Center for Youth Development and
  Intervention
University of Alabama

Mira Reichman, BA
Clinical Research Coordinator
Integrated Brain Health Clinical and
  Research Program, Department of
  Psychiatry
Massachusetts General
  Hospital/Harvard Medical
  School

Lara S. Rifkin, MA
Graduate Student
Department of Psychology
Temple University

Amy R. Sewart, PhD
Assistant Professor
Department of Psychology
California State University,
  Dominguez Hills

Colleen A. Sloan, PhD
Clinical Psychologist and Assistant
  Professor
Department of Psychology
VA Boston Healthcare System and
  Boston University School of
  Medicine

Denise M. Sloan, PhD
Associate Director and Professor
National Center for PTSD and
  Department of Psychiatry
VA Boston Healthcare System and
  Boston University School of
  Medicine

Gail Steketee, PhD, MSW
Professor Emerita
School of Social Work
Boston University

Jordan T. Stiede, MS
Graduate Student
Department of Psychology
Marquette University

Daniel R. Strunk, PhD
Professor of Psychology
Department of Psychology
The Ohio State University

Ana-Maria Vranceanu, PhD
Associate Professor of Psychology;
  Director, Integrated Brain Health
  Clinical and Research Program
Department of Psychiatry
Massachusetts General Hospital/
  Harvard Medical School

Douglas W. Woods, PhD
Dean of the Graduate School
Marquette University

Introduction

Does the Treatment Program Fit for My Case?

PHILIP C. KENDALL ■

Imagine the following private and confidential conversation between two mental health service providers. Person A and Person B are talking about Bob, Person A's 34-year-old client who meets criteria for Generalized Anxiety Disorder (GAD). The client has had a prior episode of depression, and has a variety of current complicating life circumstances including restricted physical mobility. He lives with his parents, is divorced, and has limited financial resources.

Person A says, "I've worked with anxiety issues before, including GAD, but not with much luck . . . and this guy sure has anxiety. He avoids work and friends and worries about everything. There's a catastrophe around every corner."

Person B comments, "There's this CBT program I read about. It's highly supported, and I hear good things about it."

Person A replies, "Oh yeah, I've heard of it, and I read a little bit about it, too. I hear it's effective, but is it right for Bob?

Mental health service providers hear a lot about clients who inspire the question, "Does this case fit the general finding?" In the case of Bob, the general finding is that CBT is the treatment of choice. The question is critical and cuts across clinical decision-making. How can mental health professionals sharpen their skills at making such decisions? Exactly how good are we at determining whether generally supported findings are applicable to individual clients?

Early in the development of the science of clinical psychology, Paul Meehl discussed the conditions under which one should consider a case to be an exception to a general empirical finding (see also Dawes et al., 1989). Restating his question in the context of this book, "Is this empirically supported treatment right for my case?" Or, "Does it fit for Bob?"

This is not an easy question to answer. How do we best apply general findings to an individual case? Interested readers also can pursue discussions of ergodicity.

An important and preliminary point to consider in attempting to answer this question comes from the science of decision-making: Like most people, mental health service providers are prone to making too many exceptions when considering whether an individual "fits" within a larger population. Specifically, when thinking about applying an intervention program to a specific case we are tempted to think that the case, for whatever reason, is somehow justified as an exception to the rule. "That program isn't right for Bob," we are more likely to conclude. We are prone to thinking that, for some reason or set of reasons, the circumstances of our case support departing from the empirical findings. This bias has contributed to the underutilization of empirically supported treatments.

We need not fall prey to this cognitive processing error. We can account for variations in race, ethnicity, comorbidity, culture, socioeconomic status, life circumstances, and so forth, when implementing an empirically supported treatment (EST), and we can be flexible with the EST when working with different clients. Research findings typically carry more information and more weight than the unique "features" of the individual that we are so often led to believe dictate the nonapplicability of the treatment.

As much as we may wish to deny it, as Meehl (1957) and others have shown (see Grove & Lloyd, 2006), actuarial (following the data) prediction is superior to clinical (our thinking) prediction. There is strength in properly conducted treatment evaluations, and confidence can and should be placed in the findings of these strong studies. Placing confidence in the findings of randomized controlled trials (RCTs) is wise and appropriate application of science. There is less wisdom in placing confidence in the hunches that lead us to believe a treatment program is not applicable. If we are to provide the best care, we must admit that when we claim that a program "doesn't fit for Bob," we are guessing; our hunches are not empirically supported. We humans, and mental health professionals are no exception, tend to place too much confidence in our subjective judgments. We assign them too much importance, and we tend to do so too frequently.

Thinking that we "know" why a particular treatment may not be appropriate goes beyond the data. A more humble and accurate perspective is to suspect that a certain feature of the client may be important, and to take this into account when implementing the empirically supported treatment program. Take the client's specifics into account and apply the known-to-be-effective treatment with flexibility . . . flexibility within fidelity.[1]

For example, assume for the moment that you are working with a Haitian woman who meets diagnostic criteria for a depressive disorder. You have prior training in a few approaches to treatment and you decide to follow a cognitive behavioral (CBT) approach. You have some materials from a workshop you attended on CBT for depression, and you plan to use them in the provision of services.

---

1. Please be cautious when pronouncing the phrase "flexibility within fidelity." I am arguing for flexibility in applying a program while also maintaining fidelity to the program. It is flexibility *within* fidelity (not flexibility with infidelity).

You also review some of your notes from the training. You work with the client to address depressogenic self-talk and include behavioral activation and behavioral experiments. Pleasant activities are tried out, homework tasks are assigned, and most are completed. But because the client lives in a rural environment, with limited access to several of the positive events included on the list you received in your training, you reduce the list to include only those that are potentially available to the client and supplement with several you come up with on your own. Did the treatment you provided have integrity? Was the treatment applied with flexibility?

Suppose you are working with a socially anxious Caucasian male adult, following a program such as that described by Heimberg and his colleagues (see Chapter 1). You have materials available to you and you have refreshed your understanding of the treatment manual. As you move along through the program the client is generally cooperative, displays self-awareness, and engages with the dialogue that occurs in session. You believe that progress is being made and you opt not to ask the client to do homework because he has expressed an unwillingness to do homework, and you don't want the client to be dissatisfied. At the end of treatment, the client reports some progress and you feel satisfied that some progress was made. Did the treatment you provided have integrity? Was the treatment applied with flexibility *and* fidelity?

What if you are working with a teenager who is aggressive, and you are implementing a 16-week program (à la Lochman, Chapter 11). The teen, in this instance a 14-year-old Latina with an intellectual disability, has had difficulty with some of the concepts of problem solving. You adapt the section on problem solving and extend this part of the program to help ensure that the concepts are communicated effectively; this ends up taking 20 sessions instead of 16. Did the treatment you provided have integrity? Was the treatment applied with flexibility?

Your client is an anxious 12-year-old. You are using the *Coping Cat* program and employ psychoeducation about anxiety. You provide opportunities for exposure tasks, along with homework assignments and rewards. You teach the client about self-talk, problem solving, and emotional understanding. You skip the session on relaxation training because the youth already had been taught deep breathing and relaxation, and he demonstrated that he knew it. Did the treatment you provided have integrity? Was the treatment applied with flexibility?

In short, which components of treatment are necessary to maintain fidelity? And how can these known-to-be-effective programs be implemented with flexibility, such that they are appropriate for a specific client but also faithful to the original protocol?

What follows in this book are answers to these and related questions.

REFERENCES

Butler, R., O'Day, E., & Heimberg, R. (2021). Cognitive behavioral therapy for social anxiety: Being flexible while maintaining fidelity. In P. C. Kendall (Ed), *Flexibility within fidelity: Breathing life into a manual* (pp.). Oxford University Press.

Dawes, R. Faust, D., & Meehl, P. (1989). Clinical versus actuarial judgment. *Science, 243,* 1668–1674. doi: 10.1126/science.2648573

Grove, W. M., & Lloyd, M. (2006). Meehl's contribution to clinical versus statistical prediction. *Journal of Abnormal Psychology, 115*(2), 192–194. doi.org/10.1037/ 0021-843X.115.2.192

Lochman, J., Powell, N., & Jones, S. (2021) The Coping Power program for children with aggressive behavior problems. In P. C. Kendall (Ed), *Flexibility within fidelity: Breathing life into a manual* (pp.). Oxford University Press.

Meehl, P. E. (1957). When shall we use our heads instead of the formula? *Journal of Counseling Psychology, 4,* 268–273. doi.org/10.1037/h0047554

Rifkin, L., Myerberg, L., Norris, L., Gosch, E., & Kendall, P. C. (2021). In P. C. Kendall (Ed), *Flexibility within fidelity: Breathing life into a manual.* Oxford University Press, 2021.

1

Cognitive Behavioral Therapy for Social Anxiety Disorder

Being Flexible While Maintaining Fidelity

RACHEL M. BUTLER, EMILY B. O'DAY, AND
RICHARD G. HEIMBERG ■

DECLARATION OF INTEREST

Richard G. Heimberg is a coauthor of the commercially available treatment manual reviewed in this chapter. The authors have no other conflicts of interest to report.

BACKGROUND

Social anxiety disorder (SAD) is a mental health condition marked by impairment and distress across a number of social situations. Individuals with SAD fear negative evaluation from others and typically avoid social situations due to these fears (American Psychiatric Association, 2013; Clark & Wells, 1995; Rapee & Heimberg, 1997). Social anxiety is a common and relatable experience for most people; everyone is likely to experience some level of anxiety in a social setting, such as when giving a presentation or meeting someone for the first time, at some point in their lives. Importantly, however, social anxiety exists on a continuum, ranging from mild nervousness in social settings to more severe and debilitating anxiety and avoidance of social interactions, likely resulting in impaired functioning and a diagnosis of SAD. SAD is relatively prevalent, with about 7% of adults meeting diagnostic criteria in any 12-month period (Kessler et al., 2005). Given its high prevalence both as a lived experience in people's daily lives and as a psychological disorder, SAD has become an important target of psychological intervention.

Individuals with SAD may benefit from psychological treatment targeting anxious thoughts about social situations and related patterns of avoidance.

A wealth of research over the last several decades has demonstrated that cognitive behavioral therapy (CBT) is an efficacious and effective treatment for SAD (see meta-analyses by Acarturk, Cuijpers, van Straten, & de Graaf, 2009; Barkowski et al., 2016; Mayo-Wilson et al., 2014; Powers, Sigmarsson, & Emmelkamp, 2008). Through the use of psychoeducation, cognitive restructuring, and exposure or behavioral experiments, CBT for SAD helps socially anxious individuals understand their social anxiety and how it affects their lives, learn to identify and challenge negative beliefs about themselves and their social world, and approach rather than avoid feared social situations. CBT for SAD has been shown to improve individuals' experience of social anxiety, both immediately after treatment and in the years following, indicating that treatment gains are lasting and maintained over time (for a narrative systematic review of CBT for SAD, see Kaplan, Swee, & Heimberg, 2018). For this chapter, we focus on one specific manualized protocol of individual CBT for SAD, *Managing Social Anxiety: A Cognitive Behavioral Approach*, now in its third edition (Hope, Heimberg, & Turk, 2019a, 2019b).

Individual CBT for SAD following the *Managing Social Anxiety* protocol has been shown to be efficacious in randomized controlled trials (RCTs) and effective in clinical settings. In one RCT, Ledley and colleagues (2009) found that, compared to waitlist controls, individuals with SAD who received CBT experienced substantial improvement over the course of treatment, indicated by decreases in social anxiety and social anxiety-related impairment. Goldin and colleagues (2012) similarly examined this protocol and found that CBT for SAD led to reductions in social anxiety at posttreatment and at one-year follow-up. Recently, Butler, O'Day, Swee, Horenstein, and Heimberg (2021) examined the use of this treatment protocol in a university outpatient clinic and found that after 20 weeks of treatment, individuals with SAD showed reductions in social anxiety and improvements in their quality of life. Additionally, individuals who endorsed more extreme cognitive distortions and greater use of safety behaviors before treatment showed greater improvements in their social anxiety at posttreatment. Thus, by emphasizing the importance of challenging cognitive distortions through cognitive restructuring and decreasing use of safety behaviors through exposures as core treatment components, this treatment protocol may be of most benefit to those who exhibit these features of social anxiety.

Manualized, workbook-driven protocols for CBT for SAD, such as ours, hold promise for promoting evidence-based practice across clinical settings. Not only does the protocol offer a structured framework to guide therapists through therapy sessions, but it also provides clients with their own set of resources (e.g., workbook, worksheets) to bolster what is learned in the therapy room and bring it into their daily lives. These materials include a therapist guide and session outlines to inform treatment planning, as well as a client workbook (Hope et al., 2019a, 2019b) with corresponding worksheets to translate session material into home practice. In addition, the manual and accompanying resources are accessible broadly, allowing for dissemination and implementation of its use across clinical settings and to novice and experienced clinicians alike.

These materials emphasize the importance of a client-centered approach to treatment that can be applied flexibly and adapted to the needs of the individual client: "flexibility within fidelity" (Kendall & Frank, 2018; Kendall, Gosch, Furr, & Sood, 2008). Importantly, clinicians and clients work collaboratively to identify how treatment can best match client-specific social fears and patterns of avoidance. Although key components of the treatment are required for fidelity, there is substantial flexibility built into the structure of the protocol and each component, including the number of treatment sessions, the approach to cognitive restructuring, the content of the fear and avoidance hierarchy, and the focus of exposure exercises conducted in session and as homework assignments, as well as how co-morbid psychological disorders are addressed, all of which are discussed in the following sections.

KEY COMPONENTS OF TREATMENT REQUIRED FOR FIDELITY

Our treatment protocol includes several required components. These include psychoeducation about the nature of SAD, cognitive restructuring focused on automatic thoughts, in-session exposures, homework (e.g., cognitive restructuring and exposures), and advanced cognitive restructuring focused on core beliefs. Omission of any one of these components could result in clients not receiving the full benefit of this treatment, although any specific component may be shaped to best fit the needs and abilities of the individual client.

The initial stage of treatment is psychoeducation, which involves guiding the client to a better understanding of their own social anxiety. Psychoeducation begins by orienting the client to the treatment program, distinguishing SAD from the social anxiety of everyday life, and identifying physical, cognitive, and behavioral features of social anxiety. Importantly, the therapist helps the client identify what they value in life and how this may have been adversely affected by their social anxiety; identifying individualized, valued goals related to managing one's social anxiety helps sustain motivation throughout treatment. During this phase, the therapist also learns a great deal about the client's social anxiety and associated impairment, which then guides work during later phases of treatment (e.g., cognitive restructuring and exposure). Following each psychoeducation session, homework is assigned to help the client self-monitor cognitive, behavioral, and physical features of their social anxiety, so that they can develop an awareness of how their social anxiety manifests across social situations in their daily life. The fear and avoidance hierarchy is also created collaboratively during the psychoeducation phase, based on situations the client deems anxiety-provoking and relevant to their life. Psychoeducation then moves on to examine potential genetic, environmental, and social etiological factors that the client believes may have led to the development of their social anxiety. By the end of the psychoeducation phase, the goal is for the client and therapist to have developed a common language with which to discuss aspects of social anxiety and for the client to have a good grasp on how their own social anxiety manifests and is maintained.

Cognitive restructuring is the next key component. This phase of the program begins with teaching the client about the connection between an event, beliefs about or interpretations of the event, and the emotional and behavioral consequences associated with those interpretations or beliefs. We emphasize that it is the interpretation of the event, rather than the event itself, that leads to the client's anxiety and avoidance. The therapist introduces the concept of automatic thoughts, which are defined as negative thoughts about oneself, the world, or the future that occur spontaneously in social situations (e.g., "I won't know what to say"). The therapist notes that automatic thoughts are accepted uncritically and are closely related to anxiety and other negative emotions such as shame or embarrassment, so it is crucial that the client begin to notice and challenge the validity of these automatic thoughts.

To challenge automatic thoughts, the client must first have an understanding of the frequently irrational or illogical nature of these thoughts; thus, the therapist introduces the client to a list of thinking errors that characterize the automatic thoughts of individuals with social anxiety (e.g., mind reading, all-or-nothing thinking). The client practices identifying specific thinking errors in case vignettes before moving on to examine thinking errors in their own thoughts. Typically, clients begin to notice patterns of thinking errors that show up in their automatic thoughts across social situations. After clients are able to identify their signature thinking errors, the therapist teaches the client how to use disputing questions (e.g., "What evidence do you have that . . . ?") to challenge these automatic thoughts. The client learns to use the anxious-self/coping-self dialogue, a strategy of using a disputing question to challenge an automatic thought, responding to that question, questioning the response (which may itself contain automatic thoughts), and continuing this process until the client comes to a place of diminished belief in the automatic thought. Finally, the client and therapist design a rational response (i.e., a short, meaningful coping statement related to the conclusion of cognitive restructuring) to be used during a social situation or exposure to help combat automatic thoughts in the moment when they occur. It is helpful if a certain degree of understanding is demonstrated by the client before exposures are initiated so that the client can utilize these skills in conjunction with exposures to address anticipatory anxiety, in-situation anxiety, and postsituation rumination. Throughout the cognitive restructuring portion of treatment, clients are assigned homework related to in-session content, including practice identifying thinking errors and using disputing questions and the anxious-self/coping-self dialogue to challenge automatic thoughts that arise during the week between sessions.

Once the client has demonstrated modest proficiency in cognitive restructuring, the therapist and client move on to the third component of treatment: in-session exposures. In-session exposures allow clients to confront feared social situations and to learn that their anxiety typically decreases the longer they stay in the situation, and, whether this happens or not, they are more capable of performing in the social situation than they expected. Using the fear and avoidance hierarchy, the therapist and client together identify situations for the first few exposures that elicit a moderate level of anxiety, before working up to more anxiety-provoking situations in later exposure sessions. In-session exposures are a critical treatment component for a number of reasons. They allow the therapist to observe the quality of the client's social performance and to identify and target safety behaviors that the client may be unaware they are engaging in (e.g., never asking follow-up questions for fear of appearing stupid). They can be easily structured to test automatic thoughts and beliefs (e.g., conversations go better if you never disagree with someone). Feared outcomes that are unlikely to occur in everyday life but which are nonetheless feared by the client (e.g., a rude or hostile response to a client's social approach) can be incorporated in a controlled way into in-session exposures. In-session exposures also can be designed to work on feared "downstream" behaviors that foster avoidance of earlier steps toward a goal (e.g., fears of intimate self-disclosures, which may inhibit earlier steps in relationship building, fears related to answering questions in job interviews that may inhibit applying for jobs in the first place).

Sessions during the exposure phase of treatment begin with selecting a situation for exposure in-session and then identifying automatic thoughts related to the exposure situation. Cognitive restructuring is implemented, and a rational response is identified for use during the upcoming exposure. Importantly, the client and therapist select an achievable behavioral goal for the exposure, which should be observable to both therapist and client (e.g., make eye contact, ask two questions of the interaction partner). Behavioral goals are critical, because they gradually train the client to move away from maladaptive goals (broadly stated as perfect performance without anxiety) and allow for a more objective assessment of how the client actually performed in the social situation. Once a rational response and behavioral goal are selected, the in-session exposure begins. These exposures typically consist of a role-play scenario involving the therapist or a confederate. The client is asked to rate their Subjective Units of Distress (SUD) on a scale from 0 to 100 at one-minute intervals throughout the in-session exposure. Following the exposure, the client and therapist process the exposure together ("post-exposure cognitive restructuring"), including determining whether the behavioral goal was achieved, whether the client's rated anxiety conformed to their predicted anxiety, and whether the client's negative behavioral predictions were realized. If unanticipated automatic thoughts emerged during the exposure, these can be challenged in the moment or incorporated into cognitive restructuring for future in-session exposures. New or surprising behavioral experiences (e.g., a client who believes that the other person will find them boring is surprised by the number of questions they are asked over the course of a conversation) should also be processed and incorporated into future in-session exposures.

Although in-session cognitive restructuring and exposures are key and important, the client's gains are solidified through exposure assignments to be carried out in the week between sessions. Homework assignments allow for repetition of the lessons learned in in-session exposures, which is necessary for the goals of exposures (i.e., habituation of anxiety, gathering of evidence that disconfirms the client's negative predictions, building of self-efficacy) to be achieved. Exposures outside of session also reinforce the importance of learning to approach and persist in social situations that are important to the client, irrespective of anxiety, because engaging in those social situations is consistent with their values and goals. Clients are instructed to complete a worksheet before the homework exposure that guides them through the steps of cognitive restructuring prior to entering the situation. Then, following the exposure, clients return to the worksheet and identify what they accomplished through the exposure, which is critical given that those with social anxiety often attend to negative outcomes and disqualify positive aspects of the exposure experience. The worksheet also asks clients to compare their predicted outcomes to the actual outcomes, which can lend disconfirming evidence to some of their negative automatic thoughts about the situation. Homework should always be reviewed at the beginning of the following session so that the therapist can provide positive reinforcement and feedback. Repetition of this process is necessary, because homework teaches the client the skills they need to be successful in future social situations and gives the client a sense of autonomy and confidence that they will be able to address social anxiety even when the therapist is not present.

The last major component of treatment is advanced cognitive restructuring or core beliefs work. The goal of advanced cognitive restructuring is to identify deep-seated, strongly held beliefs that the client has about themself that underlie their social anxiety and provide the engine powering automatic thoughts. Core beliefs (e.g., "I am unlovable") are distinguished from more situation-specific automatic thoughts (e.g., "They won't like me"), because they tend to elicit stronger emotions and may be more difficult to access. The therapist and client use previously completed worksheets to examine frequently occurring automatic thoughts, and the themes underlying these automatic thoughts emerge. Emotions elicited by the core beliefs are also felt and discussed. After core beliefs are identified, in-session and homework exposures should be designed that directly test or target these beliefs. Evidence from these exposures can then be used in cognitive restructuring to challenge core beliefs.

When the client is ready to conclude therapy, a termination session is conducted. During this session, the therapist and client review the skills learned over the course of treatment and discuss how the client can continue to practice and use these skills in the future. The therapist and client collaboratively re-rate the client's current level of fear and avoidance for each situation on their hierarchy, which demonstrates tangible gains the client has made over the course of treatment. Both the therapist and client go on to highlight various areas in the client's life in which they have seen improvements and the client has gained self-efficacy. Finally, the therapist and client set a few short-term goals for the client to accomplish within the month after ending therapy. This final goal-setting provides clients with an opportunity to continue working on their social anxiety as they transition out of therapy.

CLIENT-FOCUSED IMPLEMENTATION OF FLEXIBILITY WITHIN FIDELITY

Flexibility with Number of Sessions

The total number of sessions that a client completes as part of this treatment protocol is flexible and client-dependent. In the therapist guide (Hope et al., 2019b), it is suggested that the client complete 16 sessions over a 20-week period. At the beginning of treatment, clients are oriented to how they will progress through the main components of treatment and the typical number of sessions devoted to each treatment component (e.g., four sessions of psychoeducation, two sessions cognitive restructuring, seven to eight sessions of exposures, one to two sessions of core beliefs/advanced cognitive restructuring, one session for termination). However, except when operating within the confines of an RCT, therapists explain to clients that the length and pace of treatment in actuality is client-specific and may vary depending on how the client progresses through key components of treatment. For example, the therapist and client can decide how quickly they move through the protocol. Moving too slowly may bore some clients, whereas a slower pace may allow other clients to better comprehend important information, or come to accept how the information fits for them. On the other hand, moving too fast may leave some clients feeling behind and not ready for later phases of treatment. Thus, the therapist and client decide together how much time should be devoted to teaching certain concepts, such as identifying the physical, cognitive, and behavioral components of social anxiety during the psychoeducation phase; learning a specific skill such as identifying thinking errors; or practicing the anxious-self/ coping-self dialogue in the cognitive restructuring phase; or completing various exposures during the exposure phase. Whereas some clients may need to dedicate more time to understanding their own social anxiety during psychoeducation, other clients may already have a strong grasp on the components of social anxiety and how it affects their life, and they therefore can spend less time learning about social anxiety at the beginning of treatment. For example, although many clients find the psychoeducation session on potential genetic, environmental, and social etiological factors related to social anxiety interesting, the therapist could flexibly decide to remove this session if it is evident that the client has a strong grasp on how their social anxiety developed and has been maintained over time.

There is flexibility in the number of therapy sessions that can be devoted to each treatment component. Some individuals may have greater difficulty differentiating between physical, cognitive, and behavioral features of social anxiety, so additional sessions may be devoted to monitoring how social anxiety manifests for the specific client and differentiating these experiences. Alternatively, some clients may identify strongly with the cognitive component of treatment, believing that their social fears and worries are most debilitating; for these clients, therapists may want to devote a greater number of sessions to learning cognitive restructuring skills so that clients are able to confidently challenge their negative automatic thoughts before beginning exposures. Further, there may be variability in the number of exposure sessions completed, based on the different types of social situations that a client generates for their fear and avoidance hierarchy. Nevertheless, although there is flexibility, this protocol does require a minimum of four (and preferred minimum of six) exposure sessions to be conducted during treatment. If a client is predominantly fearful of public speaking situations, the majority of in-session exposures may be devoted to this specific concern. In contrast, other clients may fear a wide range of social situations (e.g., conversations, public speaking situations, dating, and eating/drinking while being observed by others), and more exposures may be needed to address the range of feared situations adequately. Although the manual emphasizes that not every social situation on the hierarchy needs to be the focus of in-session or homework exposures, it may be important to add additional exposure sessions into the therapy framework if the client's feared situations are more variable. One important note of caution, however, is that clients (or therapists!) who are anxious about doing exposures may tend to linger on earlier material as an avoidance strategy. It is important to remember that clients may not feel "ready" to begin exposures, but cognitive restructuring and other skills can continue to be refined after entering the exposure phase.

The termination of treatment is a collaborative process, determined by both therapist and client based on a variety of factors, including therapist and client availability, the client's financial resources to continue care, client readiness, and measurable improvements in social anxiety and related avoidance. Whereas many clients may feel they have gained sufficient skills and seen improvement over 20 sessions or less and are ready to terminate, other clients may benefit from a longer course of treatment. Recently, we explored whether clients who continued care in our clinic beyond 20 sessions saw additional improvements in their social anxiety symptoms compared to clients who completed 20 or fewer sessions of treatment. Those who continued treatment after 20 sessions had not experienced as much improvement as those who completed treatment at session 20 or earlier but experienced additional decreases in social anxiety from session 20 to their final assessment (Butler, O'Day, & Heimberg, 2020). A longer course of treatment may elicit meaningful improvements for some individuals with SAD using our protocol, so the number of treatment sessions should be determined flexibly, taking a collaborative approach.

Flexibility with Cognitive Restructuring

There is flexibility within the protocol in the cognitive component of treatment, in which clients are taught how to use cognitive restructuring skills to identify errors in their thinking and challenge negative automatic thoughts that exacerbate their experience of social anxiety. As highlighted previously, cognitive restructuring emphasizes that clients' interpretation of events, rather than the events themselves, lead to negative emotional and behavioral consequences, so effort is devoted to helping clients change their interpretation of events and identify more logical and realistic thoughts to counteract their anxious fears.

There are several ways that therapists may approach cognitive restructuring flexibly with a given client, based on the nature of the automatic thoughts the client brings into session. In one circumstance, if an automatic thought appears to be illogical in nature, therapists may opt to focus on highlighting the thinking errors within the automatic thought, use the anxious-self/coping-self dialogue to challenge the illogical nature of the thought, and ultimately arrive at a rational response. This type of illogical automatic thought pattern commonly arises if clients frequently engage in all-or-nothing thinking or regularly catastrophize or imagine worst-case scenarios for future events. For example, if a client has the thought, "everyone will think I'm stupid," when giving a presentation, the therapist may help the client investigate what the label "stupid" means to the client and highlight that their definition of "stupid" may not be in line with the literal definition of stupidity. The anxious-self/coping-self dialogue may illuminate, for this specific client, that the label "stupid" simply means they may have to pause to collect their thoughts from time to time during the presentation, which the therapist can argue is not the same thing as coming across as "stupid." If the therapist and client instead can generate a rational response, such as, "taking a pause to collect my thoughts during the presentation does not mean I'm stupid," the client may be able to say this to themself when anxiety peaks during the presentation and notice that their fear of looking stupid is not the same as taking a pause.

In other circumstances, an automatic thought that the client generates may actually be logical, but the feared consequences that make up the content of subsequent automatic thoughts are unlikely. In these scenarios, cognitive restructuring can be flexibly used to highlight the true likelihood of the client's feared outcome, or the gravity of the feared outcome should it occur, to disconfirm the belief. In these scenarios, cognitive restructuring and exposures together can be conceptualized as a behavioral experiment to test out whether the feared outcome is likely to actually happen, and if it does happen, whether it is something the client can tolerate. For example, a client's fear may be that in a conversation with someone, there will be silences. Because silences are a natural part of conversations, it is important to discuss the likelihood that they will occur. The therapist may be able to validate that silences may be awkward or feel uncomfortable but that they may not reflect negatively on the client or on the quality of the conversation. The therapist may challenge how long of a silence is expected by the client. Commonly, individuals with social anxiety fear that a silence will never end and the conversation will never resume. As a result, the therapist may ask the client to predict how long a silence in a conversation might last, which can be tested later in the exposure. In this case, the therapist and client together can come to a rational response that silences are normal, but they won't last more than a few seconds. They also may highlight that this is something the client could tolerate. It also may be important for the therapist to explore what a silence means to the client and use cognitive restructuring to challenge whether it is a sign that the client is a poor conversationalist (or in some other way has failed to meet a standard). Again, in these scenarios, in which a feared outcome may be somewhat likely, the therapist has an opportunity to challenge whether the feared outcome is likely to be as attached to negative consequences as the client expects.

Moreover, if a similar pattern of negative automatic thoughts recurs for clients in early sessions, therapists also have the option to flexibly incorporate more advanced cognitive restructuring/core beliefs work into treatment earlier. Examining how and why core beliefs developed may facilitate the treatment process for the client. Further, once core beliefs are identified, the therapist may be able to create exposures to directly challenge and disconfirm those core beliefs earlier in treatment. For example, if a client's underlying belief is "I am unlovable," the therapist may choose to identify disconfirming evidence for this belief as part of the early cognitive structuring process; the therapist may be able to use cognitive restructuring to broaden the client's definition of what it means to be lovable and identify people in their life or opportunities, big or small, wherein they can create positive encounters in which they are liked or enjoyed by others. The flexibility of this approach may allow gains to be made sooner in the exposure phase of treatment.

There are many other ways to teach core cognitive restructuring principles. For example, clients who have fears about small talk and the automatic thought that they "won't have anything interesting to say" can be given the homework assignment to eavesdrop on conversations around them (e.g., between coworkers, people in the grocery store checkout line, passengers on public transportation) to provide evidence that small talk is typically about common things such as the weather, rather than more unique conversational topics that need to be researched or prepared. Alternatively, therapists could ask clients whether they believe they take a competitive approach to social interactions, which may be evidenced by their automatic thoughts, and work with the client to generate more cooperative rational responses to challenge their competitive beliefs. In many scenarios, it may be beneficial to veer away from the step-by-step instructions of the anxious self/coping self dialogue to structure cognitive restructuring in session and instead help the client reinvent the cognitive restructuring process in a way that will be helpful to them. Clients may benefit from generating their own disputing questions when they think about challenging their automatic thoughts, so that they are able to easily replicate this cognitive restructuring process and generate disputing questions readily outside the therapy room.

Troubleshooting with cognitive restructuring may be needed if the therapist notices that the client feels stuck and cannot seem to generate disputing questions or alternative perspectives to challenge their original point of view. The therapist may need to pivot and provide an alternative perspective for the client to consider. Furthermore, cognitive restructuring may need to be de-emphasized for some clients. Although cognitive restructuring is an important part of treatment and can be applied flexibly in a variety of ways (as noted above), some clients have difficulty grasping the steps in the cognitive restructuring process. Such clients may benefit from devoting less time to cognitive restructuring before exposures and more time to in vivo exposures and postexposure debriefing about their anxious thoughts. For example, for clients who are lower in intellectual functioning, are highly concrete, or who have difficulty verbalizing their automatic thoughts, therapists may need to provide a rational response for clients to repeat to themselves when anxious during the exposure and begin the exposure more quickly in session. In this scenario, the therapist may devote more time following exposures to highlighting the anxious thoughts that arose during the exposure and examining how helpful the rational response was for the client, rather than determining whether their potential anxious thoughts did or did not come true. Additionally, if a client has learned English as a second language, it may be beneficial to have the client do the cognitive restructuring homework exercises in their primary language and then translate them in session with the therapist. Regardless of the shape cognitive restructuring takes, it should be flexibly and adaptably used to help the client consider alternative ways of thinking.

Flexibility with Hierarchy Creation and Use

Generating the fear and avoidance hierarchy offers another area of potential flexibility within the protocol. This process is typically a collaborative one in which the client brainstorms situations they may wish to include on the list and the therapist works with the client to refine the list and add any new items based on what the therapist knows about the client thus far. The client workbook gives a number of suggestions, which are typically helpful in jumpstarting the client's brainstorming process. Although some general ideas are given in the workbook, it is imperative that the hierarchy be a highly specific, client-centered list of feared social situations. Clients typically present to treatment because social anxiety is acutely interfering with their lives in one or more domains, and the clinician should be sure that situations from those domains are well represented on the hierarchy. For example, consider a client who seeks treatment due to the difficulty she is experiencing at work. She is required to present her work in weekly meetings and periodically consult with her boss about her progress on the projects in her purview. She finds it difficult to ask questions and thus has made several otherwise avoidable mistakes. In her personal life, she is less disturbed by social anxiety and is able to socialize with several friends and her partner. For this client, we would want to construct a hierarchy that is highly focused on social and performance situations that arise in her workplace. Items on her hierarchy might include giving a presentation in front of a small group and then a larger group, speaking with an authority figure, and asking questions or asking for help. It may be less important to include social situations outside of work, given that the client is satisfied with her functioning in that area. Thus, the hierarchy guides exposures to focus on situations that are particularly relevant to the client's current life and functioning in specific domains.

Although we may create a hierarchy that includes a range of social situations, we rarely work our way sequentially up the hierarchy when planning exposures. Typically, we begin with moderately anxiety-provoking situations on the hierarchy (e.g., a SUDS rating of 40 to 60) and work our way up to more feared situations.

We tend to focus, however, on exposures based on hierarchy items that are of most immediate relevance or value in the client's life. To continue with the above example, if the client needs to give an important presentation the following week, we would move to complete that exposure in the session, even if it is not the next item on the hierarchy. For another client who is about to begin his first semester of college, we might focus on exposures related to making friends (e.g., small talk, inviting others to get coffee) and move away from less relevant exposures for the time being. In our experience, the client tends to gain more from practicing and mastering these relevant situations through exposures than they would from continuing sequentially through other hierarchy items. We find that successful experiences in valued situations tend to generalize to other social situations.

Another important way in which we are flexible in using the hierarchy is when what we choose to do in a given exposure is largely determined, collaboratively, by what happened in the last one. Thus, you may go deeper into the first area based on the way things turn out in the initial exposure rather than moving on to another hierarchy item. Consider a case in which we start with a small talk exposure, and the client fears they will not know what to say during the conversation. Following this exposure, the client mentions that there was an "awkward silence" in which they became very uncomfortable and feared it would never end. The therapist is then likely to design the next exposure to address the client's fear of silences. In this way, automatic thoughts or feared consequences uncovered in one exposure often dictate the content of the next exposure. Altogether, adaptable use of the hierarchy involves centering it around the client's goals and values, designing exposures that directly address situations relevant to the client's current life, and adding items to the hierarchy as they reveal themselves during exposures.

Flexibility with Exposures

The therapist has a vast degree of latitude when it comes to designing exposures to target a client's particular fears of social situations. The setting of in-session exposures can be within the therapy room or in any other location that might better target the client's fears (i.e., "in-session" does not automatically equate to "in the therapy room"). For a client who fears making a mistake and embarrassing themselves while ordering at a restaurant, the therapist may go with them to several local eateries to order food. For another client who fears public speaking, the therapist may decide to gather a number of confederates and have the client give a speech in a classroom on campus. At other times, clients have walked around the campus or local neighborhood, polling strangers on a given question (e.g., "What do you think when someone blushes?"). In all of these cases, leaving the therapy room can provide additional context for the exposures and make them more realistic for the client. In other cases (e.g., making small talk), exposures within the therapy room usually suffice.

Whether the client will benefit most from one long exposure or from several short exposures is also a consideration. For some clients, the feared situation is a brief segment of a larger situation; in that case, it is much more useful for the client to gain confidence through numerous repetitions of that segment. For example, some individuals fear starting a conversation rather than maintaining the conversation once it is underway, so we repeatedly would have them approach individuals and initiate conversations rather than just role-playing a longer conversation. For someone who fears handshakes, we may have them give a handshake over and over again, in different ways (e.g., a traditional handshake, a fist bump, or a high-five), as well as with persons with different characteristics (e.g., men vs. women). For someone who fears writing in public, we might arrange for a small group to observe the client as they sign their name in increasingly smaller spaces, on increasingly formal documents, or with the "benefit" of more-or-less positive or negative comments about the quality of the client's writing. For others, a fear of awkward silences during a conversation may lead them to end conversations early. Thus, a longer conversation punctuated by several silences would likely best address that concern.

Although most in-session exposures are essentially role-play replications of a situation that might arise in the client's life (e.g., making small talk when sitting with others before a college class or business meeting), at other times, the therapist may choose instead to focus on a specific fear the client has expressed and design exposures that directly elicit that fear. For example, a client with a fear of expressing their opinion or asserting themself may find that they stay quiet or avoid expressing dissent when topics such as politics or religion arise in a conversation. Thus, a useful exposure may be to have the client argue a controversial opinion, or even an opinion opposite to their own, with a confederate in the form of a debate. For another client who presents with fears of stumbling over their words while speaking to a group, an exposure could be to read aloud complex terminology from a medical dictionary.

Understanding what the client needs to gain from the exposure is instrumental. Exposures can provide disconfirming evidence for the likelihood of a feared outcome or allow the client to gain evidence that the feared outcome, when it occurs, is not nearly as bad as they believe it to be. The therapist often has to determine which information applies best to the given client's experience. Imagine a client who fears blushing in conversations, but who, in fact, never or rarely ever blushes. For this client, exposures that provide disconfirming information about the likelihood of blushing would be useful. This could be achieved through video feedback or by eliciting feedback from the confederate. Another client who presents with fears of blushing may actually blush quite often. Exposures that allow the client to work on acceptance of their blushing and to devalue the significance of blushing would likely best serve this client, and this could be achieved by asking the confederate whether they noticed the blushing and what they thought of it. One could even survey people in the building to gain evidence about what people think when others blush. Ultimately, the client can learn that their catastrophic fears of blushing are unfounded. These same principles can be applied to other symptoms of anxiety such as shaking or sweating.

Cultural considerations can affect the type of exposures the therapist and client design. For clients who have minority identities (e.g., gender, sexual, or racial minorities), some social fears may be more realistic due to discrimination; those types of fears may be addressed in exposures, but only with great sensitivity to and validation of the client's lived experience. For example, a client may experience a macroaggression, such as being skipped over in a work meeting, and may grow to fear these situations. Another client may be anxious when meeting new people because new people often misgender them. Designing exposures with the client's values in mind, rather than with the goal of demonstrating that their fears are unlikely to come true, is most beneficial in these situations. For the first client, focusing on helping them feel confident speaking up in meetings again may be a goal of in-session exposures, but the therapist should be careful never to invalidate the client's experiences of discrimination. For the second client, determining in what contexts the client feels it is important to go forward and meet new people despite the discrimination they may face can help guide exposures. For clients who come from cultural backgrounds that value a more collectivist orientation than is the case in the United States, it also may be important to adjust the goals for in-session exposures or homework assignments, given that a greater degree of reticence when interacting with authority figures or elders may be the cultural expectation.

When planning an in-session exposure, one must determine whether it is in the client's best interest to ask for feedback from the exposure partner. For some clients, asking for feedback may be a reassurance-seeking behavior. If the client is known to excessively ask others for reassurance regarding social performance (e.g., repeatedly asking their partner whether they seemed nervous after attending a party), the therapist may not have them ask for feedback. In fact, it might be most useful to have the client sit with the uncertainty about how the interaction went, because this is likely to be their experience when interacting with others. Other clients may avoid feedback due to fears that it will be negative; in these cases, the therapist would suggest requesting feedback from the role-player in the service of overcoming that avoidance and gaining corrective information.

Flexibility with Homework

Although homework itself is vital to the success of treatment, the variability in the nature of homework given is extensive. Homework is best when it is highly specific and adapted to the client's goals and needs. For instance, it is not uncommon for therapists to find that some clients need extra practice with cognitive restructuring prior to beginning exposures. For these clients, therapists can assign additional cognitive restructuring homework for repeated practice. When assigning exposure homework, the assignment could be to replicate or expand upon the in-session exposure. After a small-talk in-session exposure, the therapist may ask the client to make small talk with one stranger each day. Alternatively, they might have the client go on a date and make small talk in that context.

Therapists can use exposure homework assignments to move clients toward their goals and values. First, the therapist should take stock of the client's important life events, goals, or desires they hope to address through treatment. An example of this may be a client who wants to develop an online presence to promote their small business; however, this client fears using social media. The therapist may then design a homework task to have the client set up an Instagram account and make posts with content related to their business. Over the course of therapy, the homework tasks could progress to interacting on social media with customers, or using social media to network with other business owners. In this way, the homework both serves to further the client's goals and lessen their social anxiety.

Flexibility with Comorbidity

Clients with comorbid psychological disorders present an interesting opportunity to apply the treatment flexibly. Many individuals with SAD also have other mental health conditions that shape their clinical presentation. Because SAD does not exist in a vacuum, it is important to be able to flexibly adapt this treatment and use a collaborative approach to suit the needs of the individual client. Although the emphasis of CBT for SAD is to target fear and avoidance of social situations, other comorbid disorders may inevitably affect and/or exacerbate a person's experiences of social anxiety.

Major depressive disorder (MDD) is the most commonly comorbid psychological disorder among individuals with SAD (with comorbidity rates ranging between 35% and 70%; Koyuncu, İnce, Ertekin, & Tükel, 2019) and may affect the course of treatment. If a client is both depressed and socially anxious, their depression may exacerbate their avoidance of social situations. When this is the case, it may be important for the therapist to flexibly attend to the client's depression, in order to increase motivation for treatment. For example, the therapist may want to incorporate education about the importance of behavioral activation into the early phases of treatment and incorporate behavioral activation into exposure work that is done between sessions. Therapists may work with clients not only to plan in vivo exposures for homework between sessions, but also to develop a schedule of basic behavioral and self-care activities to boost their daily mood. By taking this integrated approach, clients may be more willing to engage in social situations over the course of treatment and make greater gains by simultaneously addressing their depression. It is encouraging to note that those with a comorbid diagnosis of MDD are able to achieve the same rate of reduction in social anxiety over the course of CBT for SAD as those without comorbid MDD (Butler et al., 2021).

Of note, other anxiety disorders, such as generalized anxiety disorder (GAD), are commonly comorbid among individuals with social anxiety (with comorbidity rates ranging from 0.6% to 27%; Koyuncu et al., 2019), so treatment for SAD can also flexibly include a focus on other anxieties and worries across treatment components. For example, if an individual with SAD also worries about their health, family, finances, or current events (typical among those with GAD), the therapist and client may want to use cognitive restructuring to break down these other anxious thoughts or incorporate these topics into socially focused exposures during treatment.

Substance use disorders can affect the treatment of SAD. Most research has examined comorbid SAD and alcohol use disorder, which have been shown to co-occur at a lifetime prevalence rate around 2.4% (Schneier et al., 2010). If individuals with SAD use substances such as alcohol to mitigate their anxiety in social situations, this should be considered a safety behavior, because they are likely to attribute any successes to the disinhibiting effects of the alcohol, rather than their own social abilities. Thus, we tend to recommend limiting use of substances during social events so that clients can habituate to their social fears without the effects of a substance. As a part of the protocol, alcohol use is not typically addressed separately from its relation to social situations. If, however, a client feels unable to limit their substance use, and it is affecting their ability to engage in the treatment, the therapist may decide to incorporate motivational interviewing techniques to address substance use and the role it plays in the client's life (see Buckner, Ledley, Heimberg, & Schmidt, 2008, for an example). Additionally, a past substance use disorder may be relevant to a client's current social anxiety treatment if the client is in recovery and shares that they are avoiding attending group meetings (i.e., Alcoholics Anonymous [AA], Narcotics Anonymous [NA]) because of their social anxiety. Attendance and active participation in AA or other meetings may become the focus of in-session and homework exposures.

Individuals with SAD may present with an autism spectrum disorder (ASD), in which they have more difficulty reading social signals and cues in social situations. Among those with ASD, it may be important to flexibly incorporate more foundational social skills as part of the treatment. For example, social skills training may involve psychoeducation about social signaling cues, such as improving eye contact or voice inflection, or breaking down the steps in pursuing a romantic relationship if the client's goal is to date someone. It is important to note that individuals without an ASD also may benefit from learning foundational social skills, so therapists should use their own judgment on how to best incorporate social skills training flexibly throughout the protocol. Additionally, it is likely that therapists will need to include a greater number of repetitions of exposures to particular feared situations for individuals with ASD. For example, small talk exposures may require many iterations in order for the client to practice common conversational topics and improve their social signaling (e.g., eye contact, body language, voice inflection).

Some individuals with SAD may have body dysmorphic disorder (BDD), which may exacerbate their social anxiety. CBT for SAD has demonstrated effects on symptoms of BDD, thus making it possible to address these fears simultaneously (Fang, Sawyer, Aderka, & Hoffman, 2013). Certain body dysmorphic fears (e.g., being overweight, having thinning hair) may be correlated with how much a client fears being evaluated or judged by peers, which would be important to address as part of their clinical presentation. For clients with SAD and BDD, it may be useful to incorporate body-focused situations into their fear and avoidance hierarchy. For example, if a client has a fear of hair loss/balding and regularly wears a hat to hide this fear from others, the therapist may choose to design exposures in which the client must interact with others without a hat on, to challenge both BDD and SAD fears in tandem.

WHEN TREATMENT FLEXIBILITY
BECOMES NONADHERENCE

This chapter highlighted the various ways that this protocol can be adapted with flexibility to provide a collaborative approach. Despite the reasonable flexibility of this treatment, however, there are several ways in which maneuvering away from the protocol should be considered nonadherent. When considering the difference between flexibility and nonadherence, it is important to reflect that using the treatment with flexibility maintains the fundamental goals of the treatment, whereas other decisions that diverge from the premise of the treatment are nonadherent and may predict poorer treatment response.

Although clients may feel some reluctance about or discomfort with certain components of treatment, it is still imperative that they are engaged in the therapy as directed. Unwillingness to complete homework exercises (e.g., worksheets, exposures for homework between sessions) should be considered nonadherence, because homework practice is an integral and necessary part of treatment. Although clients may see some improvement in their social anxiety just by participating in sessions, noncompliance with homework limits their potential to receive the full benefits of the treatment as intended. Further, because in-session exposures are a central component of the therapy, noncompliance with exposures during sessions (i.e., not doing them) would be considered nonadherence. It is likely that clients may show some reticence to engage in exposure when first introduced to the concept, given that exposures may increase their anxiety and distress. Nevertheless, exposures are a required and necessary part of treatment, and an unwillingness to do the exposures in-session and for homework should be considered nonadherence, because exposures are the major "behavioral" component of CBT.

In addition, if a client is unwilling to pause "as-needed" medications for the purposes of exposures, this may be considered nonadherence. The client may not learn that they can engage in social situations without this safety behavior and believe that the substance, rather than the treatment, is the source of the improvements they experience in social anxiety. Similarly, if clients firmly believe that they need to change their physical appearance (e.g., plastic surgery, hair plugs) in order for change to occur in their social anxiety and take measures to pursue these alterations to their appearance during treatment, this may be considered nonadherence. Like as-needed medications, structural changes to one's physical appearance during treatment limit the ability of the client to associate any changes in their social anxiety symptoms with the treatment itself, rather than with the physical procedure or change. However, all medical interventions that occur during the course of therapy should not be considered nonadherence. A transgender or gender diverse client may elect to undergo a gender-affirming medical intervention during treatment; although gender-affirming interventions may alleviate social anxiety among transgender and gender diverse individuals (Butler et al., 2019), they would not be considered nonadherent, because the primary purpose of the intervention is related to the desire to affirm one's gender identity, not to alleviate one's social anxiety.

It is additionally important to note that therapists deviate from the protocol in other ways that result in nonadherence. Although therapists have flexibility in how they administer various parts of the protocol, they have a responsibility to guide clients through the critical session material: homework review, cognitive restructuring, planning and doing in-session exposures, and assigning at-home practice between sessions. Firstly, it is important for therapists to dedicate a portion of the session to homework review in order to reinforce the client's completion of homework. If the therapist does not review client homework, it may reduce the client's attempts to complete homework assignments, which can negatively affect treatment gains. Without a review of what the client has done between sessions, the therapist may miss opportunities to gain information that may be important to incorporate into future sessions or to know whether extra time should be devoted to a given topic. Additionally, it is important for therapists to lead clients through some form of cognitive restructuring before engaging in an in-session exposure, or after the exposure as part of the debriefing process, for the clients to get the most out of the in-session exposure experience. This practice also reinforces the importance of cognitive restructuring as a key part of exposures. Therapists may be anxious about conducting in-session exposures; nevertheless, in-session exposures are critical to the protocol. Conducting fewer than four in-session exposures over the course of treatment should be considered nonadherent. Further, during exposure sessions, it is important for therapists to reserve enough time after exposures to adequately debrief. Debriefing is an important step in the postexposure cognitive restructuring process, because it allows for a review of what went well and whether goals were met. It also offers an opportunity to challenge any negative beliefs that the client has about the exposure and to note other important automatic thoughts or reactions that occurred. Finally, failure to assign homework between sessions results in nonadherence; homework allows the client to make progress and apply skills learned in session to their own life.

CONCLUSIONS

Flexibility is encouraged in the use of the *Managing Social Anxiety* program—flexibility allows for collaborative modifications to enhance outcomes. Although the core components of psychoeducation, cognitive restructuring, in-session exposures, and homework are key to treatment success, there is room for creativity in how these components are implemented. Unique presentations, client-specific social fears, comorbidities, and difficulty understanding or using the skills of treatment are all factors that should be considered when working with a client using this program. Issues of nonadherence, such as client noncompliance or therapist stray from the manual, should be dealt with carefully so as not to adversely affect treatment outcomes for the client. Ultimately, the *Managing Social Anxiety* manual provides space for therapist creativity in implementing a treatment that will best address a client's needs.

ACKNOWLEDGMENTS

The authors wish to thank Drs. Debra Hope (University of Nebraska) and Cynthia Turk (Washburn University) for their feedback on an earlier draft of this manuscript.

REFERENCES

Acarturk, C., Cuijpers, P., van Straten, A., & de Graaf, R. (2009). Psychological treatment of social anxiety disorder: A meta-analysis. *Psychological Medicine, 39*, 241–254. https://doi.org/10.1017/s0033291708003590

American Psychiatric Association. (2013). *Diagnostic and statistical manual of mental disorders, 5th edition (DSM-5)*. American Psychiatric Publishing. https://doi.org/10.1176/appi.books.9780890425596.744053

Barkowski, S., Schwartze, D., Strauss, B., Burlingame, G. M., Barth, J., & Rosendahl, J. (2016). Efficacy of group psychotherapy for social anxiety disorder: A meta-analysis of randomized-controlled trials. *Journal of Anxiety Disorders, 39*, 44–64. https://doi.org/10.1016/j.janxdis.2016.02.005

Buckner, J. D., Ledley, D. R., Heimberg, R. G., & Schmidt, N. B. (2008). Treating comorbid social anxiety and alcohol use disorders: Combining motivation enhancement therapy with cognitive-behavioral therapy. *Clinical Case Studies, 7*, 208–223. https://doi.org/10.1177/1534650107306877

Butler, R. M., Horenstein, A., Gitlin, M., Testa, R. J., Kaplan, S. C., Swee, M. B., & Heimberg, R. G. (2019). Social anxiety among transgender and gender nonconforming individuals: The role of gender-affirming medical interventions. *Journal of Abnormal Psychology, 128*, 25–31. https://doi.org/10.1037/abn0000399

Butler, R. M., O'Day, E. B., & Heimberg, R. G. (2020). The benefits of a longer course of cognitive behavioral therapy for some patients with social anxiety disorder. *Cognitive Behaviour Therapy*. Advance online publication. https://doi.org/10.1080/16506073.2020.1829027

Butler, R. M., O'Day, E. B., Swee, M. B., Horenstein, A., & Heimberg, R. G. (2021). Cognitive behavioral therapy for social anxiety disorder: Predictors of treatment outcome in a quasi-naturalistic setting. *Behavior Therapy, 52*, 465–477. https://doi.org/10.1016/j.beth.2020.06.002

Clark, D. M., & Wells, A. (1995). A cognitive model of social phobia. In R. G. Heimberg, M. R. Liebowitz, D. A. Hope, & F. R. Schneier (Eds.), *Social phobia: Diagnosis, assessment, and treatment* (pp. 69–93). Guilford Press.

Fang, A., Sawyer, A. T., Aderka, I. M., & Hofmann, S. G. (2013). Psychological treatment of social anxiety disorder improves body dysmorphic concerns. *Journal of Anxiety Disorders, 27*, 684–691. https://doi.org/10.1016/j.janxdis.2013.07.005

Goldin, P. R., Ziv, M., Jazaieri, H., Werner, K., Kraemer, H., Heimberg, R. G., & Gross, J. J. (2012). Cognitive reappraisal self-efficacy mediates the effects of individual cognitive-behavioral therapy for social anxiety disorder. *Journal of Consulting and Clinical Psychology, 80*, 1034–1040. https://doi.org/10.1037/a0028555

Hope, D. A., Heimberg, R. G., & Turk, C. L. (2019a). *Managing social anxiety: A cognitive-behavioral therapy approach* (Client Workbook, 3rd ed.). Oxford University Press.

Hope, D. A., Heimberg, R. G., & Turk, C. L. (2019b). *Managing social anxiety: A cognitive-behavioral therapy approach* (Therapist Guide, 3rd ed.). Oxford University Press.

Kaplan, S. C., Swee, M., & Heimberg, R. G. (2018). Psychological treatments for social anxiety disorder. In O. Braddick (Ed.), *The Oxford research encyclopedia of psychology.* New York: Oxford University Press. https://doi.org/10.1093/acrefore/9780190236557.013.98

Kendall, P. C., & Frank, H. (2018). Implementing evidence-based treatment protocols: Flexibility within fidelity. *Clinical Psychology: Science and Practice, 25*, 1–12. https://doi.org/10.1111/cpsp.12271

Kendall, P. C., Gosch, E., Furr, J., & Sood, E. (2008). Flexibility within fidelity. *Journal of the American Academy of Child and Adolescent Psychiatry, 47*, 987–993. https://doi.org/10.1097/chi.0b013e31817eed2f

Kessler, R. C., Berglund, P., Demler, O., Jin, R., Merikangas, K. R., & Walters, E. E. (2005). Lifetime prevalence and age-of-onset distributions of DSM-IV disorders in the National Comorbidity Survey Replication. *Archives of General Psychiatry, 62*, 593–602. http://dx.doi.org/10.1001/archpsyc.62.6.593

Koyuncu, A., İnce, E., Ertekin, E., & Tükel, R. (2019). Comorbidity in social anxiety disorder: Diagnostic and therapeutic challenges. *Drugs in Context, 8*, 212573. https://doi.org/10.7573/dic.212573

Ledley, D. R., Heimberg, R. G., Hope, D. A., Hayes, S. A., Zaider, T. I., Van Dyke, M., Turk, C. L., Kraus, C., & Fresco, D. M. (2009). Efficacy of a manualized and workbook-driven individual treatment for social anxiety disorder. *Behavior Therapy, 40*, 414–424. https://doi.org/10.1016/j.beth.2008.12.001

Mayo-Wilson, E., Dias, S., Mavranezouli, I., Kew, K., Clark, D. M., Ades, A. E., & Pilling, S. (2014). Psychological and pharmacological interventions for social anxiety disorder in adults: A systematic review and network meta-analysis. *The Lancet Psychiatry, 1*, 368–376. https://doi.org/10.1016/s2215-0366(14)70329-3

Powers, M. B., Sigmarsson, S. R., & Emmelkamp, P. M. (2008). A meta–analytic review of psychological treatments for social anxiety disorder. *International Journal of Cognitive Therapy, 1*, 94–113. *https://doi.org/10.1521/ijct.2008.1.2.94*

Rapee, R. M., & Heimberg, R. G. (1997). A cognitive-behavioral model of anxiety in social phobia. *Behaviour Research and Therapy, 35*, 741–756. https://doi.org/10.1016/S0005-7967(97)00022-3

Schneier, F. R., Foose, T. E., Hasin, D. S., Heimberg, R. G., Liu, S. M., Grant, B. F., & Blanco, C. (2010). Social anxiety disorder and alcohol use disorder comorbidity in the National Epidemiologic Survey on Alcohol and Related Conditions. *Psychological Medicine, 40*, 977–988. https://doi.org/10.1017/S0033291709991231

2

Flexible Principles for the Treatment of Adult Worry

AMY R. SEWART AND MICHELLE G. CRASKE ■

A fundamental human experience, worry is defined as "a chain of thoughts and images, negatively affect-laden and relatively uncontrollable" (Borkovec, Robinson, Pruzinsky, & DePree, 1983), which typically focus on aversive outcomes for future events. Excessive and uncontrollable worry is reliably observed across anxiety disorders, and most evident in generalized anxiety disorder (GAD) of which it is the cardinal symptom (Olatunji, Wolitzky-Taylor, Sawchuk, & Ciesielski, 2010). The worriers' focus can be both transient and stable wherein core worries with specific themes persist across time (e.g., illness) and relatively short-term worries guided by potential life stressors shift from one topic to another (e.g., worry about upcoming plane travel). Worry, however, is a transdiagnostic phenomenon that has been observed in other disorders in which anxiety is often present, including eating (Sassaroli & Ruggiero, 2005), alcohol use (Spada & Wells, 2005), and schizophrenia spectrum disorders (Morrison & Wells, 2007). Implementing effective therapeutic strategies for worry requires an understanding of the theoretical functions of worry, as well as identifying the role this preservative cognitive style plays for a given client.

COGNITIVE AVOIDANCE MODELS OF WORRY

Worry is posited to serve in part as a cognitive avoidance response, wherein individuals engage in worry in an attempt to generate strategies to reduce the likelihood of or avoid temporally distant aversive events (Borkovec, 1994). Thus, individuals sensitive to threat detection and interpretation biases—central mechanisms of anxiety—may find themselves engaging in excessive, uncontrollable worry (MacLeod & Rutherford, 2004; Mogg & Bradley, 1998). A more recent update to our understanding of cognitive avoidance in chronic worriers has implicated intolerance of uncertainty (IU), a dispositional characteristic that results from of a set of negative beliefs about uncertainty and its implications, as a contributor to threat-related biases—specifically the tendency to interpret ambiguous situations as threatening (Dugas et al., 2007). IU has been found to be elevated in both nonclinical worriers and across disorders (Dugas et al., 2001). Regardless as to whether worry actually reduces the likelihood of future danger, worry is negatively reinforced. That is, the nonoccurrence of an anticipated negative outcome is often attributed, incorrectly, to engaging in worrying. Supporting this theory, individuals with excessive worry often believe that worry helps to: (1) determine how to avoid or prevent bad events, (2) prepare for the worst, and (3) superstitiously lessen the likelihood of bad events (Borkovec et al., 1999). As a result, some worriers may believe that they are using perseverative thinking as a problem-solving strategy—although it is often ineffective, distressing, and time-consuming. Such beliefs about worry and their relation to the development and maintenance of chronic worry has been further expanded upon in Wells's meta-cognitive model (Wells, 1995, 1999). Individuals with pathological worry exhibit a "negative problem orientation," which may interfere with solving one's problems effectively (Robichaud & Dugas, 2005).

EMOTIONAL AVOIDANCE MODELS OF WORRY

Individuals with chronic worry demonstrate avoidance of emotional experiences and related psychological arousal, in addition to deficits in emotion regulation (Mennin et al., 2005; Newman et al., 2004; Roemer et al., 2005). Specifically, those diagnosed with GAD report experiencing more intense emotional experiences coupled with a greater tendency to express negative emotions when compared to healthy controls (Mennin et al., 2005). Individuals with chronic worry also demonstrate deficits in (a) emotional clarity, (b) the ability to engage in goal-directed behaviors when distressed, (c) acceptance of emotions, (d) impulse control, and (e) access to effective regulation strategies, above and beyond negative affect (Salters-Pedneault et al., 2006). Further lending itself to negative reinforcement, engaging in worry preceding encounters with feared stimuli has been shown to dampen a worrier's somatic arousal in laboratory settings (Borkovec & Hu, 1990; Borkovec et al., 1993; Peasley-Miklus & Vrana, 2000). Worry also may serve to shift one's attention away from other emotional content (Borkovec et al., 1999; Borkovec & Roemer, 1995). Overall, these findings suggest that worry enables avoidance of distressing negative emotional states and serves as a maladaptive emotion regulation strategy, specifically through the suppression of negative affect.

CONTRAST AVOIDANCE MODEL OF WORRY

The more recent contrast avoidance model of worry hypothesizes that rather than attempting to avoid present-moment negative emotion and associated arousal through worrying, chronic worriers use worry as a means to avoid the experience of negative emotional contrasts (i.e., moving from a positive/neutral state to a negative state; Newman & Llera, 2011). Whereas aforementioned theories of worry have suggested that worry serves to dampen threat/anxiety, this model proposes that worry serves to sustain negative affect in an effort to prevent sudden shifts into negative affect and achieve emotional constancy (Llera & Newman, 2014). This theory converges with previous findings suggesting that rather than worry actually reducing anxiety, worry creates and sustains negative emotionality and prolonged physiological recovery (e.g., Brosschot, Gerin, &Thayer, 2006). Since its inception, the contrast avoidance model has been supported by studies showing negative shifts lead to greater emotional responding and impaired coping in individuals with excessive worry (e.g., Kim & Newman, 2016; Llera & Newman, 2014).

SUMMARY OF WORRY MODELS AND TREATMENT IMPLICATIONS

Each model agrees that worry is maintained by negative reinforcement—whether that be removal of threat, anxiety, negative emotional contrast, or uncertainty. There has yet to be, however, a consensus as to which models or mechanisms best account for chronic-worry psychopathology. Although traditional cognitive behavior therapy (CBT) protocols are effective for many chronic worriers (Cuijpers et al., 2014), a notable number fail to achieve lasting improvement (Borkovec & Ruscio, 2001). Treatment research on chronic worry/GAD has generally lagged behind other mood and anxiety-related disorders and information regarding moderators and mediators is scarce. Overall, treatment calls for the flexible application of science-driven therapeutic strategies—that cut across various models of worry—tailored and adapted to the individual. In other words, adhering to the scientifically supported intervention strategies while being flexible in their application ("Flexibility within fidelity," Kendall et al., 2008; Kendall & Frank, 2018). To this end, this chapter outlines various empirically supported cognitive-behavioral strategies driven by our understanding of worry-related mechanisms that may be implemented in the treatment of chronic worry. This coverage is illustrative (not exhaustive) and does not include procedures discussed in detail elsewhere (e.g., mindfulness).

COGNITIVE STRATEGIES FOR THE TREATMENT OF EXCESSIVE WORRY

Cognitive Misappraisals

Overestimation of Likelihood. Individuals with pathological worry engage in a cognitive bias described as "likelihood overestimation," wherein the odds of future negative events occurring are judged as being highly probable, more so than if odds were calculated using realistic evidence and data. Likelihood overestimation is a transdiagnostic process that serves as both a generative and maintaining factor across emotional disorders (Craske & Barlow, 2006) and as a core driver of excessive worry and related behaviors. Overestimation of likelihood is illustrated by the following examples: (a) a junior marketing executive believes with strong conviction that a mistake in their presentation will lead to their firing, (b) a father is confident that leaving his 11-year old child unattended for any period of time will lead to his child being injured, and (c) a healthy, college-aged student is convinced that not showering after grabbing the mail will result in catching a serious illness. Not surprisingly, those who perceive a high likelihood for aversive events may spend an inordinate amount of time engaging in safety behaviors—specifically generating strategies to avoid various negative outcomes through worrying—and enacting them. When individuals allocate considerable cognitive resources engaging in worry-related thoughts and behaviors, efforts to realistically appraise negative outcome likelihood are sidelined. Moreover, individuals may falsely attribute the avoidance of catastrophe to engaging in worry and related behaviors perceived to avoid disaster, thus reinforcing overestimations of threat likelihood.

Overestimation of Severity. In addition to the tendency toward likelihood overestimation, excessive worriers exhibit in severity overestimation. Also known as "catastrophizing," individuals suffering from pathological worry may perceive negative events as intolerable and devastating, when in reality these events—while certainly unpleasant and perhaps somewhat painful—are ultimately tolerable. This phenomenon is observed across anxiety disorders and for those with excessive worry serves to further reinforce the utility of avoiding perceived disaster through worry and subsequent avoidance behaviors. When an individual's attention is laser-focused on "how awful" a hypothetical event will be, a realistic evaluation of one's ability to cope with negative events is ignored. Complicating matters even further, given that many overestimated negative events have a low probability of occurring—the belief that such events are unbearable is often not directly challenged with corrective information as it would be if the event were to occur.

Metacognitive Beliefs about Worry

All individuals hold beliefs regarding its utility, as worry can indeed be an effective way to avoid potential negative outcomes. Excessive worriers have been shown to possess strong positive beliefs about the utility of worry and have high confidence in worry-related negative reinforcement contingencies (e.g., "Worrying helps me cope."; Borkovec et al., 1999). As a result, chronic worry may be maintained through an overestimation of worry's role in reducing the likelihood of future negative events. Somewhat paradoxically, chronic worriers also may simultaneously hold negative beliefs about uncontrollability and dangerousness of worry. From the metacognitive perspective, negative worry-related beliefs and related "type 2" worry (i.e., worrying about worrying) are regarded as a crucial element in the development and maintenance of generalized anxiety disorder (Wells, 1995). Such negative metacognitive beliefs also involve overestimation of likelihood, specifically that excessive worry will lead to negative mental, physical, or social consequences (e.g., "If I cannot stop my worry, I will go 'crazy'.").

Cognitive Restructuring

If one's overestimation of likelihood for negative events and their related aversiveness were to be corrected—the perceived utility of worry should diminish accordingly. As a result, the frequency and intensity of worry also should fade and be subjected to less frequent negative reinforcement. Recalibration of overestimation of threat likelihood and severity may be targeted in psychotherapy through cognitive restructuring—a process in which clients are trained to identify, evaluate, challenge, and alter maladaptive patterns of thinking. Cognitive restructuring for excessive worry follows a traditional cognitive model of anxiety treatment approach (Beck et al., 2005). The general objective with cognitive-based strategies is to teach the client how to identify maladaptive thoughts, using objective evidence, and how to then challenge these thoughts to arrive at accurate, adaptive ways of thinking (Beck et al., 2005).

Clients are first tasked with identifying their own anxious patterns of thinking. Individuals with pathological worry may feel as though anxious chatter is always present in the background of their minds, because worry is often a habitual or "automatic" event. As a result, "catching" misappraisals relating to threat and negative outcome severity may prove to be difficult at first. To assist in identifying maladaptive worries, clients may find it helpful to first monitor situations, in addition to physiological and emotional symptoms related to anxiety—such as muscle tension, irritability, or fatigue—and then question themselves to identify their own anxious patterns of thinking. Once an unrealistic, persistent worry is identified, the objective probability and severity can be evaluated.

Correcting Overestimation of Likelihood with Realistic Odds. The client is guided to understand that predictions regarding future threat, while not fact, are often seen as fact. All predictions are no more than hypotheses that may or may not be accurate, and represent one of many potential outcomes with and without negative elements. Therefore, to separate the possible from the probable, evidence for and against these hypotheses must be evaluated. Evidence of an event's likelihood is assessed by "questioning its objective probability, given consideration of all of the relevant facts, without jumping to conclusions or overgeneralizing" (Zinbarg et al., 2006). The therapist teaches the client how to independently identify objective evidence for and against worrisome thoughts and ways to generate other alternative outcomes to recalibrate over-estimation of likelihood. Clients may use a 0-to-100-point scale to rate the actual likelihood—or "real odds"—of their feared outcome occurring along with their subjective units of distress (SUDs) both before and after employing "real odds" (see Zinbarg et al., 2006 for details). Generating counterevidence may be applied similarly to challenging negative metacognitive beliefs about worry un-controllability and dangerousness (e.g., "No matter what I do, I cannot stop my worry."; see Wells, 2011 for details). If the client is responsive to this strategy, these quantitative datapoints should reflect the skill's utility through reduced ratings. However, rating reductions are not necessarily predictive of treatment response or outcomes.

Correcting Overestimation of Severity with Coping. A second cognitive strategy effective for individuals with pathological worry is challenging their overestimation of negative outcome severity. Here, the therapist highlights to the client that although some negative events may be unpleasant or uncom-fortable, this does not mean that the client is incapable of coping with them. Clients are guided to recognize that they already possess the ability to cope with painful or unpleasant events. Furthermore, while certain negative events may certainly be painful, similar to anxiety—pain fades with time. Given that a main driver of excessive worry is appraising a hypothetical negative event as insufferable, clients are assisted in re-evaluating the actual severity through decatastrophizing—or the "so what?" approach. Clients are asked to im-agine objective steps they can take to cope if the negative event were to occur, drawing from how they and others have managed difficult situations in the past. This technique can be applied to both likely (e.g., social rejection while dating) and unlikely events (e.g., death or severe physical illness to otherwise healthy individuals) that have a high predicted severity rating. Clients may use a 0-to-100-point scale to rate the perceived severity of their feared outcome occurring both before and after reassessing their ability to cope with a given negative outcome.

Correcting Positive Beliefs about Worry. A core component of metacogni-tive therapy, challenging overestimations in worry usefulness may assist clients in reducing worry frequency and severity (Wells, 2011). This challenging is achieved by highlighting that positive beliefs reinforce the use of maladaptive worry and systematically questioning the evidence for and against worry as a successful threat avoidance, coping, and problem-solving strategy. Modifying positive beliefs is posited to facilitate the use of effective, alternative means to responding to perceived external threat and cognitive phenomena (Wells, 1995). Therapists may use the Metacognitions Questionnaire 30 (MCQ-30; Wells & Cartwright-Hatton, 2004), a 30-item self-report questionnaire on trait metacognitive beliefs, judgment, and monitoring strategies to assist with identification of targets for cognitive restructuring.

Notes on Application of Cognitive Restructuring for Excessive Worry

Although guiding clients through cognitive restructuring targeting an overestimation of likelihood, the therapist remains mindful of the fact that negative events do indeed occur. The purpose of cognitive restructuring is not to replace overestimations of likelihood with underestimations—because this also would be maladaptive—rather, it is to arrive at a realistic estimation for a given hypothetical scenario. Furthermore, therapists strive to be mindful that certain estimations of likelihood and severity for negative outcomes that may be perceived by the therapist to be exaggerated may be based in a very valid personal reality. Exercising cultural humility (Hook et al., 2013) and actively asking and listening to how clients feel their various identities may inform their estimations of threat and severity of negative outcomes is critical. What if a worry involving a specific hypothetical negative event is both high likelihood and high severity? Validation of one's worry and anxiety in such cases is appropriate, as the function of worry in this case is adaptive. Worries that fit this profile are more appropriately managed through problem-solving, time management, and goal setting covered later in this chapter.

BEHAVIORAL STRATEGIES

Individuals with pathological worry engage in behavioral efforts that function as a means to (1) prevent negative outcomes from occurring, (2) control worry, (3) reduce uncertainty, and (4) alleviate worry-related distress. These behaviors may take the form of overt avoidance of situations perceived to be threatening or aversive (e.g., avoiding social situations), and engaging in safety behaviors (e.g., checking) or possessing safety objects (e.g., cell phones) while in such situations. Given that episodes of worry are often an effort to generate strategies to prevent future negative and/or intolerable events, engaging in related actions is observed in excessive worriers (Beesdo-Baum et al., 2012). For example, an excessive worrier may carry around a veritable pharmacy of over-the-counter drugs "just in case" something happens in absence of illness. Other safety behaviors related to worry include making overly detailed lists, overprotecting children, and avoiding extra responsibilities for fear of making a mistake. Although it is most oftentimes impossible to determine if such behaviors actually prevented disaster, avoidance and safety-related behaviors—along with worry—are reinforced through the nonoccurrence of negative outcomes.

Individuals who worry excessively are also likely to engage in behaviors in an attempt to silence or prevent relentless episodes of worry and associated distress. Though limiting media consumption is certainly a healthy behavior, someone may choose to no longer read or watch the news to avoid perseverating on local and global events. Similarly, procrastination also may serve as a means to avoid uncontrollable worry regarding potential catastrophes.

In an effort to reduce uncertainty, individuals may seek continual reassurance from others (e.g., asking their partner if they are upset with them when there is no apparent discord), consult multiple information sources (e.g., spending hours reviewing multiple websites about a relatively small purchase), or engage in checking behaviors (e.g., checking a flight map multiple times to ensure their partner's flight has not crashed).

Overall, these behavioral control strategies are largely maladaptive and result in further negative reinforcement of worry-related behaviors even further through alleviating worry, uncertainty, and associated emotional discomfort. Certainly, worry-related behaviors may serve multiple functions simultaneously. Avoidance and safety-related behaviors serve to perpetuate excessive worry, anxiety, and contribute to distress and impairments in functioning. Therefore, efforts to discontinue worry-related behaviors are critical treatment elements for many excessive worriers.

Removal of Safety-Related Behaviors

Individuals are encouraged to resist engaging in behaviors that are driven by worry/anxiety, and after successfully identifying such behaviors work to replace them with nonanxious responses (Zinbarg et al., 2006). Through the removal of safety-related behaviors, the individual is provided with corrective information that (1) the avoidance of catastrophe is not contingent on engaging in safety-related behaviors, (2) they are able to tolerate anxiety/distress associated with feared situations/stimuli and nonengagement in safety behaviors, and (3) anxiety, distress, and worry fade over time. Fading safety behaviors is a common component of many behavioral therapies, but has not been systematically evaluated for excessive worriers or individuals with GAD.

Behavioral Experimentation

A systematic approach to removal of safety-related behaviors may be achieved through the implementation of "behavioral experiments" wherein worry-related cognitions are tested and challenged through "real-life" experiences. For example, if a client never delegates work-related tasks due to a belief that an oversight will lead to disaster, the client is assigned to delegate work to a supervisee to test this hypothesis. Similarly, a client with socially relevant worries may avoid throwing parties out of fear that no one will attend. To test this belief, the client may be tasked with throwing a get-together to gather data on how many people indeed show up. A client who locks their car multiple times before going into a store out of fear of leaving it unlocked may be assigned to lock the car only once, go shopping, and then test to see if the car was indeed locked and not robbed.

Behavioral experiments are applied to test beliefs—both negative and positive— regarding the nature of worry itself (Wells, 1995). For example, an individual who believes that worry is uncontrollable may use stimulus control or "worry post-ponement" exercises (outlined later in this chapter) to provide evidence against uncontrollability and, as a result, decrease the strength of this belief (Wells & King, 2006). Positive beliefs relating to excessive worry, such as worry being an effective way to solve problems or that worry is an adaptive coping strategy, are also directly testable. This behavioral experiment may take the form of a worry-modulation experiment wherein individuals are directed to increase worry for one day and minimize worry on the second day (through worry postponement) so that these two days may be compared in terms of pleasantness and productivity (Wells, 2011).

Though superficially similar to exposure, behavioral experiments do not al-ways directly test the degree to which feared stimuli predict feared outcomes—the target of exposure therapy and detailed further on (Craske et al., 2014). Prior to conducting an behavioral experiment, individuals (1) clearly identify the belief they are testing, (2) rate the strength of the belief they are testing (0%–100%), (3) plan an experiment that directly tests this belief, and (4) identify any obstacles that stand in the way of hypothesis testing (e.g., needing assistance from others). Individuals then record exactly what happens while carrying out a behavioral ex-periment, and afterward reflect on the results and re-rate the strength of the belief (0%–100%).

Exposure

The fears of individuals with excessive worry are often future-oriented, dif-fuse, and lack specific anxiety-provoking triggers (Borkovec, 1994). As a result, predicted catastrophic outcomes for excessive worriers (e.g., I'm going to get fired and become homeless) are untestable within an in vivo exposure paradigm. We are able, however, to directly and systematically test an individual's ability to tol-erate the anxiety and distress associated with worry and related constructs. As previously noted, excessive worriers may believe that they are unable to tolerate the emotional consequences resulting from excessive worry, uncertainty, and/or not engaging in safety-related behaviors. Such beliefs may be present for some—but not all—excessive worriers. Furthermore, individuals who find negative af-fective states distressing may use non-imagery-based, verbal-linguistic worry to suppress uncomfortable autonomic arousal (Borkovec et al., 1991). Thus, suc-cessful affective avoidance negatively reinforces verbal-linguistic worry, as well as the continued avoidance of threatening images. Negative affect may be further moderated by deploying safety behaviors to reduce the emotional consequences of situations perceived to be threatening. Further, worry also may serve to distract individuals from other emotional content (Borkovec et al., 1999).

Applying associative learning principles to this relationship, experiencing high levels of anxiety may function as a conditional stimulus (CSs) that is predictive of "being unable to function," "going crazy," or a having "mental breakdown" (un-conditional stimulus [US]). Thus, an individual may engage in worry or safety behaviors in an attempt to control anxiety—the CS—in an attempt to avoid their predicted negative outcome or US (i.e., mental incapacitation). Exposure for excessive worry demonstrates to the client that a given CS (e.g., high anxiety) is not predictive of the identified US (e.g., mental incapacitation). To this aim, therapists work with the client to identify and operationalize what their specific feared outcome or US(s) is, and design exposure tasks to demonstrate nonoccurrence of the feared outcome (i.e., CS → noUS; see Sewart & Craske, 2020).

IMAGINAL EXPOSURE

Exposure tasks, as part of treatment for excessive worry, are designed around the ethical induction of distressing emotional states. This may be achieved through the application of imaginal exposure, wherein the client is exposed to (a) the mental image of a feared situation, and as a result exposed to (b) a heightened cognitive and psychophysiological emotional experience perceived to be intolerable (i.e., anxiety; Dugas et al., 2007). The client is then provided with corrective learning that elevated emotions induced by these images are tolerable and do not lead to predicted negative outcomes. Therapists can help clients identify these images by using a series of "what if?" questions—otherwise known as downward arrow technique—until further information can no longer be generated (van der Heiden & ten Broeke, 2009). For example, to elicit emotional distress a client may be asked to vividly imagine that they are in their bosses' office receiving a bad performance evaluation and being fired. The client then is asked to engage in minor tasks (e.g., cooking, completing a homework assignment) to demonstrate one's ability to function. It's important that tasks demonstrating ability to function not also serve as opportunities for avoidance, thus minor tasks that do not require a significant cognitive load—and as a result distraction—are suggested. Distressing images used in imaginal exposure are likely to undergo habituation after repeated presentation, demonstrating that images are no more than cognitive phenomena that possess no inherent threat. Standalone worry exposure procedures have demonstrated efficacy for the treatment of generalized anxiety disorder (Hoyer et al., 2009).

IN VIVO EXPOSURE

In addition to avoiding threatening images, individuals with pathological worry may sidestep unpredictable situations in an effort to avoid distressing emotional states brought on by worries surrounding uncertainty. As aforementioned, excessive worriers often demonstrate an intolerance of uncertainty, a dispositional characteristic corresponding with negative beliefs about uncertainty and its consequences (Robichaud et al., 2019). As a result, exposures may be designed around exposing individuals in vivo to (a) situations that possess a high level of uncertainty in an effort to expose individuals to (b) heightened cognitive and psychophysiological emotional experience perceived to be intolerable. A client may be tasked with sending an e-mail message to a boss asking for a day off, and to then sit with the uncertainty and anxiety of how their boss will react without engaging in safety behaviors. Similar to imaginal exposure, the client may then be asked to engage in minor tasks to demonstrate that they are able to function in the face of uncertainty and associated psychological/physiological states.

EXPECTANCY RATINGS PRE- AND POST-EXPOSURE

Across the anxiety disorders, fear expression during exposure (which has often been indexed by subjective units of distress or "SUDs") has not been found to be a reliable predictor of fear learning (see Craske et al., 2008). Expectancy ratings, or the degree to which a feared stimulus (i.e., CS) predicts a preidentified feared outcome (i.e., US), and their reduction pre- to post-exposure and across exposure trials provide a more theoretically appropriate measure of extinction learning. Because this is a recently new and novel approach to exposures, there is limited data to confirm its utility above and beyond the use of SUDs and is supported by mostly experimental studies (see Craske et al., 2014 for review). Prior to exposure, clients provide an expectancy rating for a given feared outcome on a 0-to-100-point scale, where 0 represents the belief that the feared outcome is *not at all likely to happen* and 100 is *entirely certain the feared outcome will happen*. This rating can be assessed by asking the question, "How likely is it that what I am/you are most worried about will occur?" Using the same rating anchors, the postexposure expectancy level also can be assessed by asking the question, "Imagine you repeated the same exposure practice. How likely is it that what I was/you were most worried about before will occur this time?" (Sewart & Craske, 2020). As with SUDs, reductions in expectancy ratings or lack thereof should indicate when repeated presentations of a given feared stimulus/situation is warranted. (For further information on the application of inhibitory learning principles in exposure therapy, see Sewart & Craske, 2020.)

Stimulus Control

Pathological worry is often prompted by a broad range of, as opposed to invariant, stimuli (e.g., not receiving a response to a text within an expected time frame, receiving a bill in the mail). In addition, distinct from other anxiety-related disorders, the feared outcome—or unconditional stimulus (US)—continually shifts within and across episodes of worry (e.g., social rejection, illness, failure). As a result, the phenomenon of worry is pervasive and presents in a variety of everyday situations, allowing for continuous opportunities for negative reinforcement. As a result, individuals with excessive worry are described as having poor discriminative stimulus control wherein a large array of stimuli and contexts prompt worry-laden episodes (Borkovec et al., 2004). Therefore, efforts to restrict situations in which worry is permitted to occur is helpful in gaining control over excessive perseveration. Stimulus control or worry postponement procedures were pioneered by Borkovec, Wilkinson, Folensbee, and Lerman (1983) to help clients achieve greater stimulus discrimination. They consist of four general rules: (a) identify worrisome and unpleasant thoughts and learn to distinguish those from other more pleasant thoughts; (b) establish a 30-minute "worry period" to occur at the same time and in the same location; (c) delay spontaneous worry to the worry period and instead focus on the present moment; and (d) use the 30-minute worry period to worry about concerns and problem solve to reduce or eliminate concerns. Standalone stimulus control procedures have demonstrated significant reductions in daily worrying (Borkovec et al., 1983; McGowan & Behar, 2013).

Problem Orientation

When faced with current "real-world" problems, individuals with excessive worry display deficiencies in problem orientation, including appraisal of one-self as a problem-solving agent, perceptions of problems, and expectations re-garding problem-solving outcomes (D'Zurilla & Nezu, 2010; Robichaud & Dugas, 2005). Problem orientation is distinct from problem-solving skills (e.g., defining the problem and formulating problem-solving goals), which excessive worriers generally demonstrate knowledge of (Dugas et al., 1997). Excessive worriers may avoid solving problems due to the perception that problems are threatening or aversive, doubt their abilities as a problem-solving agent, and possess pessimism regarding problem-solving outcomes (Robichaud et al., 2019). The effects of a chosen solution may be unpredictable, which further leads to difficulty in effec-tively managing problems in individuals with a low tolerance for uncertainty. As a result, many pathological worriers exhibit a "negative problem orientation" and do not apply appropriate problem-solving skills. This, in turn, leaves the problem unsolved and increases the incidence of future worry. Thus, targeting problem-solving deficits observed in excessive worriers consists of improving both problem orientation and the application of problem-solving skills (see Robichaud et al., 2019). Active problem solving serves as a useful "alternative" to excessive worry.

Strategies to enhance problem orientation include (1) learning to identify problems before it is too late, (2) recognizing that problems are a normal part of everyday life, and (3) shifting one's view toward seeing problems as opportunities rather than threats (see Robichaud et al., 2019). For problem solving, individuals are trained to properly define a problem in discrete and clear terms in order to facilitate the formulation of related goals and potential solutions. In addition, ex-cessive worriers may be guided through how to strategically brainstorm alterna-tive, concrete solutions to problems. From these alternative solutions, excessive worriers are then guided through how to systematically chose the best—not perfect—solution. Solutions are then implemented and the effectiveness of the applied solution is then verified (Robichaud et al., 2019).

A result of ineffective application of problem-solving strategies and negative problem orientation is difficulty with time management. Further adding to time management difficulties, excessive worriers may feel the need to take on extra tasks out of personal responsibility and also desire that every outcome be "per-fect." To manage time more efficiently, clients may be encouraged to (1) delegate responsibility of tasks, (2) say "no" to overcommitting to tasks, (3) stick to an agenda, and (4) avoid perfectionism (Zinbarg et al., 2006). Time management also may be facilitated by organizing daily tasks and prioritizing activities that are time sensitive. Such strategies help clients avoid feeling overwhelmed with everyday issues.

Evidence on Cognitive Behavior Therapy Effectiveness

The aforementioned strategies originate from evidence-based theoretical understandings of excessive worry and generalized anxiety. That said, there has been limited standalone evaluation of these therapeutic approaches or dismantling studies seeking to assess individual components of manualized treatments. Thus, it is difficult to say with confidence which single strategies are essential and for whom are they especially effective, and which strategies are ultimately disposable. Overall, CBT is an empirically supported treatment for generalized anxiety disorder (Chambless & Ollendick, 2001), resulting in significant declines in worry-related symptoms and observed long-term maintenance of treatment gains (Covin et al., 2008; Cuijpers et al., 2014; Hunot et al., 2007). Although the exact features that constitute "CBT" vary a bit from protocol to protocol, they do not include "free association," "hypnosis," or strategies not described in this chapter. At this time, achieving treatment fidelity for CBT for excessive worry requires (a) cognitive restructuring—wherein targets can range from challenging overestimation of likelihood, severity of negative outcomes, or metacognitive beliefs about worry; (b) exposure, either in vivo or imaginal, as a means to provide extinction learning around feared outcomes involving uncertainty or aversive emotional experiences; (c) behavioral experimentation through which worry-related cognitions are tested and challenged through "real-life" experiences, which may involve stimulus control/worry postponement; (d) explicit removal of safety behaviors throughout all components of treatment; and (e) incorporation of strategies to enhance problem orientation. Using a case formulation-driven approach, these elements can be flexibly applied in a systematic, responsive, and data-driven manner to target the deficits present in the individual.

Overall, CBT packages have been evaluated in clinical trials and found to be superior to waitlist and nonspecific therapy control conditions (Borkovec & Ruscio, 2001; Cuijpers et al., 2014). Furthermore, some limited evidence suggests CBT is more effective than standalone applied relaxation (Cuijpers et al., 2014). Metacognitive therapy (MCT) and intolerance of uncertainty therapy (IUT)—both variants of traditional CBT—also demonstrate general efficacy in treating generalized anxiety disorder (Ladouceur et al., 2000; Normann et al., 2014). There is, however, a general dearth of research comparing active treatments.

Recent research suggests that individuals with a longer course of GAD may respond better to more focused treatments (e.g., cognitive therapy or self-control desensitization), whereas those with a shorter course may respond better to cognitive and behavioral techniques when delivered in combination (Fisher & Newman, 2013). Individuals with intrusive and dominant interpersonal problems were observed to respond better to behavioral therapy than interventions that include cognitive elements (Newman et al., 2017). These findings suggest a personalized approach may be more beneficial for more complex presentations of worry (i.e., long duration, interpersonal problems; Newman et al., 2020). With an overall lack of information to guide treatment-making decisions, a strong case formulation-driven approach (Persons, 2006) is suggested for the treatment of chronic worry. Selected interventions are guided by theory, the results of ongoing assessment (e.g., Penn State Worry Questionnaire; Molina & Borkovec, 1994), and may take a hypothesis-testing approach to each individual case.

REFERENCES

Beck, A. T., Emery, G., & Greenberg, R. L. (2005). *Anxiety disorders and phobias: A cognitive perspective*. Basic Books.

Beesdo-Baum, K., Jenjahn, E., Höfler, M., Lueken, U., Becker, E. S., & Hoyer, J. (2012). Avoidance, safety behavior, and reassurance seeking in generalized anxiety disorder. *Depression and Anxiety, 29*(11), 948–957.

Borkovec, T. D. (1994). The nature, functions, and origins of worry. In G. C. L. Davey & F. Tallis (Eds.), *Wiley series in clinical psychology. Worrying: Perspectives on theory, assessment and treatment* (pp. 5–33). John Wiley & Sons.

Borkovec, T. D., Alcaine, O. M., & Behar, E. (2004). Avoidance {Theory} of {Worry} and {Generalized} {Anxiety} {Disorder}. *Generalized Anxiety Disorder: {Advances} in Research and Practice, 2004,* 77–108.

Borkovec, T. D., Hazlett-Stevens, H., & Diaz, M. L. (1999). The role of positive beliefs about worry in generalized anxiety disorder and its treatment. *Clinical Psychology & Psychotherapy: An International Journal of Theory & Practice, 6*(2), 126–138.

Borkovec, T. D., & Hu, S. (1990). The effect of worry on cardiovascular response to phobic imagery. *Behaviour Research and Therapy, 28*(1), 69–73.

Borkovec, T. D., Robinson, E., Pruzinsky, T., & DePree, J. A. (1983). Preliminary exploration of worry: Some characteristics and processes. *Behaviour Research and Therapy, 21*(1), 9–16.

Borkovec, T. D., & Roemer, L. (1995). Perceived functions of worry among generalized anxiety disorder subjects: Distraction from more emotionally distressing topics? *Journal of Behavior Therapy and Experimental Psychiatry, 26*(1), 25–30. https://doi.org/10.1016/0005-7916(94)00064-s

Borkovec, T. D., Wilkinson, L., Folensbee, R., & Lerman, C. (1983). Stimulus control applications to the treatment of worry. *Behaviour Research and Therapy, 21*(3), 247–251.

Borkovec, T. D., Lyonfields, J. D., Wiser, S. L., & Deihl, L. (1993). The role of worrisome thinking in the suppression of cardiovascular response to phobic imagery. *Behaviour Research and Therapy, 31*(3), 321–324.

Borkovec, T. D., & Ruscio, A. M. (2001). Psychotherapy for generalized anxiety disorder. *The Journal of Clinical Psychiatry, 62,* 37–42.

Borkovec, T. D., Shadick, R. N., & Hopkins, M. (1991). *The nature of normal and pathological worry.* In R. M. Rapee & D. H. Barlow (Eds.), *Chronic anxiety: Generalized anxiety disorder and mixed anxiety-depression* (pp. 29–51). Guilford Press.

Brosschot, J. F., Gerin, W., & Thayer, J. F. (2006). The perseverative cognition hypothesis: A review of worry, prolonged stress-related physiological activation, and health. *Journal of Psychosomatic Research, 60*(2), 113–124.

Chambless, D. L., & Ollendick, T. H. (2001). Empirically supported psychological interventions: Controversies and evidence. *Annual Review of Psychology, 52*(1), 685–716.

Covin, R., Ouimet, A. J., Seeds, P. M., & Dozois, D. J. A. (2008). A meta-analysis of CBT for pathological worry among clients with GAD. *Journal of Anxiety Disorders, 22*(1), 108–116.

Craske, M. G., & Barlow, D. H. (2006). *Mastery of your anxiety and worry.* Oxford University Press.

Craske, M. G., Kircanski, K., Zelikowsky, M., Mystkowski, J., Chowdhury, N., & Baker, A. (2008). Optimizing inhibitory learning during exposure therapy. *Behaviour Rresearch and Therapy, 46*(1), 5–27.

Craske, M. G., Treanor, M., Conway, C. C., Zbozinek, T., & Vervliet, B. (2014). Maximizing exposure therapy: An inhibitory learning approach. *Behaviour Research and Therapy, 58*, 10–23.

Cuijpers, P., Sijbrandij, M., Koole, S., Huibers, M., Berking, M., & Andersson, G. (2014). Psychological treatment of generalized anxiety disorder: A meta-analysis. *Clinical Psychology Review, 34*(2), 130–140.

D'Zurilla, T. J., & Nezu, A. M. (2010). Problem-solving therapy. *Handbook of Cognitive-Behavioral Therapies, 3*, 197–225.

Dugas, M. J., Freeston, M. H., & Ladouceur, R. (1997). Intolerance of uncertainty and problem orientation in worry. *Cognitive Therapy and Research, 21*(6), 593–606.

Dugas, M. J., Gosselin, P., & Ladouceur, R. (2001). Intolerance of uncertainty and worry: Investigating specificity in a nonclinical sample. *Cognitive Therapy and Research, 25*(5), 551–558.

Dugas, M. J., Savard, P., Gaudet, A., Turcotte, J., Laugesen, N., Robichaud, M., Francis, K., & Koerner, N. (2007). Can the components of a cognitive model predict the severity of generalized anxiety disorder? *Behavior Therapy, 38*(2), 169–178.

Fisher, A. J., & Newman, M. G. (2013). Heart rate and autonomic response to stress after experimental induction of worry versus relaxation in healthy, high-worry, and generalized anxiety disorder individuals. *Biological Psychology, 93*(1), 65–74.

Hook, J. N., Davis, D. E., Owen, J., Worthington Jr, E. L., & Utsey, S. O. (2013). Cultural humility: Measuring openness to culturally diverse clients. *Journal of Counseling Psychology, 60*(3), 353.

Hoyer, J., Beesdo, K., Gloster, A. T., Runge, J., Höfler, M., & Becker, E. S. (2009). Worry exposure versus applied relaxation in the treatment of generalized anxiety disorder. *Psychotherapy and Psychosomatics, 78*(2), 106–115.

Hunot, V., Churchill, R., Teixeira, V., & de Lima, M. S. (2007). Psychological therapies for generalised anxiety disorder. *Cochrane Database of Systematic Reviews, 1*.

Kendall, P. C., Gosch, E., Furr, J. M., & Sood, E. (2008). Flexibility within fidelity. *Journal of the American Academy of Child and Adolescent Psychiatry, 47*(9), 987–993. https://doi.org/10.1097/CHI.0b013e31817eed2f

Kendall, P. C., & Frank, H. E. (2018). Implementing evidence-based treatment protocols: Flexibility within fidelity. *Clinical Psychology: Science and Practice, 25*(4), e12271.

Kim, H., & Newman, M. G. (2016, October). Emotional contrast avoidance in generalized anxiety disorder and major depressive disorder: A comparison between the perseveration processes of worry and rumination. Paper presented at the 50th Annual Meeting of the Association for Behavioral and Cognitive Therapies, New York, NY.

Ladouceur, R., Dugas, M. J., Freeston, M. H., Léger, E., Gagnon, F., & Thibodeau, N. (2000). Efficacy of a cognitive–behavioral treatment for generalized anxiety disorder: Evaluation in a controlled clinical trial. *Journal of Consulting and Clinical Psychology, 68*(6), 957.

Llera, S. J., & Newman, M. G. (2014). Rethinking the role of worry in generalized anxiety disorder: Evidence supporting a model of emotional contrast avoidance. *Behavior Therapy, 45*(3), 283–299.

MacLeod, C., & Rutherford, E. (2004). *Information-processing approaches: Assessing the selective functioning of attention, interpretation, and retrieval.* In R. G. Heimberg, C. L. Turk, & D. S. Mennin (Eds.), *Generalized anxiety disorder: Advances in research and practice* (pp. 109–142). The Guilford Press.

McGowan, S. K., & Behar, E. (2013). A preliminary investigation of stimulus control training for worry: Effects on anxiety and insomnia. *Behavior Modification, 37*(1), 90–112.

Mennin, D. S., Heimberg, R. G., Turk, C. L., & Fresco, D. M. (2005). Preliminary evidence for an emotion dysregulation model of generalized anxiety disorder. *Behaviour Research and Therapy, 43*(10), 1281–1310.

Mogg, K., & Bradley, B. P. (1998). A cognitive-motivational analysis of anxiety. *Behaviour Research and Therapy, 36*(9), 809–848.

Molina, S., & Borkovec, T. D. (1994). *The Penn State Worry Questionnaire: Psychometric properties and associated characteristics.*

Morrison, A. P., & Wells, A. (2007). Relationships between worry, psychotic experiences and emotional distress in patients with schizophrenia spectrum diagnoses and comparisons with anxious and non-patient groups. *Behaviour Research and Therapy, 45*(7), 1593–1600.

Newman, M. G., Castonguay, L. G., Borkovec, T. D., & Molnar, C. (2004). Integrative psychotherapy. In R. G. Heimberg, C. L. Turk, & D. S. Mennin (Eds.), *Generalized anxiety disorder: Advances in research and practice* (pp. 320–350). The Guilford Press.

Newman, M. G., Jacobson, N. C., Erickson, T. M., & Fisher, A. J. (2017). Interpersonal problems predict differential response to cognitive versus behavioral treatment in a randomized controlled trial. *Behavior Therapy, 48*(1), 56–68.

Newman, M. G., & Llera, S. J. (2011). A novel theory of experiential avoidance in generalized anxiety disorder: A review and synthesis of research supporting a contrast avoidance model of worry. *Clinical Psychology Review, 31*(3), 371–382.

Newman, M. G., Zainal, N. H., & Hoyer, J. (2020). Cognitive-behavioral therapy (CBT) for Generalized Anxiety Disorder (GAD). In L. Gerlach & A. T. Gloster (Eds.), *Generalized anxiety disorder and worrying: A comprehensive handbook for clinicians and researchers* (pp. 203–230). John Wiley & Sons.

Normann, N., van Emmerik, A. A. P., & Morina, N. (2014). The efficacy of metacognitive therapy for anxiety and depression: A meta-analytic review. *Depression and Anxiety, 31*(5), 402–411.

Olatunji, B. O., Wolitzky-Taylor, K. B., Sawchuk, C. N., & Ciesielski, B. G. (2010). Worry and the anxiety disorders: A meta-analytic synthesis of specificity to GAD. *Applied and Preventive Psychology, 14*(1–4), 1–24.

Peasley-Miklus, C., & Vrana, S. R. (2000). Effect of worrisome and relaxing thinking on fearful emotional processing. *Behaviour Research and Therapy, 38*(2), 129–144.

Persons, J. B. (2006). Case formulation–driven psychotherapy. *Clinical Psychology: Science and Practice, 13*(2), 167–170.

Robichaud, M., & Dugas, M. J. (2005). Negative problem orientation (Part II): Construct validity and specificity to worry. *Behaviour Research and Therapy, 43*(3), 403–412.

Robichaud, M., Koerner, N., & Dugas, M. J. (2019). *Cognitive behavioral treatment for generalized anxiety disorder: From science to practice.* Routledge.

Roemer, L., Salters, K., Raffa, S. D., & Orsillo, S. M. (2005). Fear and avoidance of internal experiences in GAD: Preliminary tests of a conceptual model. *Cognitive Therapy and Research, 29*(1), 71–88.

Salters-Pedneault, K., Roemer, L., Tull, M. T., Rucker, L., & Mennin, D. S. (2006). Evidence of broad deficits in emotion regulation associated with chronic worry and generalized anxiety disorder. *Cognitive Therapy and Research, 30*(4), 469–480.

Sassaroli, S., & Ruggiero, G. M. (2005). The role of stress in the association between low self esteem, perfectionism, and worry, and eating disorders. *International Journal of Eating Disorders, 37*(2), 135–141.

Sewart, A. R., & Craske, M. G. (2020). *Inhibitory learning.* In J. S. Abramowitz & S. M. Blakey (Eds.), *Clinical handbook of fear and anxiety: Maintenance processes and treatment mechanisms* (pp. 265–285). American Psychological Association.

Spada, M. M., & Wells, A. (2005). Metacognitions, emotion and alcohol use. *Clinical Psychology & Psychotherapy, 12*(2), 150–155.

van der Heiden, C., & ten Broeke, E. (2009). The when, why, and how of worry exposure. *Cognitive and Behavioral Practice, 16*(4), 386–393.

Wells, A. (1995). Meta-cognition and worry: A cognitive model of generalized anxiety disorder. *Behavioural and Cognitive Psychotherapy, 23*(3), 301–320.

Wells, A. (1999). A metacognitive model and therapy for generalized anxiety disorder. *Clinical Psychology & Psychotherapy: An International Journal of Theory & Practice, 6*(2), 86–95.

Wells, A. (2011). *Metacognitive therapy for anxiety and depression.* Guilford Press.

Wells, A., & Cartwright-Hatton, S. (2004). A short form of the metacognitions questionnaire: Properties of the MCQ-30. *Behaviour Research and Therapy, 42*(4), 385–396.

Wells, A., & King, P. (2006). Metacognitive therapy for generalized anxiety disorder: An open trial. *Journal of Behavior Therapy and Experimental Psychiatry, 37*(3), 206–212.

Zinbarg, R. E., Craske, M. G., & Barlow, D. H. (2006). *Mastery of your anxiety and worry (MAW): Therapist guide.* Oxford University Press.

3

Post-Traumatic Stress Disorder Treatment with Adults

Making Modifications While Maintaining Fidelity

COLLEEN A. SLOAN, SCOTT LITWACK,
AND DENISE M. SLOAN ■

A variety of evidence-based treatment approaches for post-traumatic stress disorder (PTSD) are available. Although these treatments are manual-based, knowing how and when to flexibly use these treatment protocols is key to reducing treatment dropout and maximizing treatment outcomes. In this chapter, consistent with the approach known as "flexibility within fidelity" (Kendall & Beidas, 2007; Kendall & Frank, 2018), we provide an overview of evidence-based treatment approaches for PTSD, describe the core underlying theories of these treatments, and then discuss conditions under which flexible delivery can be considered and how the treatments can be modified. Throughout the chapter we emphasize the importance of considering the underlying theory of the PTSD treatments when deciding when, how, and whether to make adaptations.

EVIDENCE-BASED TREATMENT FOR POST-TRAUMATIC STRESS DISORDER

There have been meaningful advances in the treatment of PTSD over the past 40 years, with several effective treatment protocols available for adults with PTSD. These treatments include Prolonged Exposure (PE; Foa et al., 2019), Cognitive Processing Therapy (CPT; Resick et al., 2017), cognitive behavioral therapy, exposure-based treatment, and cognitive therapy. Although acknowledged as a treatment, most PTSD treatment guidelines do not include Eye Movement Desensitization and Reprocessing Therapy (Shapiro, 2018) as a first line or recommended treatment approach because PTSD outcomes are generally small in magnitude (e.g., American Psychological Association [APA], 2017).

Although a variety of empirically supported programs are recommended for the treatment of PTSD (APA, 2017; Department of Veterans Affairs/Department of Defense, 2017; International Society in Trauma Stress Studies, 2018; National Institute for Health and Care Excellence, 2018), there is a central theme: Each is trauma-focused. That is, each protocol focuses on changing behaviors and thoughts resulting from the trauma experience. These treatments aim to change avoidance (e.g., avoidant behavior; negative cognitions), the factors known to maintain symptoms of PTSD. Two main theories underlie trauma-focused treatment approaches: (a) emotional processing theory and (b) information processing theory.

Theories of Post-Traumatic Stress Disorder

Emotional Processing Theory. Emotional Processing Theory of PTSD (EPT; Foa & Kozak, 1986) posits that individuals possess a fear network or "program" that is biologically functional to escape danger or threat. Within this network, associations exist that connect fear stimuli or cues (e.g., vicious animal) with fear responses (e.g., increased physiological arousal), as well as the meaning (e.g., vicious animals are threatening). When this network becomes activated by a "real" threat, such as a vicious animal, the individual response is considered adaptive, because escaping from a vicious animal may keep an individual alive and prevent harm. This fear network becomes maladaptive, however, when individuals experience traumatic events from which they are unable to recover and the network becomes overgeneralized and activates in situations where no "real" objective threat is present.

Maladaptive fear networks contain problematic network connections, wherein innocuous cues present at the time of the trauma become associated with threat, thus prompting fear response with attached meaning (e.g., feeling fearful when in presence of any animal after being attacked by vicious animal). Therefore, exposure-based trauma-focused treatment (rooted within EPT) aims to access the problematic fear network via behavioral exposure, in order to extinguish pathological fear response (i.e., fear that is out of proportion to the actual danger present in a given stimulus). Extinguishing pathological fear response is accomplished by repeatedly exposing a person to the stimulus (e.g., trauma memory, crowded grocery store) in the absence of danger so that the person learns that their feared situations and trauma memories are no longer dangerous. In other words, exposure activates the fear network, while simultaneously providing realistic, objective information regarding (a) the probability of harm and (b) the anticipated cost of experiencing the distress itself (e.g., "I'll go crazy if I experience anxiety.").

Prolonged Exposure (Foa et al., 2019) relies exclusively on EPT to conceptualize PTSD and utilizes two types of exposure in treatment—imaginal and in vivo.

Imaginal exposure, or revisiting a trauma memory, is conducted on the trauma memory itself and aims to enhance an individual's ability to access all details of the memory, promote emotional engagement, and facilitate an individual's own narrative of a traumatic event. In vivo exposures are conducted with situations, objects, places, and people an individual has been avoiding since the trauma to help facilitate habituation of distress when in the presence of these cues, while also aiming to increase an individual's sense of competency. Both imaginal and in vivo exposures directly target avoidance of trauma-related memories and relevant cues and promote trauma recovery via changing behavior, which in turn facilitates changes in trauma-related cognitions. Other recommended trauma-focused treatments also incorporate imaginal exposure and/or in-vivo exposures. For instance, written exposure therapy (Sloan & Marx, 2019) includes imaginal exposure via having clients repeatedly write about their trauma memory.

Information Processing Theory. Information-processing theory has been a foundation for understanding the development and maintenance of PTSD (Lang, 1979). This theory proposes that information about emotion-laden events, such as traumatic events, are stored in networks of information about the stimuli or situation, information about the person's responses to the stimuli, and the meaning of both the stimuli and responses. The cognitive model of PTSD more specifically proposes that PTSD is developed as a result of extreme negative appraisals of the trauma and/or the subsequent events that lead to a current sense of threat as well as a disruption in the autobiographical memory surrounding the trauma and its associations (Ehlers & Clark, 2000). Based on such a model, a number of cognitive therapies have been developed to treat PTSD, with CPT being the most widely implemented and studied to date (VA/DoD, 2017).

Cognitive therapies for PTSD begin with identifying the specific beliefs that maintain symptoms via an examination of the subjective impact that the traumatic event has on a person's life. This typically includes identifying specific beliefs about elements of the traumatic event including both the internal experience of the individual (e.g., emotions, physiological experiences) and the external environment and stimuli (e.g., sensory input such as noises and smells), as well as changes in the client's beliefs about underlying dimensions, such as safety, trust, and power. This examination of impact also may involve the explicit, detailed recounting of the event(s) in order to bring to light beliefs about the event itself and/or one's response to the event that are being avoided with or without awareness, and, in turn, maintaining symptoms.

Cognitive restructuring is the primary tool used in cognitive therapy for PTSD and involves identifying and challenging inaccurate, exaggerated, and/or unhelpful thoughts about the traumatic experiences themselves, one's reaction to the traumatic events both immediately and long-term, as well as broader beliefs about oneself, others, and the world in general that the individual has developed since the traumatic experiences. A number of strategies are commonly used to help with such challenges, including evaluating evidence for and against identified beliefs, incorporating more information at the micro- and macrolevels of the experience, and identifying assumptions and patterns of problematic thinking.

Socratic questioning is used by therapists during sessions to help guide the discussion toward active self-reflection and challenging of beliefs (e.g., "What's the evidence that the grocery store is dangerous?"). The goal is to develop alternative beliefs that are more accurate, balanced, and helpful. The adoption of such alternative beliefs is intended to lead to decreased negative appraisals of oneself, others, and the world, and in turn to reduce internal and behavioral avoidance and improve one's quality of life.

USING POST-TRAUMATIC STRESS DISORDER TREATMENTS FLEXIBLY TO MAXIMIZE OUTCOMES

Flexibility with Exposure-Based Treatments for Post-Traumatic Stress Disorder

The exposure-based treatment for PTSD that has received the most empirical support for its use is PE (APA, 2017; VA/DoD, 2017). This section draws from available literature evaluating PE and offers evidence-based guidelines and recommendations regarding when and how to conduct the intervention flexibly and with fidelity. Note that many of the suggestions made here also apply to other exposure-based treatments for PTSD. As is true for case conceptualization, the theory of the development and maintenance of PTSD is critical when considering making modifications to exposure-based treatment protocols. In general, modifications to the protocol are made to increase client engagement in treatment and maximize treatment outcome.

Brown and colleagues (2019) highlight mechanisms of change including emotion activation, within-session pathological fear extinction, between-session extinction, and PTSD-related negative cognitions, and indicate that modifications made to the treatment protocol should aim to enable or enhance these mechanisms. These authors also cite research findings indicating that within-session pathological fear extinction is less relevant, because it is not related to treatment outcome. Therefore, the following will focus on modifications in exposure therapy to promote emotion activation and facilitate change in PTSD-related negative cognitions. Although promotion of between-session extinction is specific to exposure therapy, relevant modifications function to enhance between-session compliance, which is necessary for cognitive therapies as well; as such, we will discuss modifications to promote between-session compliance more broadly later in this chapter.

FLEXIBILITY TO ADDRESS UNDERENGAGEMENT AND PROMOTE EMOTION ACTIVATION

According to EPT, emotion activation must occur to access one's fear network, promote extinction, and correct faulty beliefs and meanings. When difficulties arise that interfere with emotion processing, they must be addressed to facilitate response to treatment and recovery from trauma. Brown and colleagues (2019) suggest revisiting rationale and reiterating psychoeducation, as inadequate under-standing or "buy-in" are possible interfering factors. Either in conjunction with this or separately, exploring faulty beliefs about engagement is also recommended. For example, does the client believe that he/she/they will "lose it" if they engage? Efforts to help shift these beliefs via reiterating psychoeducation and rationale may be useful. Additionally, engaging in general, nontrauma-related emotional exposures (e.g., exposure to sadness- or anxiety-related cues) also may be helpful to increase clients' "buy-in" through direct experience. Finally, therapist prompts during imaginal exposure may prove useful. Generally speaking, the therapist avoids engaging with clients during imaginal exposure, so as to not distract or dis-rupt clients' engagement. However, when clients are displaying underengagement (e.g., little to no affect; monotone voice; fast pace when recalling painful details), therapists may use prompts including asking about physiological symptoms, thoughts, and emotions, and may work to help the client remain engaged in the "worst" moments of the memory. For instance, a therapist may ask a client, "In this moment, what do you feel in your body?" or "What is running through your mind when the gun is pointed at you?" The strategy is essential, but it can be implemented with flexibility.

FLEXIBILITY IN DELIVERING IMAGINAL AND IN VIVO EXPOSURE

Clients may have difficulty with in vivo exposures but not with imaginal exposures or vice versa. Although clinicians may be able to use content discussed earlier to address some of these challenges effectively, this section provides additional recommendations to increase client willingness to continue in treatment and to engage effectively with exposure. These recommendations may be particularly helpful when clients present with a history of multiple traumatic events, across trauma types, and when the client and the therapist have difficulty with collabora-tively identifying initial treatment targets.

Imaginal exposure. It is generally recommended to start imaginal exposure on the event that is most distressing to the client. Therapists are encouraged to engage in honest, direct discussion regarding the benefits of this approach, be-cause it likely will give the client the "most bang for their buck" (i.e., lead to the greatest generalization of decreasing avoidance and fear of less distressing events). At the same time, clients may not be willing to engage with their most distressing memory, but may be willing to start with a memory that is less distressing. Therapists are encouraged to engage in a discussion about the costs and benefits of each approach and collaboratively decide the best course of action with their clients. Although starting with a less distressing event may temporarily reinforce avoidant behavior, it also may empower the client to make their own decision and reduce the likelihood of premature treatment dropout. Additionally, when clients benefit from exposure on less distressing memories, this builds mastery; in turn, clients may internalize increased competency, which better enables them to continue with treatment. Thus, it may be best to develop a hierarchy of traumatic memories to use for imaginal exposures rather than focus on the most distressing trauma memory.

Specific adjustments can be made when conducting imaginal exposure. The specific instructions for imaginal exposure specify that clients close their eyes, speak out loud and in present tense, and provide explicit details. As a general rule, therapists aim to conduct imaginal exposure with these instructions and coach and reinforce clients when difficulties arise. However, the PE protocol (Foa et al., 2019) allows for "titrating" exposures in order to make them more tolerable to clients. For example, the therapist might ask the client to recall a memory with eyes open initially, gradually working toward client recalling with eyes closed. Similarly, clients may initially recall the event in past tense, again gradually working toward recalling in present tense; therapists may choose to have clients write out a traumatic memory before recalling verbally. Although session-duration considerations will be discussed in detail later, it is worth mentioning here that clients may evidence difficulty tolerating imaginal exposure for the recommended 40 minutes. When this occurs, the therapist and client may choose to shorten the duration; indeed, shortening imaginal exposure sessions has found to be unrelated to treatment outcome (e.g., Nacasch et al., 2015; van Minnen & Foa, 2006). The therapist and client have a thoughtful discussion regarding these modifications, with attention to considering the possible role of avoidance (i.e., avoidance of engaging in imaginal exposure) and determining the best path forward to keep the client engaged in and benefitting from treatment.

In vivo exposure. In addition to recommendations that function to promote between-session extinction (discussed later), modifications to the actual implementation of in vivo exposures may be useful. First, it is recommended that clients start in vivo exposure with a situation on their hierarchy that is moderately distressing, generally an exposure that the client rated via Subjective Units of Distress Scale (SUDS) of approximately 40 (on a scale from 0 to 100). Simultaneously, therapists carefully consider what specific exposures will help facilitate mastery and sense of competency as quickly as possible. Accordingly, the therapist and client may thoughtfully choose an item ranked at or lower than 40 SUDS on the hierarchy to facilitate effective engagement and success. Relatedly, and consistent with the PE protocol (Foa et al., 2019), in vivo exposures also can be "titrated." For example, a therapist and client may choose to assign an exposure task, but make a slight adjustment to reduce the SUDS rating. For instance, the client first looking at pictures of military fatigues, then client looking at their own military fatigues, followed by client wearing military fatigues. Other options that might help with titration include incorporation of "coaches." For instance, a therapist may assign a client to go to a store first with a friend/coach, then alone while friend waits in car, then alone without friend but available via phone, then alone without friend at all. When clients repeatedly struggle with engagement despite these adjustments, therapists may choose to first engage in an in vivo assignment with their client, and then assign the client to continue without the therapist for homework (perhaps with some of the aforementioned modifications, but with the ultimate goal that the client will complete alone).

PTSD-related negative cognition. In many instances, what is referred to as exposure therapy does not directly incorporate traditional cognitive therapy strategies. That is, the goal of exposure therapy is to create opportunities that naturally challenge a client's trauma-related beliefs through direct experience and foster corrective learning. Cognitive therapy directly asks clients to specifically attend to their thoughts and challenge them using cognitive restructuring skills.

The details elicited via imaginal exposure facilitate a shift in clients' perceptions about the traumatic event itself, their behavior at the time of the event, and sense of responsibility. Likewise, in vivo exposure helps clients change their beliefs regarding objective safety and incompetency via their direct experience. In fact, PE has been found to reduce trauma-related cognitions effectively even without adding a cognitive restructuring component to treatment (Foa & Rauch, 2004). Nevertheless, Craske and colleagues (2014) have identified ways to enhance exposure therapy for anxiety disorders and PTSD by more explicitly attending to the cognitions that maintain symptoms. These authors recommend strategies that attend to: (1) expectancy violation, (2) deepened extinction, (3) occasional reinforced extinction, (4) removal of safety signals, (5) variability, (6) retrieval cues, (7) multiple contexts, and (8) affect labeling. For example, if a client has difficulty engaging in in vivo exposure due to specific fear-related belief of "losing control and lashing out at others," enhancing in vivo exposure by explicitly attending to this belief and focusing on corrective learning after exposure completion may be useful. Indeed, the Dialectical Behavior Therapy Prolonged Exposure (DBT PE) integrated protocol for PTSD (Harned & Schmidt, 2019) uses enhanced exposure tracking, relying on therapy tools that specifically evaluate cognitive factors such as the cost and probability estimates related to the exposure experience. Explicit attention in the context of exposure may prove useful to facilitating change in inaccurate PTSD-related negative cognitions (e.g., "People can't be trusted." "The world is a dangerous place.").

Flexibility with Cognitive Treatments for Post-Traumatic Stress Disorder

The core components of cognitive restructuring for PTSD include identifying thoughts and feelings in response to events, challenging one's thoughts, and generating alternative ways of viewing situations (e.g., Resick et al., 2002). Cognitive Processing Therapy is by far the most empirically supported cognitive treatment for PTSD, so we will describe it and the potentially helpful flexibilities. The flexibilities described here are, however, relevant for other cognitive treatments for PTSD.

CPT involves clients sharing their beliefs about why the traumatic event occurred and ways in which it has changed their thinking about themselves, others, and the world, as well as some degree of sharing about the trauma experience to uncover potentially maladaptive beliefs related to the trauma. Therapists use Socratic questioning to help clients critically examine and challenge extreme, rigid, inflexible, and inaccurate beliefs that have been learned through or reinforced by traumatic experiences. Therapists introduce multiple worksheets that guide clients through learning various techniques for how to challenge beliefs. Clients first complete worksheets in session collaboratively with therapists to reinforce learning how to complete them, and then clients complete worksheets independently between sessions. Maladaptive beliefs about the traumatic experience (assimilated) are targeted first in treatment, followed by the targeting of broader beliefs that have been extremely altered after the trauma (overaccommodated). Therapists provide clients psychoeducation related to common themes (e.g., trust) and ask clients to identify and challenge maladaptive beliefs that they may have related to these themes (e.g., "If I trust anyone, I will get hurt.").

Although adaptations of CPT over the past two decades have involved more general aspects of treatment structure (e.g., frequency of sessions), changes to the core process of cognitive restructuring have been implemented in response to working with individuals with PTSD who have cognitive, educational, and language limitations (Galovski et al., 2020). To increase effectiveness of response in individuals with ongoing memory, attention, or problem-solving deficits (e.g., related to traumatic brain injury, low intelligence level), adaptations can include simplifying and reorganizing cognitive restructuring worksheets (Jak et al., 2019). For example, Jak and colleagues (2019) adapted the "Challenging Questions" Worksheet in CPT from eleven to seven questions, five of which have response choices instead of the standard open-ended prompts. Additionally, cultural adaptations to language and, in particular, metaphors, have been implemented in a number of settings including in the Middle East, as well as with refugees in the United States (e.g., Bass et al., 2013; Weiss et al., 2015). This includes the incorporation of pictures in place of words (e.g., Kaysen et al., 2013) and the memorization of forms and concepts, so that clients with literacy limitations can practice cognitive restructuring and culturally adapted phrasing, such as using the term "small work" instead of "homework" (Bass et al., 2013). Furthermore, clinical examples of maladaptive beliefs and cognitive restructuring have regularly been adapted to the specific culture in which the treatment is being implemented. In their adaptation of CPT for Spanish-speaking Latinx clients seen in a diverse community mental health clinic, Valentine and colleagues (2017) incorporated clinical examples that focused on traumatic experiences most common to this population, namely community violence, domestic violence, physical assault, and gang violence.

Additional changes have been made to some aspects of the basic structure of CPT when adapting the treatment for traumatized populations in low resource settings and with trauma survivors who are illiterate. For instance, oral completion of assignments has been implemented when literacy levels made the use of written assignments impossible (e.g., Bass et al., 2013).

Flexibility with Trauma-Focused Treatments

We have described ways in which flexibility can be used in the delivery of specific treatment components of exposure- and cognitive-based treatments for

PTSD. Other approaches for clients suffering with PTSD are referred to as trauma focused, and we next describe modifications that can be made to maximize outcomes in trauma-focused treatment more generally.

Flexibility with Between-Session Practice

A key component of most cognitive behavioral interventions is homework, otherwise known as between-session practice. In both PE and CPT, homework compliance is associated with greater reduction in PTSD symptoms (Brown et al., 2019; Cooper et al., 2017; Resick et al., 2017), suggesting that attention to this particular component is important for positive change and essential for treatment fidelity. Client compliance with homework assignments is variable, however, and increasing compliance may require employing additional strategies. These strategies include exploring and addressing faulty beliefs interfering with compliance, exploring and addressing ambivalence, and revisiting rationale. Addressing faulty beliefs lends itself well to CPT in particular, because therapists may ask clients to complete worksheets on beliefs about the treatment itself. Relatedly, therapists may assess clients' perceptions regarding the intensity of homework assignments involving in vivo exposures and alter the intensity to align more with client willingness to engage in the exposures. Therapists also might consider use of motivation enhancement strategies, as well as offer between-session support (check-in phone calls) to increase compliance and motivation. Lastly, behavioral strategies also can be used; therapists can reinforce any evidence of compliance, even if not "perfect," and can work to shape behavior toward more effective engagement. For example, if a client is unwilling to listen to an imaginal recording daily, the therapist can ask for commitment to listen three times per week. Likewise, if a client is unwilling to complete CPT worksheets daily, the therapist can ask the client to complete the worksheets less frequently. Problem-solving, including planning around anticipated barriers, also may be useful. Proactively addressing any barriers decreases the ease with which clients can avoid between-session practice assignments. Therapists also may consider inviting clients to call with "good news" or between-session task successes to reinforce compliance.

Refusal: Flexibility When Addressing Unwillingness

Therapists and clients are encouraged to have thoughtful discussions regarding available treatment options, client willingness, barriers, and necessity of specific treatment components. For instance, clients engaged in PE may request to focus only on imaginal exposure rather than both imaginal exposure and in vivo exposures. Importantly, there is no evidence to support that delivering PE in such a piecemeal fashion is efficacious (Brown et al., 2019). If clients are unwilling to engage in a particular required treatment component, the therapist and client may collaboratively choose another trauma-focused treatment approach. In CPT, the therapist and client collaboratively choose whether or not to include a trauma narrative account, because this component is no longer considered a required component of the CPT protocol (Resick et al., 2017).

Flexibility Based on Client Identity and Type of Trauma

There has been discussion and debate within the field of mental health and trauma regarding the differentiation between traumatic stressors and minority stressors (e.g., identity-based discrimination), with particular focus on Criterion A (APA, 2013) traumatic stressors and non-Criterion A stressors specifically impacting minoritized groups, such as racial, ethnic, sexual, and gender minority communities. We will not attempt to reconcile nor add to this debate here, but we do believe it is important to draw from relevant literature (e.g., Williams et al., 2014; Livingston et al., 2019) and recommend that trauma therapists carefully consider the diverse identities of their clients, to educate themselves on relevant cultural factors associated with these identities, assess for minority stress (e.g., Hendricks & Testa, 2012), and incorporate minority stress models into case conceptualizations and treatment. Therapists are best when they understand the ways in which minority stress may complicate traumatic stress and clinical presentation, as well as ways in which minority stress may contribute to negative trauma-related cognitions and nontrauma-related negative cognitions (e.g., internalized stigma) and adaptive versus maladaptive avoidance (e.g., Black man avoiding police officers vs. avoiding leaving the house).

Logistical Flexibility

ATTENDING TO CLIENT-ENVIRONMENT FACTORS

Given the importance of between-session adherence, therapists are wise to consider evaluating the factors outside of the therapy room that may be affecting treatment. Therapists and clients benefit from thoughtful discussions regarding if and when to include family members or other important people in clients' lives. The therapist and the client may agree to schedule an additional session, wherein a client's partner is present in the session. This session can be used to provide the client's family member with information about the symptoms of PTSD and the goals of trauma-focused treatment. Engaging the family member can be helpful to ensure that the family member does not engage in accommodating behaviors (e.g., bringing food into the home so the client can avoid going out of the house) and instead serve as an additional support to the client in completing assignments between sessions. In addition, the therapist may inquire about the client's physical home environment and assess for the presence of safety cues (e.g., home security systems, weapons), while also incorporating an appreciation for objectively dangerous environments in which clients may live. Overall, logistical modifications aim to enhance the client's ability to successfully both attend sessions and complete between-session tasks.

FLEXIBILITY WITH SESSION FREQUENCY

Trauma-focused treatments are typically recommended to be delivered twice per week and this is the schedule of delivery of sessions that has been evaluated in studies examining efficacy and effectiveness of trauma-focused treatments (e.g., Resick et al., 2017; Foa et al., 2019). Delivering treatment twice per week is suggested to minimize avoidance behavior in which clients with PTSD are likely to engage. Relatedly, more frequent initial sessions may encourage homework compliance. Increasing homework compliance is especially important when conducting in vivo exposures as well as practicing and mastering cognitive restructuring skills.

There is evidence that delivering trauma-focused treatment in a massed format (e.g., five times per week) is associated with treatment outcome similar to the standard format of delivery but with significantly better treatment retention (Sciarrino, Warnecke, & Teng, 2020). Delivering treatment in a massed format would be a particularly desirable delivery method in an intensive outpatient program or residential program.

Despite the standard recommendations to deliver treatment twice per week, it is not always feasible or possible to deliver treatment sessions twice per week. Some clinics are not able to accommodate twice-per-week sessions due to the high number of clients in need of services in combination with the availability of providers. In such instances, sessions can be scheduled weekly. Given the focus on completing homework assignments to practice cognitive restructuring skills, listen to imaginal recordings, and conduct in vivo exposures, spacing sessions less frequently than once a week is likely to dampen the effects of the treatment. Indeed, Gutner and colleagues (2016) found that a shorter amount of time between sessions was associated with better treatment outcomes for both PE and CPT. These investigators also found that the more time between sessions, the greater the likelihood that clients will prematurely drop out of treatment. These matters are given careful attention as one decides on the frequency with which treatment sessions will be delivered.

There are instances in which sessions might be scheduled less frequently than once per week. For instance, if the client or the therapist will be out of town on vacation or due to a client's work demands (e.g., business trips). A discussion about planned absences should occur at the start of treatment. It is important to have consistent sessions that occur at least once a week at the beginning phase of trauma-focused treatment, when dropout is most likely to occur (Gutner et al., 2016). Spacing sessions two weeks apart might be considered toward the end of treatment as a way to phase out treatment and allow clients more time to practice skills they learn during treatment. Another possibility is to propose a compromise with clients who state they can only attend sessions weekly. Specifically, the therapist can suggest that sessions are held twice a week for just the first week or two, during the phase of treatment that is typically the most challenging because clients are starting exposures and/or learning how to challenge their cognitive distortions. After this first week or two, sessions can occur once per week.

FLEXIBILITY WITH NUMBER AND DURATION OF SESSIONS

The treatment protocols for evidence-based trauma-focused approaches are very clear regarding the number and duration of sessions included in the protocols. There is, however, growing evidence that clients may not need as many sessions and as long of a duration of sessions as prescribed in the treatment manual to achieve good outcomes. For instance, there are now several studies indicating that 90-minute sessions of PE are not necessary; 60-minute sessions result in treatment outcomes that are comparable to 90-minute sessions (Foa et al., 2020; Nacasch et al., 2015; van Minnen & Foa, 2006). The shorter PE sessions are the result of decreasing the amount of time dedicated to imaginal exposures. When PE was initially developed it was assumed that at least 40 minutes of imaginal exposure was needed for successful treatment outcome, but accumulating evidence suggests that only 20 minutes of imaginal exposure is needed. These findings have practice implications, given that 90-minute sessions may be difficult to accommodate in clinic settings, and may not be possible for clients.

There is growing evidence that the number of sessions indicated in trauma-focused treatment manuals can be flexible. For instance, van Minnen and Foa (2006) found that clients in PE had a 50% reduction in baseline PTSD symptoms at the seventh session of PE and no further reduction of symptoms was observed after the seventh session. Similarly, Sloan and Marx reported that five sessions of 30-minute imaginal exposures conducted using written narratives is sufficient for successful treatment outcome (Sloan et al., 2012) and is not inferior to treatment outcome compared with the more time-intensive CPT (Sloan et al., 2018). Variability in optimal treatment dose also has been reported for CPT. The CPT protocol consists of 12, one-hour sessions, but there is support for using a variable length format, which adjusts the number of sessions to accommodate client needs (Galovski et al., 2012; Resick et al., 2020). Taken together, the findings underscore the importance of evaluating treatment progress, and ending treatment once the desired treatment outcome is obtained rather than a rigid delivery of a proscribed number of sessions regardless of treatment gain.

FLEXIBILITY WITH DELIVERY FORMAT

The most common format for delivering trauma-focused treatments is in person. There may be times, however, when it is not possible or desirable to deliver treatment in person. Indeed, there is increasing demand for telehealth delivery of psychological therapies. Treatment offered remotely might be the only option for clients who would otherwise need to travel a considerable distance or who may have health issues that make it very difficult or impossible to travel. The COVID-19 global pandemic also has necessitated the need to deliver treatment remotely (Rosen et al., 2020). In general, remote delivery of treatment can increase the reach of evidence-based treatments to clients in need of these treatments and can lead to greater treatment retention. There is a growing body of evidence that delivering trauma-focused treatment remotely is as effective as delivering treatment in person (e.g., Morland et al., 2014; Yuen et al., 2015). The studies conducted to date, however, have examined telehealth delivery using videoconferencing. The effectiveness of trauma-focused treatment delivered via telephone is currently unknown.

In addition to delivering treatment via telehealth, there is evidence that treatment delivered in the client's home may increase a client's engagement and retention in treatment. This literature finds that delivering trauma-focused treatment in the client's home is just as effective as delivering treatment in the clinic. Moreover, treatment dropout rates are substantially lower when treatment is delivered in the client's home (e.g., Morland et al., 2019; Peterson et al., 2019). For instance, Resick and colleagues (2020) found dropout rates to be 21% for individuals who completed CPT with the provider presenting to their home compared with a dropout rate of 33% for those who completed CPT via telehealth, and 44% for participants who completed CPT in the therapist's office.

Taken together, the findings indicate that flexibility in *where* treatment is conducted affects the likelihood that clients will complete trauma-focused treatment. Giving clients choices on how and where treatment is delivered will improve treatment retention. Nevertheless, where treatment is delivered should be carefully considered. For example, it may not be in the client's best interest to receive care in their home if they are isolating themselves within their home; alternatively, a therapist and client may agree to initiate treatment at the client's home or remotely with an explicit plan to shift the location of treatment to the clinic office, which would build on the client's developing competency.

FLEXIBILITY DUE TO CRISIS SITUATIONS

Clients with PTSD often present to treatment sessions reporting a recent crisis that they want to be the focus of the session rather than continuing the trauma-focused treatment session. In addition, clients can experience an increase in suicidal ideation or symptom exacerbation, which may necessitate setting aside the planned trauma-focused treatment session to address the issue. It can, at times, be appropriate to conduct several emergency or crisis sessions during the course of trauma-focused treatment. It is important, however, to evaluate whether an emergency session is needed, as well as to track the number of emergency sessions that are conducted. If a client needs repeated emergency sessions (i.e., more than three during the course of treatment or multiple crisis sessions in a row) during the course of trauma-focused treatment, then trauma-focused treatment should be stopped in order to manage the recurring clinical emergencies.

Therapists are wise to evaluate whether or not a trauma-focused treatment session should be set aside due to a recent crisis event. The occurrence of such events is likely to be frequent during the course of treatment, especially if it develops into a reinforcing pattern of avoidance. It is often in the best interest of the client to continue to progress with trauma-focused treatment sessions rather than to intermittently cease trauma-focused sessions to address recurring "crises." One strategy to manage such recurring events is to set aside the last 10 to 15 minutes of a session to discuss them. This strategy will address the client's desire to discuss pressing life events, while still progressing with trauma-focused treatment. In addition, therapists may reinforce treatment compliance by offering additional between-session contact (e.g., phone calls) to address stressors if a client follows through with all of their trauma-focused assignment.

Flexibility Due to Comorbid Mental Health Conditions

Approximately 80% of individuals with PTSD are diagnosed with a comorbid mental health disorder in their lifetime (Foa et al., 2009). A common concern among clinicians is whether trauma-focused treatments can be implemented with clients who have comorbid conditions, such as substance use disorder. Importantly, successful treatment responses from CPT and PE have been found for individuals who have a variety of comorbid conditions, including substance use disorders (e.g., Kaysen et al., 2014; Foa et al., 2013) depression (e.g., Larsen et al., 2020), anxiety (e.g., Lloyd et al., 2014), and personality disorders (e.g., Holder et al., 2017). Decisions about whether to use the standard protocols for trauma-focused therapies or to consider sequential treatment or adaptations are best when based on a number of factors. A thorough conceptualization of the relationship between the comorbid conditions is necessary, and attention should be given to the timing of symptom development, the severity of symptoms of each disorder, and the apparent function of the maladaptive cognitions or behaviors of the comorbid condition. For example, a standard trauma-focused protocol would be more indicated if the comorbid condition developed or was clearly exacerbated after the trauma (e.g., substance use disorder emerging after the trauma), the function of the behaviors tied to the comorbid condition are conceptually related to trauma symptoms (e.g., alcohol is used mostly in the evenings to manage trauma-related sleep problems), and the severity of the comorbid condition does not indicate the necessity for a sequential approach (e.g., severity of alcohol use does not indicate the necessity for a detox and the client has shown recent ability to limit or abstain from alcohol use).

Standard trauma-focused therapies have been found to be effective for many clients with comorbid conditions, but there are others who do not experience meaningful improvement, and there is some evidence that comorbid conditions may decrease the likelihood of a fully effective treatment response (Foa et al., 2013). Integrated treatments designed to target PTSD and comorbid conditions have been developed in hopes of improving these outcomes. These integrated treatment protocols address a broad range of comorbidities including but not limited to depression, substance use disorders, Borderline Personality Disorder, chronic pain, and traumatic brain injury. Many of these treatments supplement trauma-focused treatments with additional structure and skills. Although some add additional components prior to the introduction of CPT or PE (Galovski et al., 2016), more commonly, comorbid treatments target both disorders in an integrated manner. For example, Harned and Schmidt (2019) integrated dialectical behavior therapy for Borderline Personality Disorder with PE in a staged, principle-driven treatment.

When considering integrated treatments and the desire for fidelity, it is critical that the core procedures of the PTSD treatments are maintained, and that any adaptations are principle-driven and based in clear case conceptualizations. Additionally, when considering adding components from other treatments, it is important that clinicians are sensitive to the potential cognitive, emotional, and logistical burden clients may experience when focusing on a broader set of symptoms. Treatments that are conceptually grounded in a common theory and integrated to use common interventions (e.g., primarily behavioral interventions targeting both disorders) are more likely to be effective without increasing burden. For example, Norman and colleagues (2019) developed a treatment for PTSD and SUD that integrates PE with cognitive behavioral relapse prevention skills for SUD across 12 sessions; Otis and colleagues (2009) integrated components of CPT with components of CBT for chronic pain management into a 12-session treatment.

CONCLUSIONS

Trauma-focused treatments for PTSD are manual-based protocols that have been found to be effective, but these protocols are effective when used flexibly. Modifications to the protocols rely on an understanding of the theory underlying the treatment, so that the protocols are implemented flexibly without comprising their fidelity. The examples provided illustrate how and when PTSD treatments can be modified with the ultimate goal of maximizing treatment outcomes.

REFERENCES

American Psychiatric Association. (2013). Anxiety Disorders. In *Diagnostic and statistical manual of mental disorders* (5th ed.). Author. https://doi.org/10.1176/appi.books.9780890425596.dsm05

American Psychological Association. (2017). *Clinical practice guideline for the treatment of PTSD*. Author.

Bass, J. K., Annan, J., Murray, S. M., Kaysen, D., Griffiths, S., Cetinoglu, T., Wachter, K., Murray, L. K., & Bolton, P. A. (2013). Controlled trial of psychotherapy for Congolese survivors of sexual violence. *New England Journal of Medicine, 368*(23), 2182–2191. doi:10.1056/nejmoa1211853

Brown, L. A., Zandberg, L. J., & Foa, E. B. (2019). Mechanisms of change in prolonged exposure therapy for PTSD: Implications for clinical practice. *Journal of Psychotherapy Integration, 29*(1), 6–14. https://doi-org.ezproxy.bu.edu/10.1037/int0000109

Cooper, A. A., Kline, A. C., Graham, B., Bedard Gilligan, M., Mello, P. G., Feeny, N. C., & Zoellner, L. A. (2017). Homework "dose," type, and helpfulness as predictors of clinical outcomes in prolonged exposure for PTSD. *Behavior Therapy, 48*, 182–194. http://dx.doi.org/10.1016/j.beth.2016 .02.013

Craske, M. G., Treanor, M., Conway, C. C., Zbozinek, T., & Vervliet, B. (2014). Maximizing exposure therapy: An inhibitory learning approach. *Behaviour Research and Therapy, 58*, 10–23. https://doi.org/10.1016/j.brat.2014.04.006

Department of Veterans Affairs and Department of Defense (VA/DoD; 2017). *VA/DoD clinical practice guideline for the management of posttraumatic stress disorder and acute stress disorder*. Author.

Ehlers, A., & Clark, D. M. (2000). A cognitive model of posttraumatic stress disorder. *Behaviour Research and Therapy, 38*(4), 319–345. https://doi.org/10.1016/s0005-7967(99)00123-0

Foa, E. B., Acierno, R. Muzzy, W., Rosenfield, D., & Bredemeier, K. (Oct, 2020). *90-minute versus 60-minute sessions of prolonged exposure for the treatment of PTSD.* Presentation at the 5th Annual San Antonio Combat PTSD Conference.

Foa, E. B., Hembree, E., Rothbaum, B. O., & Rauch, S. A. M. (2019). Prolonged exposure *therapy for PTSD: Emotional processing of traumatic experiences therapist guide* (2nd ed.). Oxford University Press.

Foa, E. B., Keane, T. M., Friedman, M. J., & Cohen, J. A. (Eds.). (2009). *Effective treatments for PTSD: Practice guidelines from the International Society for Traumatic Stress Studies* (2nd ed.). The Guilford Press.

Foa, E. B., & Kozak, M. J. (1986). Emotional processing of fear: Exposure to corrective information. *Psychological Bulletin, 99*(1), 20–35. https://doi.org/10.1037/0033-2909.99.1.20

Foa, E. B., & Rauch, S. A. M. (2004). Cognitive changes during prolonged exposure versus prolonged exposure plus cognitive restructuring in female assault survivors with posttraumatic stress disorder. *Journal of Consulting and Clinical Psychology, 72*(5), 879–884. https://doi.org/10.1037/0022-006X.72.5.879

Foa, E. B., Yusko, D. A., McLean, C. P., Suvak, M. K., Bux, D. A., Jr, Oslin, D., O'Brien, C. P., Imms, P., Riggs, D. S., & Volpicelli, J. (2013). Concurrent naltrexone and prolonged exposure therapy for patients with comorbid alcohol dependence and PTSD: A randomized clinical trial. *JAMA, 310*(5), 488–495. https://doi.org/10.1001/jama.2013.8268

Galovski, T. E., Blain, L. M., Mott, J. M., Elwood, L., & Houle, T. (2012). Manualized therapy for PTSD: Flexing the structure of cognitive processing therapy. *Journal of Consulting and Clinical Psychology, 80*(6), 968–981. https://doi.org/10.1037/a0030600

Galovski, T. E., Harik, J. M., Blain, L. M., Elwood, L., Gloth, C., & Fletcher, T. D. (2016). Augmenting cognitive processing therapy to improve sleep impairment in PTSD: A randomized controlled trial. *Journal of Consulting and Clinical Psychology, 84*(2), 167–177. https://doi.org/ 10.1037/ccp0000059.

Galovski, T., Nixon, R., & Kaysen, D. (2020). *Flexible applications of cognitive processing therapy*. Academic Press.

Gutner, C. A., Gallagher, M. W., Baker, A. S., Sloan, D. M., & Resick, P. A. (2016). Time course of treatment dropout in cognitive-behavioral therapies for posttraumatic stress disorder. *Psychological Trauma: Theory, Research, Practice and Policy, 8*(1), 115–121. https://doi.org/10.1037/tra0000062

Gutner, C. A., Suvak, M. K., Sloan, D. M., & Resick, P. A. (2016). Does timing matter? Examining the impact of session timing on outcome. *Journal of Consulting and Clinical Psychology, 84*(12), 1108–1115. https://doi.org/10.1037/ccp0000120

Harned, M. S., & Schmidt, S. C. (2019). Integrating PTSD treatment into DBT: Clinical application and implementation of the DBT Prolonged Exposure protocol. In M. Swales (Ed.), *Oxford Handbook of Dialectical Behaviour Therapy* (pp. 797–814). Oxford University Press.

Hendricks, M. L., & Testa, R. J. (2012). A conceptual framework for clinical work with transgender and gender nonconforming clients: An adaptation of the Minority

Stress Model. *Professional Psychology: Research and Practice, 43*(5), 460–467. https://doi-org.ezproxy.bu.edu/10.1037/a0029597

Holder, N., Holliday, R., Pai, A., & Suris, A. (2017). Role of borderline personality disorder in the treatment of military sexual trauma-related posttraumatic stress disorder with cognitive processing therapy. *Behavioral Medicine, 43*(3), 184–190. http://dx.doi.org.visn1kis.idm.oclc.org/10.1080/08964289.2016.1276430

International Society for Traumatic Stress Studies (ISTSS; 2018). *ISTSS PTSD prevention and treatment guidelines: Methodology and recommendations.* Retrieved from http://www.istss.org/getattachment/Treating-Trauma/New-ISTSS-Prevention-and-Treatment-Guidelines/ISTSS_PreventionTreatmentGuidelines_FNL-March-19-2019.pdf.aspx

Jak, A. J., Jurick, S., Crocker, L. D., Sanderson-Cimino, M., Aupperle, R., Rodgers, C. S., Thomas, K. R., Boyd, B., Norman, S. B., Lang, A. J., Keller, A. V., Schiehser, D. M., & Twamley, E. W. (2019). SMART-CPT for veterans with comorbid post-traumatic stress disorder and history of traumatic brain injury: A randomised controlled trial. *Journal of Neurology, Neurosurgery, and Psychiatry, 90*(3), 333–341. https://doi.org/10.1136/jnnp-2018-319315

Kaysen, D., Lindgren, K., Zangana, G. A. S., Murray, L., Bass, J., & Bolton, P. (2013). Adaptation of cognitive processing therapy for treatment of torture victims: Experience in Kurdistan, Iraq. *Psychological Trauma: Theory, Research, Practice, and Policy, 5*(2), 184–192. https://doi.org/10.1037/a0026053

Kaysen, D., Schumm, J., Pedersen, E. R., Seim, R. W., Bedard-Gilligan, M., & Chard, K. (2014). Cognitive processing therapy for veterans with comorbid PTSD and alcohol use disorders. *Addictive Behaviors, 39*(2), 420–427. https://doi.org/10.1016/j.addbeh.2013.08.016

Kendall, P. C., & Beidas, R. S. (2007). Smoothing the trail for dissemination of evidence-based practices of youth: Flexibility within fidelity. *Professional Psychology: Research and Practice, 58*, 13–20.

Kendall, P. C., & Frank, H. E. (2018). Implementing evidence-based treatment protocols: Flexibility within fidelity. *Clinical Psychology: Science and Practice, 25*(4), doi: 10.1111/cpsp.12271

Lang, P. J. (1979). Presidential address, 1978. A bio-informational theory of emotional imagery. *Psychophysiology 16*(6), 495–512. https://doi.org/10.1111/j.1469-8986.1979.tb01511.x.

Larsen, S. E., Mackintosh, M. A., La Bash, H., Evans, W. R., Suvak, M. K., Shields, N., Lane, J. E. M., Sijercic, I., Monson, C. M., & Wiltsey Stirman, S. (2020). Temporary PTSD symptom increases among individuals receiving CPT in a hybrid effectiveness-implementation trial: Potential predictors and association with overall symptom change trajectory. *Psychological Trauma: Theory, Research, Practice, and Policy.* Advance online publication. https://doi.org/10.1037/tra0000545

Livingston, N. A., Berke, D. S., Ruben, M. A., Matza, A. R., & Shipherd, J. C. (2019). Experiences of trauma, discrimination, microaggressions, and minority stress among trauma-exposed LGBT veterans: Unexpected findings and unresolved service gaps. *Psychological Trauma: Theory, Research, Practice, and Policy, 11*(7), 695–703. https://doi-org.ezproxy.bu.edu/10.1037/tra0000464

Lloyd, D., Nixon, R. D., Varker, T., Elliott, P., Perry, D., Bryant, R. A., Creamer, M., & Forbes, D. (2014). Comorbidity in the prediction of Cognitive Processing Therapy treatment outcomes for combat-related posttraumatic stress disorder. *Journal of Anxiety Disorders, 28*(2), 237–240. https://doi.org/10.1016/j.janxdis.2013.12.002

Morland, L. A., Mackintosh, M. A., Glasman, L. H., Wells, S. Y., Thorp, S. R., Rauch, S. A. M., Cunningham, P. B., Tuerk, P. W., Grubbs, K. M., Golshan, S, Sohn, M. J., & Acierno, R. (2019). Home-based delivery of variable length prolonged exposure therapy: A comparison of clinical efficacy between service modalities. *Depression and Anxiety, 37*, 346–355. https://doi.org/10.1002/da.22979

Morland, L. A., Mackintosh, M. A., Greene, C. J., Rosen, C. S., Chard, K. M., Resick, P., & Frueh, B. C. (2014). Cognitive processing therapy for posttraumatic stress disorder delivered to rural veterans via telemental health: A randomized noninferiority clinical trial. *The Journal of Clinical Psychiatry, 75*(5), 470–476. https://doi.org/10.4088/JCP.13m08842

Nacasch, N., Huppert, J. D., Su, Y. J., Kivity, Y., Dinshtein, Y., Yeh, R., & Foa, E. B. (2015). Are 60-minute prolonged exposure sessions with 20-minute imaginal exposure to traumatic memories sufficient to successfully treat PTSD? A randomized noninferiority clinical trial. *Behavior Therapy, 46*(3), 328–341. https://doi.org/10.1016/j.beth.2014.12.002

National Institute for Health and Care Excellence (NICE; 2018). *Guideline for posttraumatic stress disorder*. National Institute for Health and Clinical Practice.

Norman, S. B., Trim, R., Haller, M., Davis, B. C., Myers, U. S., Colvonen, P. J., Blanes, E., Lyons, R., Siegel, E. Y., Angkaw, A. C., Norman, G. J., & Mayes, T. (2019). Efficacy of Integrated Exposure Therapy vs Integrated Coping Skills Therapy for Comorbid Posttraumatic Stress Disorder and Alcohol Use Disorder: A randomized clinical trial. *JAMA Psychiatry, 76*(8), 791–799. https://doi.org/10.1001/jamapsychiatry.2019.0638

Otis, J. D., Keane, T. M., Kerns, R. D., Monson, C., & Scioli, E. (2009). The development of an integrated treatment for veterans with comorbid chronic pain and posttraumatic stress disorder. *Pain Medicine, 10*(7), 1300–1311. https://doi.org/10.1111/j.1526-4637.2009.00715.x

Peterson, A. L., Mintz, J., Moring, J., Nabity, P., Bira, L., Young-McCaughan, S., Hale, W. J., McGeary, C. A., Litz, B. T., McGeary, D. D., Velligan, D. I., Macdonald, A., Mata-Galan, E., Holliday, S. L., Dillon, K. H., Yarvis, J. S., Roache, J. D., & Resick, P. A.; for the STRONG STAR Consortium. (2019, October). *In-office, in-home, and telebehavioral-health cognitive processing therapy for combat-related PTSD: Preliminary results of a randomized clinical trial.* Plenary presentation given at the San Antonio Combat PTSD Conference, San Antonio, TX.

Resick, P.A., Monson, C. M., & Chard, K. M. (2017). *Cognitive Processing Therapy for PTSD. A comprehensive manual.* Guilford Press.

Resick, P. A., Nishith, P., Weaver, T. L., Astin, M. C., & Feuer, C. A. (2002). A comparison of cognitive-processing therapy with prolonged exposure and a waiting condition for the treatment of chronic posttraumatic stress disorder in female rape victims. *Journal of Consulting and Clinical Psychology, 70*(4), 867–879. https://doi.org/10.1037//0022-006x.70.4.867

Resick, P. A., Wachen, J. S., Dondanville, K. A., LoSavio, S. T., Young-McCaughan, S., Yarvis, J. S., Pruiksma, K. E., Blankenship, A., Jacoby, V., & Peterson, J. (Oct, 2020). *Variable-Length Cognitive Processing Therapy for Posttraumatic Stress Disorder in active duty military: Outcomes and predictors. Keynote presentation* at the 5th Annual San Antonio Combat PTSD Conference.

Rosen, C. S., Morland, L. A., Glassman, L. H., Marx, B. P., Weaver, K., Smith, C. A., Pollack, S., & Schnurr, P. P. (2020). Virtual mental health care in the Veterans Health Administration's immediate response to coronavirus disease-19. *American Psychologist, 76*(1), 26–38. https://doi.org/10.1037/amp0000751

Sciarrino, N. A., Warnecke, A. J., & Teng, E. J. (2020). A systematic review of intensive empirically supported treatments for Posttraumatic Stress Disorder. *Journal of Traumatic Stress,* 10.1002/jts.22556. Advance online publication. https://doi.org/10.1002/jts.22556

Shapiro, F. (2018). *Eye Movement Desensitization and Reprocessing (EMDR) Therapy* (3rd ed.). Guilford Press.

Sloan, D. M., & Marx, B. P. (2019). *Written Exposure Therapy for PTSD: A brief treatment approach for mental health professionals.* American Psychological Press.

Sloan, D. M., Marx, B. P., Bovin, M. J., Feinstein, B. A., & Gallagher, M. W. (2012). Written exposure as an intervention for PTSD: A randomized clinical trial with motor vehicle accident survivors. *Behaviour Research and Therapy, 50*(10), 627–635. https://dx.doi.org/10.1016%2Fj.brat.2012.07.001

Sloan, D. M., Marx, B. P., Lee, D. J., & Resick, P. A. (2018). A brief exposure-based treatment vs Cognitive Processing Therapy for Posttraumatic Stress Disorder: A randomized noninferiority clinical trial. *JAMA Psychiatry, 75*(3), 233–239. https://doi.org/10.1001/jamapsychiatry.2017.4249

Valentine, S. E., Borba, C. P., Dixon, L., Vaewsorn, A. S., Guajardo, J. G., Resick, P. A., Wiltsey Stirman, S., & Marques, L. (2017). Cognitive Processing Therapy for Spanish-speaking Latinos: A formative study of a model-driven cultural adaptation of the manual to enhance implementation in a usual care setting. *Journal of Clinical Psychology, 73*(3), 239–256. https://doi.org/10.1002/jclp.22337

van Minnen, A., & Foa, E. B. (2006). The effect of imaginal exposure length on outcome of treatment for PTSD. *Journal of Traumatic Stress, 19*(4), 427–438. https://doi.org/10.1002/jts.20146

Weiss, W. M., Murray, L. K., Zangana, G. A., Mahmooth, Z., Kaysen, D., Dorsey, S., Lindgren, K., Gross, A., Murray, S. M., Bass, J. K., & Bolton, P. (2015). Community-based mental health treatments for survivors of torture and militant attacks in Southern Iraq: A randomized control trial. *BMC Psychiatry, 15,* 249. https://doi.org/10.1186/s12888-015-0622-7

Williams, M. T., Malcoun, E., Sawyer, B. A., Davis, D. M., Nouri, L. B., & Bruce, S. L. (2014). Cultural adaptations of prolonged exposure therapy for treatment and prevention of posttraumatic stress disorder in African Americans. *Behavioral Sciences, 4,* 102–124. https://doi.org/10.3390/bs4020102

Yuen, E. K., Gros, D. F., Price, M., Zeigler, S., Tuerk, P. W., Foa, E. B., & Acierno, R. (2015). Randomized controlled trial of home-based telehealth versus in-person prolonged exposure for combat-related PTSD in veterans: Preliminary results. *Journal of Clinical Psychology, 71*(6), 500–512. https://doi.org/10.1002/jclp.22168

4

Being Flexible While Maintaining Fidelity in Cognitive Behavioral Therapy of Depression

DANIEL R. STRUNK, ABBY ADLER MANDEL, AND IONY D. EZAWA ■

One of the most extensively studied psychological therapies for depression is cognitive therapy, also referred to as cognitive behavioral therapy (CBT), as developed by Beck and colleagues (1979). At the heart of this form of CBT are the efforts of therapists and clients working together to help clients identify and correct unrealistic negative thoughts and beliefs theorized to promote negative emotions and maintain depression. Evidence from randomized clinical trials (RCTs) comparing CBT to psychotropic medication shows comparable therapeutic effects, with long-term outcomes of discontinued CBT being comparable to continued medication in the years following initial treatment (Strunk et al., 2017). Compared to some other manual-based treatments, CBT for depression is considerably more flexible, offering therapists considerable discretion about the timing and use of various interventions. In providing CBT, therapists make decisions about the selection and personalization of interventions based on their conceptualization of each case. The original treatment manual (Beck et al., 1979) included suggestions for using interventions to target specific symptoms. Later publications have elaborated on approaches to developing a more formal case conceptualization, highlighting the importance of identifying clients' core beliefs (Beck, 1995). We suspect therapists vary in how they select interventions and personalize CBT. Researchers have tried to identify effective approaches to personalizing CBT; however, evidence to inform their decision-making is not yet entirely adequate for many of the decisions they face (Whisman, 2008). In the absence of more informative findings, what is the best practice for providing CBT for depression? What forms of flexibility or personalization are recommended? What flexibility is possible while still ensuring that one is providing the treatment that has demonstrated its therapeutic benefits in RCTs? In this chapter, we discuss the considerable flexibility that is a part of CBT for depression, expert recommendations on what is required to maintain fidelity to the treatment, and recommendations (informed by research when possible) about how the flexibility of the treatment can be used to maximize positive treatment outcomes.

THE FLEXIBILITY OF COGNITIVE BEHAVIORAL THERAPY FOR DEPRESSION

Treatment manuals vary considerably in the extent to which they are highly prescribed or more flexible. As we noted earlier, the treatment manual for CBT for depression has considerable flexibility. To illustrate some of the ways that this treatment is flexible (cf. Kendall et al., 2008; Kendall & Frank, 2018), we consider some of the decisions (large and small) that therapists face over the course of treatment. Before describing efforts to identify the core elements necessary for maintaining fidelity, we highlight 10 illustrative areas of flexibility.

Flexibility through Treatment Goals

Very early in treatment, therapists often work with their clients to identify a set of treatment goals. These goals ensure the therapist and client have identified the changes that the client sees as an important part of overcoming depression and achieving a successful outcome. The goals are highly personal. Goals can include improving self-confidence, better managing stressful events, improving personal relationships, adopting a healthier lifestyle, or making a change in one's career. Clients and therapists collaborate to identify the changes they think would be most important to achieve. This sets the stage for a treatment that will be highly personalized to address each client's goals.

Flexibility in Introducing the Model in Cognitive Behavioral Therapy

Early in treatment, therapists introduce the CBT model, highlighting how unrealistic negative thoughts contribute to negative emotions and depressive symptoms. In doing so, therapists illustrate the model with an example from the patient's own life. Depending on the client's presentation, therapists can make various choices about how to elicit an example and how in-depth to go in showing the application of the CBT model in that case. This first example is also one for which it is especially important to get feedback, to elicit the client's thoughts about the use of the model. Depending on the feedback given, the therapist can take various steps to address any questions or concerns the client may have.

Flexibility in Session Focus

One of the major features of CBT that contributes to its flexibility is the fact that the content of sessions is not prescribed. Therapists are not to follow a session-by-session schedule of topics. Instead, an agenda is set collaboratively at each session, with topics selected that are important to the client and likely to help the client achieve a positive outcome. In fact, some CBT experts have suggested that therapists tend to be less effective when they go into a session knowing what they plan to cover. Therapists may have possibilities in mind, but it is important that the focus of sessions is determined through a collaborative process that considers the needs of each client, which makes each client's course of CBT unique.

Flexibility in Using Cognitive Strategies

Therapists can show flexibility in the use of cognitive strategies in various ways over the course of CBT. Flexibility is needed in addressing the heterogenous content of the thoughts (self-talk) people with depression report. Although there are common themes (e.g., being inadequate or unlovable), it is central to CBT to focus on each client's specific thoughts and what those thoughts mean to them. One of the core tasks of CBT is to help clients cultivate the skill of developing alternative responses to automatic thoughts. Therapists can take advantage of the room for flexibility in how they go about doing this. Several standard questions for generating alternative responses tend to work in a variety of situations (e.g., "What is the evidence for and against this thought?"). But therapists also can craft individualized questions that may be particularly useful in helping a client arrive at a new perspective in a specific situation. Asking good questions is a cardinal skill for therapists providing CBT.

When a client appears unreceptive to a clinical strategy or a strategy is not initially successful, flexibility may be needed. Some have suggested that rigid manuals promote an inflexible response, essentially asking therapists to double down on the strategies that were just used without alteration. Others have suggested that a willingness to shift strategies while still adhering to the principles of the treatment is key. For example, a therapist working with a client who does not see any evidence that conflicts with the negative views or self-talk might shift tactics and try a different line of questioning to explore the possibility that the views are overly negative (e.g., asking what the client would tell a friend in their situation). Competent delivery of CBT often involves being flexible, while still adhering to the principles of the treatment. There are several advantages to therapists showing clients they are willing to try alternative approaches within the CBT framework. It shows that the principles of the treatment are flexible and can be used to address a wide variety of situations. It models persistence and creativity in using the skills of CBT. This strategy also shows the client that their therapist is being attentive to their individual needs and responsive to their feedback.

In our clinical training and supervision efforts, we have observed that trainees are often ready to abandon an approach too readily. When CBT strategies do not meet with initial success, therapists sometimes look to very different strategies from other therapeutic approaches to find something they think will be positively received. Although we recognize that it is important to be responsive to clients' needs, too readily writing off a strategy can also be problematic. Cases that involve greater complexity tend to require ongoing work to help a client find ways to use strategies successfully. Abandoning an effort prematurely may mean that a client never works through the difficulties and may mistakenly conclude that CBT strategies could not work for them.

Cognitive strategies also can be adapted to suit clients with writing difficulties or visual impairments. Finally, the speed with which the therapist and client progress along each step in the cognitive restructuring process can be adjusted to suit each client and the pace at which they develop the relevant skills.

Flexibility in Intervention Selection

Although cognitive strategies tend to get considerable emphasis in CBT, the treatment involves behavioral strategies as well. The degree to which cognitive versus behavioral strategies are used early in treatment is another way in which CBT offers flexibility. Perhaps influenced by the design of Jacobson and colleagues' component analysis (1996), a popular misconception about CBT is that behavioral strategies are always to be used extensively early in treatment and cognitive strategies are only to be used much later. In fact, the manual allows therapists considerable latitude in determining when to introduce these strategies and how much therapy time will be spent on each. The degree to which behavioral strategies such as self-monitoring are an ongoing focus varies considerably. For some clients, therapy begins with a heavy emphasis on behavioral strategies that continues for several weeks. For other clients, behavioral strategies may get much less emphasis, with thought records and associated cognitive change strategies being a major focus from the first session. The timing and use of strategies involved in identifying and re-evaluating core beliefs has similar flexibility. Although these strategies tend to be used later in treatment, therapists have great discretion in deciding when and to what extent they get attention in sessions.

Flexibility in Bolstering Cognitive Change

Not only can therapists be flexible with the timing and extent to which the major intervention procedures are used in CBT, they also can be flexible with the strategies they use to bolster clients' alternative responses to negative thoughts and beliefs. Clients who generate alternatives but find it difficult to believe them may benefit from behavioral experiments that allow them to test the validity of these alternatives in their own lives. For example, a client who predicts that reaching out to others will be followed by social rejection may need to test this view by taking a series of social risks. When alternative responses are insufficient, obtaining experiential evidence can be a useful supplement. Therapists can consider the conceptualization of the case and a client's responses to previous efforts to identify alternatives when considering when and how to integrate behavioral experiments into their work.

Flexibility in Developing Independence

Another kind of flexibility relates to the nature of the collaborative endeavor between client and therapist. Early on in treatment therapists often take a stronger leading role in introducing clients to cognitive strategies and helping them to see how these strategies can be applied in their own lives. As treatment progresses, therapists increasingly get out of the way, allowing clients to take a greater role and helping them to establish confidence in their ability to apply the strategies of CBT without their therapist. The rate of this progression is individualized in an effort to best serve clients.

Flexibility in Focus (the Present, the Therapeutic Relationship, or the Past)

In CBT, therapists tend to focus on the present (or recent events), developing and rehearsing strategies for coping with such events. However, the focus on the present is an additional area of flexibility. When there is a rupture in the working relationship, therapists can shift the focus to these ruptures, using this as another context for highlighting the benefits of the strategies taught in CBT. Alternatively, when the client's past experiences appear important to making progress in the current situation, the therapist can shift focus to address these experiences. The extent to which the therapist shifts focus to the relationship or to past experiences depends very much on the client and the therapist's view of the extent to which such shifts would be helpful. Some have suggested that therapists think of the area of focus as represented by a three-legged stool. Therapists tend to focus on the present leg unless or until there is an indication that a shift of focus to the therapeutic relationship leg or the leg representing the client's past would be useful.

Homework Flexibility

Therapists can work with clients to tailor homework assignments to their needs. Homework can involve standard assignments such as self-monitoring of moods and activities or using thought records, but these assignments also can be tailored to clients' specific needs. For example, therapists may work with clients to customize self-monitoring forms to track a client's specific behavioral goals. Or, clients might choose to fill out a custom thought record on their smart phone.

Therapists also can use the principles of CBT to help a client develop an even more customized assignment. For example, for a client who has struggled to get out of bed in the morning, the therapist and client might work to develop a specific multistage plan to use a series of cognitive behavioral strategies to get out of bed and engage in a morning routine.

Flexibility in Relapse Prevention Efforts

Near the conclusion of CBT, therapists shift to a discussion of relapse prevention. As part of this effort, therapists elicit potentially challenging stressors that the client might face in the future. Then, the clients can anticipate and rehearse the use of CBT strategies to manage these stressors. The process calls for flexibility in identifying various kinds of stressors that clients may face, in thinking through the strategies that a client will find most useful in various circumstances, and in helping the client to take the lead in thinking through these challenges.

MAINTAINING FIDELITY IN COGNITIVE BEHAVIORAL THERAPY FOR DEPRESSION

As evident in this illustrative list of 10 areas, CBT for depression is an intervention with many opportunities for flexibility. In addition to the considerable ways in which therapists can be flexible in providing CBT, there are features required to maintain fidelity.

Researchers have introduced several constructs to help address this topic. One of the most important is *adherence*, the extent to which therapists engage in manual-prescribed behaviors (Waltz et al., 1993; Rodriguez-Quintana & Lewis, 2018). The Collaborative Study Psychotherapy Rating Scale (CSPRS; Hollon et al., 1988) is likely the most influential measure of adherence to CBT for depression. Items assess the extent to which therapists engage in recommended behaviors (e.g., reporting cognitions, distancing, evaluating evidence). Higher adherence scores indicate greater use of manual-prescribed behaviors. However, the exact level of these behaviors that is required for fidelity has not been determined.

Measures such as the CSPRS require observers to review and rate recordings of CBT sessions. Adherence ratings have been used for research purposes but are generally not used for providing clinical feedback. One key reason for this is that it is unclear how well different raters agree on what would reflect various levels of adherence. To promote reliability, raters working as part of the same team are trained to make ratings similarly. It is unclear to what extent, however, the mean level of adherence can be meaningfully compared when ratings are made by different raters or from raters working in different groups. Ultimately, this problem might be addressed by use of standardized rater training materials or approaches to assessing adherence that do not rely so strongly on observers (Imel et al., 2014; Stirman et al., 2021). Additional research is needed to pursue these possibilities.

Another complication is the need to think carefully about different aspects of adherence. If a therapist does not use some clinical strategies with much frequency, can that therapist offset their low adherence in one area by using other strategies? Is use of any specific strategies required for an adherent session or for an adherent course of CBT? Should some strategies be used more in some circumstances? The research literature has yet to answer some of these questions and has only limited evidence relevant to answering the others. Partly because research involving observer ratings of therapy sessions is labor intensive, only a limited body of studies have involved examining adherence in CBT for depression. In most studies, the researchers have focused on the question of whether adherence is related to outcome. Even among researchers using the CSPRS, however, there have been different approaches to scoring measures of adherence. Factor analyses of adherence ratings have suggested that adherence to CBT is not best represented by a single overall adherence factor (Strunk et al., 2012). Therefore, it is likely important to not just assess whether a therapist is adherent, but whether the therapist is adherent to specific aspects of the treatment (e.g., using cognitive methods, using behavioral methods). Several studies have found one or more aspects of adherence predicted therapeutic outcomes (Feeley et al., 1999; Strunk, Brotman, & DeRubeis, 2010). However, with different approaches to scoring adherence measures, different approaches to assessing adherence (e.g., at which sessions), and different approaches to analyzing the relation of adherence and outcome, research findings have been mixed (see Webb et al., 2010). Partly for this reason, our understanding of which aspects of adherence are generally important and which may be most important in specific contexts remains limited. In addition, several experts have suggested that it may be important to distinguish the extent to which therapists use manual-prescribed therapeutic methods from the quality with which those methods are delivered.

For this reason, the construct that most often has been used to assess whether CBT is being provided with fidelity is *therapist competence*. Like adherence, competence often has been assessed using observer ratings of session recordings. Although there are a few variations, the Cognitive Therapy Scale (CTS; Beck Institute for Cognitive Behavior Therapy, 2020) has been the most widely used measure of competence (but see Muse & McManus [2013] for a review of alternatives). Competence items are intended to assess the quality of the therapist contributions. So, unlike adherence, competence measures do not necessarily simply reflect greater use of intervention strategies prescribed by the treatment manual. Moderate use of CBT strategies delivered expertly would presumably reflect greater competence than very high use of CBT strategies used poorly. In addition, because competence reflects a more complex judgment, there is a common view that raters of competence would ideally be trained as CBT therapists and perhaps even have demonstrated competence themselves.

Unfortunately, competence assessments do not appear to be consistently reliable. As reviewed elsewhere (Schmidt et al., 2018), one study reported intraclass correlation coefficients < .10. A conference focused on competency held in 1998 obtained similarly low estimates (R. J. DeRubeis, personal communication, 2002).

Other studies have reported adequate reliability with raters who have trained together to achieve agreement. In a particularly troubling analysis, another study suggested that reliable estimates of therapist competence might require as many as 60 ratings (Dennhag et al., 2012). These findings suggest the common practice of relying on a very small number of ratings may be problematic.

What about evidence for a relation between competence and outcome? The evidence for such a relationship is mixed. A meta-analytic estimate of the competence-outcome relationship across diverse problems and treatments suggested a mean effect size of .07 (Webb et al., 2010). A more recent estimate from a sample of 43 therapists working in the Improving Access to Psychological Therapies Program in the United Kingdom failed to find a simple relationship between competence and outcome (Branson et al., 2015). In our own study focused on CBT for depression conducted as part of a clinical trial, we found evidence for a modest relationship between competence and session-to-session symptom change early in treatment. Interestingly, the relationship appeared to be considerably larger among clients who had characteristics suggesting they would be more complex to treat (Strunk, Brotman, DeRubeis, & Hollon, 2010). A nonrandomized comparison suggested that a workshop followed by ongoing supervision focused on CBT for depression appeared to improve therapist competence and achieve modest improvement in therapeutic outcomes relative to treatment as usual (Simons et al., 2010).

When CTS scores are used to judge competence, a cut-off score often is used. Although we are aware of no empirical basis for a specific cut-off score for demonstrating competence, requiring a score of 40 or greater has been most common (though the Beck Institute has more recently suggested 44). It is unlikely that the use of a cut-off score does much to address the concerns that have been raised about the use of competence scores. Despite these limitations, competence as assessed by the CTS remains the most commonly and carefully evaluated standard for evaluating whether CBT is being provided with fidelity. For this reason, we continue to cautiously use these assessments as aids in training, supervision, and in the context of research on CBT.

One approach to providing a treatment with fidelity is to ensure that it includes *core components* (i.e., those components that cannot be bypassed or ignored; Kendall et al., 2008). Examples of components commonly considered to be core would be: setting agendas for sessions, a collaborative approach, self-monitoring of moods and activities, teaching cognitive methods to re-evaluate negative thoughts and beliefs, and using homework assignments. The CTS does not clearly identify aspects of CBT as core components insofar as one can achieve a relatively high total score even if a score of zero is given on any one item. Rather, the CTS emphasizes aspects of treatment that are generally important. How much a treatment is compromised by less competent delivery of each aspect of CBT is not clear. Complicating matters further, some items of the CTS are quite general (e.g., the item assessing the therapist's strategy for change), allowing for therapists to achieve high scores using different intervention strategies (see Schmidt et al., 2018).

WHAT ARE THE LIMITS OF FLEXIBILITY?

How flexible can a therapist be in providing CBT for depression without losing fidelity to the treatment? This question is a difficult one to answer in a way that would lead to universal agreement. For the sake of illustration, we lay out two contrasting views. A more conservative view is that the manual used in clinical trials is the definitive source for guiding therapists on questions of flexibility (Wilson, 1996). The manual is meant to describe how a treatment that was found to be beneficial was provided. Although a manual may not be entirely sufficient for allowing one to deliver a treatment competently, it is meant to describe how the treatment is to be delivered sufficiently so that those with adequate clinical training could provide the treatment in line with the delivery of the treatment in clinical trials. When specific issues are not addressed by the manual, therapists might look for information about whether these issues came up in clinical trials and, if so, how they were addressed.

A more permissive view that allows for greater flexibility is that therapists maintain fidelity to the manual so long as their work is informed by the theory underlying the treatment and the conceptualization of each individual case. With a permissive approach, treatment developers and others can propose new strategies to use in a treatment without the cumbersome process of testing the new strategies or the revised treatment package. This view allows for the possibility that therapists could use intervention strategies not specifically mentioned in the treatment manual or make adaptations to prescribed strategies, so long as they are in line with the CBT conceptualization. Several CBT experts have advanced the cause of a more central role for case conceptualization in CBT (Persons, 2008). Judy Beck (1995) introduced new tools such as a cognitive conceptualization diagram, which were incorporated into CBT as provided in some more recent trials. Nonetheless, it is also important to note that the validity of key aspects of conceptualization have not been fully demonstrated (Bieling & Kuyken, 2003). The greater flexibility of this permissive approach may be an advantage for disseminating a treatment because it may be easier to get therapists to adopt a new treatment if it comes with such flexibility. Such a flexible approach, however, necessarily weakens the degree of confidence one can have that a treatment will offer the therapeutic effects that have been demonstrated in multiple clinical trials. We highlight these two views for the sake of illustration, recognizing that positions between them are possible.

EMPIRICALLY INFORMED FLEXIBILITY AND LIMITS ON FLEXIBILITY

Cognitive Behavioral Therapy has been practiced for several decades, and it is both thoroughly studied and strongly supported as a psychological therapy for depression. We hope that our field will work toward developing more empirically informed forms of flexibility and empirically informed ways of limiting flexibility (the latter by finding what strategies are most promising in what contexts). We highlight two examples of recent research findings that could inform the nature of therapists' efforts to be flexible in providing CBT.

The first has to do with session frequency. In clinical trials, CBT often has been provided as an acute treatment for 12 to 16 weeks. Sessions are provided weekly or twice weekly with tapering to weekly sessions. In a recent trial, Bruijniks and colleagues (2020) randomized clients to CBT versus Interpersonal Therapy (IPT) and to once versus twice weekly sessions. Those in the twice weekly conditions were less likely to drop out of treatment and experienced greater improvements in depressive symptoms. To our knowledge, this is the only study of CBT for depression to examine session frequency experimentally. Interestingly, this study suggests that therapists might enhance outcomes simply by working to provide twice weekly sessions (a practice that we suspect is not all that common). If so, this gives therapists a reason to consider being less flexible than they might have otherwise been with session frequency.

The second example has to do with providing CBT in combination with psychotropic medication. RCTs of CBT for depression have tended to test CBT over a fixed duration, such as 16 weeks. In this context, CBT provided in combination with medication appears to lead to slightly greater symptom reductions than either treatment alone (Forand, DeRubeis, & Amsterdam, 2013). A more critical test of combined treatment, however, would evaluate its long-term effects. In a recent trial (DeRubeis et al., 2020), chronic and recurrent patients with depression were randomized to medication alone or medication combined with CBT. In an effort to achieve a stable positive outcome, treatment was provided for up to two years. Following a positive clinical outcome, patients were randomized to continued medication or discontinuing medication and followed for three years. In this context, CBT did not enhance the probability of achieving a sustained recovery. This study suggests that the value of combined treatment may be fairly limited in terms of long-term outcomes. Rather than being flexible in offering CBT for patients who are or are not also receiving psychiatric medication, this finding suggests that therapists could maximize the impact of CBT on long-term outcomes by focusing on providing CBT alone.

ANOTHER CONTEXT FOR FLEXIBILITY: CULTURAL ADAPTATIONS AND CULTURAL COMPETENCE

We have not yet commented on therapist flexibility in working with clients from different cultural backgrounds. We wanted to address these issues separately and more extensively as they are of special importance. We live in a world in which therapists are increasingly likely to work with clients with backgrounds that differ from their own. To work effectively with people from different cultures, therapists often are advised to take several steps. A starting point is for therapists to work to become aware of and attentive to their own attitudes toward people with different backgrounds.

To help ensure quality care for all clients, psychologists have suggested that CBT therapists and treatment protocols be sensitive to the diverse needs of different clients. One approach to doing so is to focus on the cultural competence of therapists providing CBT. In line with this idea, therapists are encouraged to strengthen their ability to understand and effectively communicate and interact with individuals from different cultures. Part of this notion includes increasing knowledge about and skills to work with individuals from other cultures, but cultural competence also includes awareness of one's own culture and attitudes toward cultural differences (Sue et al., 1982; Sue, 2001).

Other psychologists have suggested that because of the unique needs of clients from minority groups, CBT should be adapted to be as effective as possible for clients from various backgrounds. In line with this reasoning, several culturally adapted forms of CBT have been created and tested. One notable example includes an effort from Miranda and colleagues (2006) in which CBT for depression was adapted for low-income, minority women. In this study, CBT was provided in keeping with its basic principles (with a focus on developing skills for identifying and re-evaluating negative thoughts). Yet, the treatment was adapted by modifying its delivery (i.e., providing child care and transportation), introducing psychoeducational sessions, adding culturally related examples, and delivering the protocol in the client's native language. Similar to this effort, other CBT adaptations also have aimed to use core principles of CBT for depression while making changes to make the therapy more easily accessed, understood, and relatable to individuals from different cultures. In a meta-analysis of 56 RCTs of psychological therapies for depression, Ünlü Ince and colleagues (2014) examined the association between ethnic/racial minority status and outcome. Minority status was not associated with differential outcome. Nonetheless, in a recent meta-analysis of culturally adapted (mostly incorporating language and treatment delivery adaptations) and nonadapted psychological treatments (predominantly CBT) for depression, Chowdhary and colleagues (2014) found a moderate difference in favor of the adapted treatments.

Although there is general agreement on the importance of both cultural competence and treatments that are sensitive to the diverse needs of clients, there is not agreement on a precise definition of cultural competence or what methods are most important in providing culturally competent care. In line with this limitation, it is still unclear whether and how treatments should be adapted (Whaley & Davis, 2007). Our group recently conducted a study of therapists' views of the importance of cognitive change strategies when working with African American versus White clients (Ezawa & Strunk, 2021a). Therapists presented with vignettes of African American clients rated cognitive change strategies as significantly less important than therapists presented with White clients. In a study of CBT, we found that therapists did in fact use less cognitive change strategies when working with African American clients as compared to White clients, but we found no difference in symptom change or dropout rates (Ezawa & Strunk, 2021b). It will be important for future research to determine whether the cognitive strategies that are central to CBT need to be used to a different degree or in a different manner when working with diverse client groups.

CONCLUSION

Cognitive Behavioral Therapy for depression is a treatment with tremendous flexibility. From the focus of the sessions, to efforts to understand the content of clients' cognitions, to identifying means of re-evaluating those cognitions, competent CBT requires multifaceted flexibility on the part of therapists. Of course, competent CBT also requires therapists to be faithful to the treatment strategies, guiding principles, and core components. Both the principles of CBT and the specific intervention strategies used in CBT allow for considerable flexibility. Perhaps what is most central to this treatment is the therapist and client collaborating to help clients to appreciate how their unrealistic negative thoughts and beliefs serve to promote negative affect and perpetuate their experience of depression. By learning a set of flexible cognitive behavioral strategies, clients can develop the ability to identify these cognitive processes and re-evaluate them, developing more accurate and adaptive views to reduce their experience of depression.

REFERENCES

Beck, J. S. (1995). *Cognitive therapy: Basics and beyond*. Guilford.

Beck, A. T., Rush, A. J., Shaw, B. F., & Emery, G. (1979). *Cognitive therapy of depression*. Guilford.

Beck Institute for Cognitive Behavior Therapy. (2020). Cognitive Therapy Rating Scale. Retrieved from https://beckinstitute.org/wp-content/uploads/2015/10/CTRS-12-2011_portrait-Cognitive-Therapy-Rating-Scale-1.pdf

Bieling, P. J., & Kuyken, W. (2003). Is cognitive case formulation science or science fiction? *Clinical Psychology: Science and Practice, 10*, 52–69. https://doi.org/10.1093/clipsy.10.1.52

Branson, A., Shafran, R., & Myles, P. (2015). Investigating the relationship between competence and patient outcome with CBT. *Behaviour Research and Therapy, 68*, 19–26. https://doi.org/10.1016/j.brat.2015.03.002.

Bruijniks, S. J., Lemmens, L. H., Hollon, S. D., Peeters, F. P., Cuijpers, P., Arntz, A., Dingemanse, P., Willems, L., van Oppen, P., Twisk, J. W. R., van den Boogaard, M., Spijker, J., Bosmans, J., & Huibers, M. J. H. (2020). The effects of once-versus twice-weekly sessions on psychotherapy outcomes in depressed patients. *The British Journal of Psychiatry, 216*, 222–230. https://doi.org/10.1192/bjp.2019.265

Chowdhary, N., Jotheeswaran, A. T., Nadkarni, A., Hollon, S. D., King, M., Jordans, M. J. D., Rahman, A., Verdeli, H., Araya, R., & Patel, V. (2014). The methods and outcomes of cultural adaptations of psychological treatments for depressive disorders: A systematic review. *Psychological Medicine, 44*, 1131–1146. https://doi.org/10.1017/S0033291713001785

Dennhag, I., Gibbons, M. B. C., Barber, J. P., Gallop, R., & Crits-Christoph, P. (2012). How many treatment sessions and patients are needed to create a stable score of adherence and competence in the treatment of cocaine dependence? *Psychotherapy Research, 22*, 475–488. https://doi.org/10.1080/10503307.2012.674790

DeRubeis, R. J., Zajecka, J., Shelton, R. C., Amsterdam, J. D., Fawcett, J., Xu, C., Young, P. R., Gallop, R., & Hollon, S. D. (2020). Prevention of recurrence after recovery from a major depressive episode with antidepressant medication alone or in combination with cognitive behavioral therapy: Phase 2 of a 2-phase randomized clinical trial. *JAMA Psychiatry, 77*, 237–245. https://doi.org/10.1001/jamapsychiatry.2019.3900

Ezawa, I. D., & Strunk, D. R. (2021a). *Working with Black vs. White patients: An experimental test of therapists' decisions in providing cognitive behavioral therapy for depression*. Manuscript in preparation.

Ezawa, I. D., & Strunk, D. R. (2021b). *Differences in the delivery of cognitive behavioral therapy for depression when therapists work with Black and White patients*. Manuscript submitted for publication.

Jacobson, N. S., Dobson, K. S., Truax, P. A., Addis, M. E., Koerner, K., Gollan, J. K., Gortner, E., & Prince, S. E. (1996). A component analysis of cognitive-behavioral treatment for depression. *Journal of Consulting and Clinical Psychology, 64*, 295–304. https://doi.org/10.1037/0022-006X.64.2.295

Feeley, M., DeRubeis, R. J., & Gelfand, L. A. (1999). The temporal relation of adherence and alliance to symptom change in cognitive therapy for depression. *Journal of Consulting and Clinical Psychology, 67*, 578–582. https://doi.org/10.1037/0022-006X.67.4.578

Forand, N. R., DeRubeis, R. J., & Amsterdam, J. D. (2013). The combination of psychotherapy and medication in the treatment of mental disorders. In M. J. Lambert (Ed.), *Bergin and Garfield's handbook of psychotherapy and behavior change* (6th ed., pp. 735–774). Wiley.

Hollon, S. D., Evans, M. D., Auerbach, A., DeRubeis, R. J., Elkin, I., Lowery, A., & Piasecki, J. (1988). Development of a system for rating therapies for depression: Differentiating cognitive therapy, interpersonal psychotherapy and clinical management pharmacotherapy. Unpublished manuscript, Vanderbilt University, Nashville.

Imel, Z. E., Baldwin, S. A., Baer, J. S., Hartzler, B., Dunn, C., Rosengren, D. B., & Atkins, D. C. (2014). Evaluating therapist adherence in motivational interviewing by comparing performance with standardized and real patients. *Journal of Consulting and Clinical Psychology, 82*, 472–481. http://dx.doi.org/10.1037/a0036158

Kendall, P. C., & Frank, H. (2018). Implementing evidence-based treatment protocols: Flexibility within fidelity. *Clinical Psychology: Science and Practice, 25*, 1–12. https://doi.org/10.1111/cpsp.12271.

Kendall, P. C., Gosch, E., Furr, J. M., & Sood, E. (2008). Flexibility within fidelity. *Journal of the American Academy of Child and Adolescent Psychiatry, 47*, 987–993. https://10.1097/CHI.0b013e31817eed2f

Miranda, J., Green, B. L., Krupnick, J. L., Chung, J., Siddique, J., Beslin, T., & Revicki, D. (2006). One-year outcome of a randomized clinical trial treating depression in low-income minority women. *Journal of Consulting and Clinical Psychology, 74*, 99–111. https://doi.org/10.1037/0022-006X.74.1.99

Muse, K., & McManus, F. (2013). A systematic review of methods for assessing competence in cognitive-behavioural therapy. *Clinical Psychology Review, 33*, 484–499. https://doi.org/10.1016/j.cpr.2013.01.010

Persons, J. B. (2008). *The case formulation approach to cognitive-behavior therapy (guides to individualized evidence-based treatment)*. Guilford.

Rodriguez-Quintana, N., & Lewis, C. C. (2018). Observational coding training methods for CBT treatment fidelity: A systematic review. *Cognitive Therapy and Research, 42,* 358–368. https://doi.org/10.1007/s10608-018-9898-5

Schmidt, I. D., Strunk, D. R., DeRubeis, R. J., Conklin, L. R., & Braun, J. D. (2018). Revisiting how we assess therapist competence in cognitive therapy. *Cognitive Therapy and Research, 42,* 369–384. https://doi.org/10.1007/s10608-018-9908-7

Simons, A. D., Padesky, C. A., Montemarano, J., Lewis, C. C., Murakami, J., Lamb, K., DeVinney, S., Reid, M., Smith, D. A., & Beck, A. T. (2010). Training and dissemination of cognitive behavior therapy for depression in adults: A preliminary examination of therapist competence and client outcomes. *Journal of Consulting and Clinical Psychology, 78,* 751–756. doi:10.1037/a0020569

Stirman, S. W., Gutner, C. A., Gamarra, J., Suvak, M. K., Vogt, D., Johnson, C., Wachen, J. S., Dondanville, K. A., Yarvis, J. S., Mintz, J., Peterson, A. L., Young-McCaughan, S., Resick, A. L. (2021). A novel approach to the assessment of fidelity to a cognitive behavioral therapy for PTSD using clinical worksheets: A proof of concept with cognitive processing therapy. *Behavior Therapy, 52,* 656–672. https://doi.org/10.1016/j.beth.2020.08.005

Strunk, D. R., Adler, A. D., & Hollon, S. D. (2017). Cognitive therapy of depression. In R. J. DeRubeis & D. R. Strunk (Eds.), *The Oxford handbook of mood disorders* (pp. 411–422). Oxford University Press.

Strunk, D. R., Cooper, A. A., Ryan, E. T., DeRubeis, R. J., & Hollon, S. D. (2012). The process of change in cognitive therapy for depression when combined with antidepressant medication: Predictors of early inter-session symptom gains. *Journal of Consulting and Clinical Psychology, 80,* 730–738. https://doi.org/10.1037/a0029281

Strunk, D. R., Brotman, M. A., & DeRubeis, R. J. (2010). The process of change in cognitive therapy for depression: Predictors of early inter-session symptom gains. *Behaviour Research and Therapy, 48,* 599–606. https://doi.org/10.1016/j.brat.2010.03.011

Strunk, D. R., Brotman, M. A., DeRubeis, R. J., & Hollon, S. D. (2010). Therapist competence in cognitive therapy for depression: Predicting subsequent symptom change. *Journal of Consulting and Clinical Psychology, 78,* 429–437. https://doi.org/10.1037/a0019631

Sue, D. W. (2001). Multidimensional facets of cultural competence. *The counseling psychologist, 29*(6), 790–821. https://doi.org/10.1177/0011000001296002

Sue, D. W., Bernier, J. E., Durran, A., Feinberg, L., Pedersen, P., Smith, E. J., & Vasquez-Nuttall, E. (1982). Position paper: Cross-cultural counseling competencies. *The Counseling Psychologist, 10,* 45–52. https://doi.org/10.1177/0011000082102008

Ünlü Ince, B., Riper, H., van 't Hof, E., & Cuijpers, P. (2014). The effects of psychotherapy on depression among racial-ethnic minority groups: A metaregression analysis. *Psychiatric Services, 65,* 612–617. https://doi.org/10.1176/appi.ps.201300165

Waltz, J., Addis, M. E., Koerner, K., & Jacobson, N. S. (1993). Testing the integrity of a psychotherapy protocol: Assessment of adherence and competence. *Journal of Consulting and Clinical Psychology, 61,* 620–630. https://doi.org/10.1037/0022-006X.61.4.620

Webb, C. A., DeRubeis, R. J., & Barber, J. P. (2010). Therapist adherence/competence and treatment outcome: A meta-analytic review. *Journal of Consulting and Clinical Psychology, 78*, 200–211. https://doi.org/10.1037/a0018912

Whaley, A. L., & Davis, K. E. (2007). Cultural competence and evidence-based practice in mental health services: A complementary perspective. *American Psychologist, 62*, 563–574. https://doi.org/10.1037/0003-066X.62.6.563

Whisman, M. A. (Ed.). (2008). *Adapting cognitive therapy for depression: Managing complexity and comorbidity.* Guilford.

Wilson, G. T. (1996). Manual-based treatments: The clinical application of research findings. *Behaviour Research and Therapy, 34*, 295–314. https://doi.org/10.1016/0005-7967(95)00084-4

5

Empirically Supported Treatment for Obsessive-Compulsive Disorder

Core Elements and Adaptive Applications

MARTIN E. FRANKLIN AND SARAH G. TURK KARAN ■

EVIDENCE FOR THE EFFICACY OF TREATMENT

The first question to be considered is which treatment should be chosen as the first-line intervention for obsessive-compulsive disorder (OCD) across the developmental spectrum. As it turns out, the adult and pediatric literatures are highly convergent with respect to this: Cognitive-Behavioral Therapy (CBT) involving Exposure Plus Response Prevention (ERP) is the treatment with the most empirical support, and its effects appear to be both robust and durable (see Öst et al., 2015, 2016 for meta-analytic reviews). ERP has been found efficacious as an initial treatment both alone and in combination with serotonergic medications and in comparison to pill placebo (e.g., Foa et al, 2005; Pediatric OCD Treatment Study Team, 2004), relative to waitlist and other psychosocial control conditions such as relaxation (e.g., Freeman et al., 2014; Marks et al., 1980; Piacentini et al., 2011), and as an augmentative treatment for medication partial responders (e.g., Franklin et al., 2011; Simpson et al., 2008, 2013). Responder rates across multiple studies conducted around the world have been reported at 60% to 90% of study participants, with an OCD symptom reduction rate of about 50% to 80% (e.g., Abramowitz, 1996, Abramowitz et al., 2005; Foa & Kozak, 1996). Accordingly, it is scientifically justifiable to say that ERP is efficacious for the majority to the vast majority of treatment completers; studies that have included follow-up data attest to the durability of gains in most patients who responded well to ERP initially (see Öst et al., 2015, 2016). That said, response to ERP remains neither universal nor complete, so more effort is needed to improve outcomes for every potential OCD patient.

Randomized controlled trials (RCTs) such as those cited above were designed to emphasize internal validity in order to establish efficacy, and suffice it to say that over the past three decades the efficacy of ERP has been well established. Certain design elements of efficacy trials, however, such as careful sample selection, use of treatment manuals that prescribe implementation of specific procedures, and careful assessment of study protocol adherence do not resemble how treatment is likely to be conducted in practice settings, thus leaving unanswered questions regarding the generalizability of RCT outcomes to such settings (e.g., Persons & Silberschatz, 1998; Westen et al., 2004). Effectiveness and dissemination research have since been conducted on ERP in the wake of the aforementioned efficacy work, and thus far it appears that findings achieved in efficacy trials are generalizable to clinical practice settings outside the academic medical context where the treatments were designed and tested (e.g., Franklin et al., 2000; Torp et al., 2015). That said, dissemination of ERP to clinical settings that emphasize external over internal validity remains the next frontier, with efforts needed to ensure that this efficacious treatment will be made more readily available to patients with OCD. Collectively, the efficacy and effectiveness/dissemination studies support the use of ERP for patients with OCD across the developmental spectrum in myriad clinical and research settings. Given this evidence, we might ask ourselves: What are the core elements of this effective intervention? How might it be best to promote adherence to the essential aspects of treatment? And where is it best to be flexible?

Before taking on these issues, we first review the data on predictors and moderators of differential ERP outcomes, because these variables offer advance notice about which patients may experience difficulty achieving optimal treatment outcomes. The mechanism by which treatment outcomes are realized is through associated between-session patient nonadherence, which has emerged as a strong predictor of CBT outcome in and of itself (Simpson et al., 2011). Unfortunately, the moderator/predictor literature in OCD is relatively underdeveloped and underpowered statistically. Some recent efforts have been made to collapse across treatment trials to provide sufficient sample sizes to generate hypotheses about prediction and moderation, and those studies will be emphasized.

PREDICTORS AND MODERATORS OF DIFFERENTIAL OUTCOMES

In the investigation of ERP efficacy and potential predictors of outcome conducted by Simpson and colleagues (Maher et al., 2012; Simpson et al., 2011, 2012), in addition to patient between-session adherence, three other factors significantly predicted differential outcome: hoarding subtype, working alliance, and treatment expectancy. Notably, patient adherence mediated all three of these predictors (Simpson et al., 2011). Maher and colleagues (2012) replicated the finding for hoarding status and working alliance, and provided evidence suggesting that readiness for treatment predicted outcome, with patient adherence again serving as the mediator of this relationship. Additional factors that were examined, such as treatment expectancy, readiness to change, and work impairment did not differentially predict outcome (Maher et al., 2012). These collective findings clearly suggested that factors that compromise between-session adherence will likely attenuate ERP's benefits, which then translates readily into advice for the clinician conducting ERP: emphasize homework completion, ask about it at the beginning of each session, and troubleshoot early whenever homework completion appears to be compromised.

Initial OCD symptom severity and mental health comorbidity often are suggested to be associated with ERP outcomes. However, moderator/predictor analyses from a recent multisite randomized controlled trial examining ERP and risperidone as augmentative treatments for adult patients who have evidenced a partial response to selective serotonin reuptake inhibitors (SSRIs) did not support a significant association between ERP outcomes and either pretreatment OCD symptom severity or pretreatment depressive symptoms (Wheaton et al., 2015). That said, outcomes for the ERP group were again found to be associated with patient adherence to the ERP protocol (Wheaton et al., 2016). Note, between-session adherence to response prevention instructions in particular was strongly associated with outcome: the more adherence to the manual-based treatment the better the outcome. When applying treatment, this point should be strongly emphasized.

Taking advantage of the improved statistical power afforded by meta-analytic approaches, Knopp and colleagues (2013) examined data from 39 published RCTs of adults with OCD that included a psychosocial treatment including ERP. Hoarding, unemployment, being single, pretreatment OCD severity, and pretreatment anxiety levels were each associated with outcomes. The authors duly note that some of these variables did not emerge as predictive in individual studies yet did so here, perhaps linked to the statistical methods and associated improvements in power achieved by aggregating the data.

With respect to pediatric OCD specifically, Ginsburg, Kingery, Drake, and Grados (2008) reviewed the data on prediction and moderation of differential outcomes and identified baseline OCD symptom severity and family psychopathology as predictors of poorer response to CBT. In the multisite Pediatric OCD Treatment Study I (POTS Team, 2004), the presence of comorbid tic symptoms moderated pharmacotherapy treatment response; that is, it predicted poorer outcome to sertraline (SER) alone but not to the treatment conditions that included CBT (CBT alone or COMB; see March et al., 2007). That finding was not replicated in a large open study conducted in Norway that focused on prediction of CBT response (Torp et al., 2015). A comprehensive examination of the POTS I data set published after Ginsburg and colleagues' systematic review (Garcia et al., 2010) identified several predictors of response to all treatments: lower OCD symptom severity, less OCD-related impairment, greater insight, fewer comorbid externalizing symptoms, and lower levels of family accommodation were associated with better outcomes regardless of treatment condition. With respect to predicting response to specific treatments, only a family history of OCD emerged; although family history attenuated outcome somewhat across all treatment conditions, those with a family history had a sixfold decrease in effect size for CBT monotherapy compared to those without such a history. The mechanism by which this moderation occurred has yet to be elucidated, although examination of family variables in another RCT may prove helpful. Peris and colleagues (2012) examined data from Piacentini and colleagues' (2011) RCT and found that families with lower levels of parental blame and family conflict, as well as higher levels of family cohesion at baseline, were more likely to have a child who responded favorably to family-based CBT. These findings indicate that, in general, family environment and family history of OCD are important clinical considerations when treating OCD, as is family accommodation of OCD symptoms.

CORE ELEMENTS OF EXPOSURE PLUS RESPONSE PREVENTION REQUIRED TO MAINTAIN FIDELITY

Recent ERP manuals for both adults (Foa, Yadin, & Lichner, 2012) and youth (Franklin, Freeman, & March, 2019) emphasize the importance of core treatment elements: (1) psychoeducation regarding OCD theory and the treatment procedures that flow from understanding of its core psychopathology; (2) development of OCD-symptom hierarchies to guide treatment; (3) in vivo and imaginal exposure; (4) response prevention instructions; and (5) training in relapse prevention. Accordingly, treatment fidelity procedures used in clinical trials and extended for use in clinical supervision outside the context of randomized trials underscore the need to emphasize implementation of these core procedures. The core procedures have an empirical foundation. Foa and colleagues (1984) conducted an ERP randomized dismantling study in which the elements of exposure, response prevention, and their combination were evaluated. In that study, EX alone (expose to feared stimuli but OK to ritualize) and RP alone (reduce rituals but without needing to expose to feared stimuli) were both less efficacious and less durable than their combination (ERP). These findings set the stage for the current emphasis on leaning into situations that provoke distress while *simultaneously* reducing and ultimately eliminating compulsions and other forms of avoidance (Franklin, Freeman, & March, 2019).

To maximize ERP outcomes it is important to ensure that other procedures are not used instead of the core elements. For example, in their review of the ERP literature, Foa, Franklin, and Moser (2002) recommended that cognitive strategies be used in support of exposure rather than to replace it. In fidelity monitoring and clinical supervision on exposure-based sessions, therefore, it is important that therapists start exposures early enough in session so as to leave sufficient time for their completion and for the postexposure processing that often allows the therapist to promote the cognitive changes, particularly the emphasis on corrective information, thought to be essential to maximize ERP outcomes (Foa & Kozak, 1985, 1986). Benito and colleagues (2020) reported that patient outcomes were enhanced when therapists persisted in response to patient avoidance or refusal of planned exposure; patients whose therapists changed (weakened) treatment procedures in response to their avoidant style tended to experience less robust treatment responses.

The importance of adherence to response prevention instructions during ERP has received further empirical support. Wheaton and colleagues (2016) found that a patient adherence rating that corresponded to approximately 75% or higher resistance to compulsive urges was significantly and strongly associated with optimized posttreatment outcome. This empirical finding translates to pithy advice for clinicians: Keep a close eye on successful response prevention and adapt when it appears that it is falling below the 75% resistance rate.

MEASUREMENT OF THERAPIST AND PATIENT TREATMENT ADHERENCE AND FIDELITY

In addition to the necessity of therapists adhering to ERP protocols to promote treatment efficacy, patients must adhere to their between-session assignments to achieve peak treatment benefits (Simpson et al., 2011; Maher et al., 2012). Indeed, out-of-session solo practice reinforces and helps generalize the work that therapists do with patients during sessions (Abramowitz et al., 2002). Given that ERP requires patients to face their fears, record their levels of anxiety, and attempt to refrain from engaging in any behaviors/rituals that comfort them, maintaining adherence is often challenging. To accurately measure between-session adherence, Simpson and colleagues (2010) developed the Patient EX/RP Adherence Scale (PEAS). The PEAS includes three core features: simplicity, quality/quantity, and a complete assessment of adherence. Simplicity refers to the ease of implementing the PEAS into each therapy session. Quality/quantity refers to the fact that the PEAS addresses the quality and quantity of the patient's adherence to the EX/RP homework between sessions. The PEAS evaluates patient adherence in full because the PEAS assesses the patient's exposures as well as response prevention between sessions. The PEAS format involves a three-item scale assessing the percentage of exposures attempted, the quality of exposures attempted, and the percentage of rituals resisted. All items refer to the exercises that the therapist gave to the patient to complete between sessions, and each item is rated on a seven-point Likert scale. Simpson and colleagues (2010) indicated that the PEAS has interrater reliability and is relatively easy to administer. A strong relationship was demonstrated between the quantity and quality of exposures that the patient attempted, as well as between the quality of exposures and the quantity of responses (compulsions) prevented (Simpson et al., 2010).

Simpson and colleagues (2011) and Maher and colleagues (2012) extended the work of Simpson and colleagues (2010) by using the PEAS to investigate whether a relationship exists between OCD patients' between-session adherence to EX/

RP and their treatment outcome. Both Simpson and colleagues (2011) and Maher and colleagues (2012) found evidence indicating that between-session patient adherence significantly predicted a lower OCD severity posttreatment. Additionally, data suggested that the degree of between-session adherence was significantly related to the degree of improvement and to the likelihood of a positive treatment response. The benefits of between-session adherence early in the treatment process also were emphasized, given that higher PEAS scores during sessions five through nine (out of a total of 18 sessions) predicted lower posttreatment Y-BOCS scores (Simpson et al., 2011). This information is critical clinically, in that it provides a timeline by which good adherence should be achieved to ensure optimized outcomes. Patients who are not getting to that point need to be reinstructed before continued nonadherence begins to erode outcomes.

Although flexibility in tailoring evidence-based practices (EBPs)—such as ERP—to each patient is crucial, effective administration of EBPs simultaneously requires the therapist to adhere to the treatment protocols (Abramowitz et al., 2003). Adherence refers to whether and how well the therapist employs specified procedures during treatment (Barber et al., 2007; Öst et al., 2015). Maintaining treatment fidelity helps the patient to get the most out of the therapy. Examination of these variables has been unfortunately limited in OCD specifically, but there is important information to be gleaned from research endeavors made in the field more broadly speaking. Accordingly, consideration of the work of Beidas and Kendall (2010) and Beidas and colleagues (2015) in examining therapist adherence in particular is warranted.

When comparing Beidas and colleagues (2015) to Beidas and Kendall (2010), it is important to emphasize that Beidas and colleagues (2015) was an observational study that included self-report measures, whereas Beidas and Kendall (2010) was a review of various studies for which some included self-report measures while others involved independent rating. Therefore, Beidas and Kendall (2010) developed a method of scaling their data to compare the studies effectively. Additionally, many community-based therapists in the Beidas and colleagues (2015) study reported using CBT techniques in addition to other strategies, which poses the questions: How much emphasis did they put on CBT techniques? And, which aspects of CBT were they using?

The Beidas and Kendall (2010) review employed the systems-contextual (SC) perspective to examine studies focusing on trained service providers' dissemination and implementation (DI) of EBP. They focused on how therapist training influences providers' knowledge and behavior as well as how a therapist's environment impacts their utilization of interventions. This reflects the SC perspective because of the focus on the influences of organizational, client, and therapist variables (Sanders & Turner, 2005; Turner & Sanders, 2006). The studies that Beidas and Kendall (2010) analyzed employed various designs, but they all consisted of therapists treating clinical/at-risk populations.

Beidas and Kendall's (2010) analyses enabled them to conclude that training impacts therapists' knowledge, attitudes, and to a lesser degree behaviors. Therapists' attitudes tended to improve following the completion of EBP training in all of the studies. This attitude improvement was maintained at follow-up for all of the therapists and treatment modalities (Beidas & Kendall, 2010). Additionally, across studies, therapists' perceived and declarative knowledge tended to increase following their completion of EBP training. Increased knowledge, however, does not necessarily entail improved treatment administration (Beidas & Kendall, 2010). Previously, various researchers reported that the "gold standard" of EBP training included clinical supervision, a workshop, and a manual (e.g., Sholomskas et al., 2005). However, Beidas and Kendall (2010) provided evidence suggesting that this gold standard may be insufficient, given that many therapists who completed training programs that met the gold standard did not display proficiency in adherence, skill, or competence. Beidas and Kendall (2010) specified that training programs that involve active learning, as well as address all levels of the SC model, are crucial in yielding improvements in therapist adherence (e.g. Sanders, Tully, et al., 2003), which then improves patient outcome (e.g. Miller et al., 2004).

To make matters more complex, a disparity occurred between therapists' perceived confidence in their skills versus their actual skills: Their confidence was higher than their true skill level (Beidas & Kendall, 2010). This difference poses two major issues: (1) The patients do not receive the most effective treatment, and (2) perceived proficiency decreases the likelihood that the therapists will obtain further training in EBP (Beidas & Kendall, 2010; Miller & Mount, 2001). Treatment fidelity is of utmost importance for EBP because, without it, patients will not be able to maximally benefit from the treatment (Elliot & Mihalic, 2004).

Similar to Beidas and Kendall's (2010) focus on the SC model, Beidas and colleagues (2015) investigated the contribution of organizational and individual factors on therapists' self-reported usage of cognitive-behavioral, psychodynamic, and family therapy. We will only focus on their findings relative to CBT for the present purpose, because CBT is the recommended EBP for OCD. This study was cross-sectional and observed 19 pediatric mental health agencies. Organizational factors tended to influence the use of EBPs more than individual factors (Beidas et al., 2015). Evidence suggested, however, that age and attitude were individual factors that did contribute to the likelihood of employing CBT. Unsurprisingly and replicating prior research (Aarons, 2005), therapists with more open attitudes were more likely to administer the empirically supported treatment (i.e., CBT). Inconsistent with previous research (Aarons, 2004), older therapists were more likely to employ CBT than younger therapists (Beidas et al., 2015).

Organizational factors accounted for 23% of the overall variation for CBT, as opposed to the 16% variance accounted for by individual factors. Beidas and colleagues (2015) evaluated and categorized the agencies based on their cultures and climates and found that organizations with more resistant cultures (organizations that expect therapists to be apathetic) and those with more functional climates (therapists have confidence in their abilities to complete their job with efficacy) were more likely to use CBT techniques. Therapists working in functional climates tended to be more likely to implement CBT (Beidas et al., 2015), which contrasts with Beidas and Kendall's (2010) finding that therapists' perceptions of their abilities to provide therapy effectively did not tend to predict improved treatment administration.

Beidas and colleagues (2015) additionally examined implementation climate and implementation leadership, which are both of great importance to the present chapter. Therapists, supervisors, and administrators from each organization completed the Implementation Climate Scale to provide information about the organization's degree of emphasis on EBPs (Beidas et al., 2015). Only therapists filled out the Implementation Leadership Scale (Aarons, Ehrhart, & Farahnak, 2014), which was based on their direct supervisor's behaviors regarding the implementation of EBP (Beidas et al., 2015). Surprisingly, implementation climate and implementation leadership were not predictive of EBP usage (Beidas et al., 2015). It is possible, however, that more complex mediational or interactive factors could account for this, but Beidas and colleagues (2015) did not evaluate such factors.

Much of this information can be useful to therapists, supervisors, and researchers working in clinical practice settings. Indeed, clinician training and attitudes are important to take into account when providing ERP in diverse clinical settings. Fortunately, data from both adult and pediatric OCD indicates that excellent outcomes comparable to those achieved in RCTs can be realized in clinical practice settings (see Franklin et al., 2000).

Evidence documents that ERP can be delivered successfully in a variety of clinical settings in which the therapists and even supervisors are not necessarily ERP developers or experts (e.g., Torp et al., 2015; Valderhaug et al., 2007; Warren & Thomas, 2001). In these settings, however, promotion of therapist use of and adherence to the core ERP procedures should be emphasized and re-emphasized. Recording of sessions where possible or even having the supervisor join in on some sessions may further adherence. ERP manuals are typically built upon many years of scientific observations regarding optimal ordering of techniques and even precise wording of how best to convey core treatment concepts. At the same time, no manual can be entirely exhaustive, so there needs to be sufficient flexibility built in to allow clinicians to meet the needs of specific patients. This delicate balance between fidelity and flexibility is crucial for successful implementation: There is a reason that procedures have been laid out as they have, yet common and even uncommon stumbling blocks are encountered, and the clinician would be well served to use empirically grounded knowledge for when the road less traveled should be attempted. Here we provide examples of the latter, without losing sight of the former.

FLEXIBILITY TO PROMOTE CLIENT-FOCUSED IMPLEMENTATION

Contemporary ERP manuals emphasize the following core procedures: (1) psychoeducation; (2) hierarchy development; (3) in vivo and imaginal exposure; (4) response prevention; and (5) relapse prevention. We shortly will discuss situations in which clinical circumstances dictate a deviation or modification of the protocol from the way these procedures are described in the manual or customarily implemented—being flexible while maintaining fidelity (Kendall & Beidas, 2007; Kendall & Frank, 2018). Our effort is to demonstrate the need for flexibility at times, even when maintaining fidelity to the treatment on the whole. It is strongly preferred that when such leeway is taken that it is guided by scientifically valid reasoning rather than employed more arbitrarily; clinical supervision is an ideal context in which to check in on the justification when the core procedures are modified in their implementation. Note that the following examples are simply that, examples, and that there are many other reasons why clinicians may adapt the manual to meet clinical need or to avert the development of problems in treatment known to have negative effects on outcome. Therapist experience appears to play a role in how comfortable clinicians are in being flexible, and how successful they are likely to be when they are (see Huppert et al., 2001, on adult panic disorder). In our experience there is great value in encouraging protocol adherence, yet at the same time teaching junior clinicians when to bypass potential roadblocks that they can see coming. The following is simply an explication of some of these attempts.

Psychoeducation. ERP interventions are grounded theoretically upon Mowrer's Two-Factor Theory (1939, 1960), which emphasizes the critical role of negative reinforcement brought on by compulsions in the maintenance of obsessions and associated anxiety. An elaboration upon this theory took cognitive factors into account (e.g., activation of "fear structures"), and emphasized the importance of setting up exposure exercises as opportunities to provide corrective information (Foa & Kozak, 1985, 1986). Collectively these theoretical accounts are emphasized in most ERP manuals, and the process of habituation is thought to be evidence that the fear has been both activated and remediated. OCD, however, is a heterogeneous condition, and not all associated clinical observations necessarily fall neatly under these theoretical umbrellas. For example, there is now growing empirical evidence that the decay slopes associated with disgust and not-just-right presentations of OCD are as robust as what is typically seen in OCD with feared consequences (see Schwartz, 2018, for a review); accordingly, there may be a disconnect between what is told to such patients about how and why exposure works and their own psychological experiences. In such circumstances, it would seem that telling patients to wait for within- and between-session habituation when this is unlikely to occur fully is akin to Waiting for Godot, and perhaps opens an avenue to between-session nonadherence: If I am given the impression that I am supposed to feel better in due time and yet I don't, my willingness to engage in exposure might be subsequently diminished. Here then is an opportunity to anticipate a potential roadblock in patient adherence, so other theoretical explanations for how "Not Just Right" OCD works may help avert this roadblock. In such cases, perhaps greater emphasis should be placed on acceptance-based explanations (see Twohig et al., 2015) or on other theoretical accounts that emphasize learning principles but rely less on habituation (e.g., Inhibitory Learning, Craske et al., 2014), because these accounts would better match the experiences of such patients and hence promote continuation of exposures despite incomplete habituation. Some manuals already have incorporated some of these suggested theoretical modifications depending on the characteristics of patients' specific characteristics, but for many if not most ERP manuals, habituation is still invoked as the overarching goal of exposure. It is important to recognize that this still may be the case for most OCD patients, which is why it is advanced as such. However, for the minority of OCD patients for whom this is not true, it is critical to flex the theoretical underpinning of exposure so it better matches their own personal experiences.

Hierarchy Development. A staple of ERP is the development of treatment hierarchies to provide a map for treatment. Such hierarchies list an array of fear-relevant stimuli and rank-order them to provide an estimate of how difficult a given exposure might be when conducted. For the ranking of these stimuli, the original Subjective Units of Distress Scale (SUDS) presented by Wolpe (rate your anxiety from 0 to 100) often is used, although it has been modified for ease of use with youth (such as 0–10 scales as presented in Franklin et al., 2019) and to decrease rumination about providing completely accurate information such as might be seen in OCD patients suffering from maladaptive perfectionism (e.g., those who spend several minutes getting to the conclusion that their SUDS is a 56.5). The SUDS or Fear Thermometer ratings should allow patients to quickly rank-order possible exposure stimuli from low to medium to high levels of fear and convey to therapists what to expect when confronting fear-invoking situations and stimuli. Most of the time this procedure works well, especially when therapists convey to patients that these ratings are simply estimates of how much fear is likely to be experienced, rather than a close representation of what *will* be experienced when the patient actually engages in a given exposure. In many ERP protocols, patients are taught to use the scale as a rough guide for whether to move further up the hierarchy if actual fear is low or to break the exposure down into manageable steps if actual fear is too high.

There are times in the provision of clinical care when the hierarchy itself becomes problematic, sometimes because patients give very high ratings for many items as a way to convey that they do not wish to engage in exposures. In such cases the language used to rank exposures may need to be modified to better reflect the purpose of the procedure. For example, Abramowitz and others (e.g., Jacoby & Abramowitz, 2016) have suggested shifting language away from ranking the patient's subjective level of fear, which might convey to the patient that they cannot and should not attempt to tolerate high levels of anxiety. Instead, the recommendation in such circumstances may be made to ask patients to rate their "willingness" to engage in an exposure rather than how anxious they would expect to be, were they to do so. This modification is convergent with the principles and procedures of Inhibitory Learning wherein violation of patient expectancies in exposure exercises is considered more relevant than maximizing anxiety levels and waiting for them to habituate. Clinicians who encounter patients who may be using SUDS as a way to convey that they do not wish to proceed with exposure to anxiety-evoking thoughts and situations might be more fully engaged in conversations around willingness, which may allow for aversion of another roadblock in treatment.

A subgroup of patients for whom using SUDS to craft stimulus hierarchies can prove problematic are those with autism spectrum disorders (ASDs). The rates of OCD comorbidity in ASD are quite high, but the use of SUDS to rank hypothetical exposures to feared stimuli may well prove to be a gap too large to breach. Many with ASD have difficulty with such abstractions, and asking such patients to rank anxiety on a numeric scale could lead to frustration, noncompliance, and unwillingness to engage in the treatment process. In such cases, there may well be workarounds: borrowing from the pain literature, visual depictions of faces experiencing various levels of anxiety, or possibly even color-coded levels of fear (shades of blue to crimson red) may offer methods of hierarchy ranking that would be more palatable or preferable to the patients while still affording the clinician a way to at least generate an estimate of fear in a given situation. Other modifications of instruction are likely to be needed when treating OCD in those who have ASD, but finding other ways to glean these fear estimates from patients efficiently in setting up the treatment is a common place where flexibility will be needed to maintain fidelity to the protocol.

Imaginal and In Vivo Exposure. Most ERP manuals move relatively quickly from the provision of psychoeducation and the creation of OCD treatment hierarchies into the administration of in vivo exposure, which can be augmented by imaginal exposure for patients who report that they have specific consequences they fear will ensue if they refrain from compulsions and other forms of avoidance. Treatment should progress from low-level exposures onto increasingly challenging ones, until such time that the therapist believes the patient is ready to summit, that is, confront the most difficult items on the hierarchy. All exposure manuals are convergent in vigorously encouraging therapists to reach these peak exposures well before the end of the acute phase of treatment, so as to provide multiple opportunities for repetition and thus mastery of the main fears. When patients progress according to plan there are few reasons to deviate from the protocol; when patients struggle to climb the stimulus hierarchy, however, there may be a need to engage in treatment in a more flexible manner. One suggestion would be to bring Motivational Interviewing (MI) procedures to bear when patients are declining exposures, doing them and then undoing them, or not following through on exposure homework despite doing their due diligence with therapist-assisted exposure. MI is not customarily embedded formally in ERP manuals, but we do know—if not expect—that patients will at times struggle with proceeding up the stimulus hierarchy. Clinically, this situation may prompt more discussion in treatment about patient's reasons for and against doing the treatment as prescribed, as well as the pros and cons of continuing to experience OCD symptoms at their current level of severity. MI has been brought to bear with a wide variety of clinical problems including OCD (e.g., Simpson et al., 2011; Tolin & Maltby, 2008). Moving over to MI likely will require a temporary stay from the usual progression up the stimulus hierarchy as encouraged in the ERP manual, but at the same time partial adherence, especially between sessions, is a known risk factor for attenuated outcome. Accordingly, suspending ERP temporarily to marshal the motivational resources that will be needed to propel the ERP forward would seem clinically indicated. Such a decision will take the therapist off the ERP path temporarily, but if the course the patient is on is headed toward the jagged rocks then a course correction may well be the most prudent way to get the therapy back on track.

Response Prevention. The importance of response prevention, which essentially boils down to refraining from acting on urges to ritualize or avoid, is core and strongly emphasized in ERP manuals. That said, patient difficulties with successfully meeting the necessary goal of resisting most if not all said urges is a very common problem in treatment, especially early on. The goal may well be implementation of successive approximations, that is, rewarding and reinforcing efforts in the right direction then raising the bar. The recent paper that addressed patient nonadherence to response prevention makes clear, however, that patient outcomes are compromised if, during ERP, patients are falling below the 75% resistance ratio. Accordingly, moving up the exposure hierarchy without paying sufficient attention to successful response prevention is strongly contraindicated. Here again, MI could be brought to bear, again as an extra intervention rather than a core ERP procedure. If the issue is less one of motivation than of becoming overwhelmed by fear when resisting urges to ritualize, it may well be that some time must be allocated in treatment to figuring out with the patient how to implement RP successfully. For example, a child (pre-Covid19) was having great difficulty refraining from urges to ritualize immediately upon coming home from a stressful day at school. Contamination accumulated at school was the prime source of discomfort, but it also appeared that the stress of the school day more broadly speaking lowered the patient's resistance. Further encouragement to refrain, which is convergent with the ERP manual, appeared unlikely to be successful given the severity of the rituals engaged in upon returning home: The patient would change all of his now-contaminated clothing in the garage, dump these into a metal bin, and walk naked through the house straight to the bathroom, where he would then engage in an hour-long ritualized shower. As an alternative, the therapist worked with the patient diligently to design additional procedures that would likely make it easier to refrain from this ritual. Together they came up with "Frog Hour," wherein the patient would leave his bookbag on the side of the house rather than enter the garage, then proceed straight to the local wooded area that included several large ponds. The patient, who loved nature, would then go searching for wildlife at the ponds, categorize and chronicle what he found, then return home after about an hour. The reduction in stress that came from this nature ride was palpable, and the patient then found himself in a better position to refrain from the stripping ritual and the compulsive shower. The irony of the process was not lost on the patient: He spent an hour wallowing in pond muck in order to then come home to then refrain from washing extensively—but the patient's main sources of contamination were the bodily fluids of other students, which were in short supply in the remote woods. The therapist immediately saw the improved engagement of the patient and encouraged him to bring his "Critter Journal" to every subsequent session. Reviewing the Critter Journal was the way that the therapist and patient kicked off the sessions, and it allowed them to have bigger conversations about living life in accordance with one's values and interests rather than at the mercy of OCD. These theoretical deviations, clearly more convergent with Acceptance and Commitment Therapy (ACT) rather than with ERP per se, were seen as a means to promote ERP adherence between sessions, rather than a threat to the integrity of the intervention. Critter Journal and acceptance-based discussions may not generalize to the treatment of other patients, but in this case, may have helped the therapist avoid the common pitfall of between-session nonadherence to response prevention instructions.

Relapse Prevention. Conveying core concepts in treatment is essential, because it is from theoretical understanding that the capacity to serve as one's own therapist is derived, and ultimately that is the objective in ERP. Accordingly, the language selected to convey this information needs to be tailored to the patient, especially if the prescribed methods of doing so from the ERP manual were not found especially illuminating or helpful. In the context of an RCT examining the relative and combined efficacy of medication and ERP (Foa et al., 2005), one of us (MEF) was assigned an ERP patient. The patient was not especially academically minded and did not take immediately or well to some of the dry ways that concepts were conveyed in the manual. Accordingly, rather than risk disengagement or compromised understanding, the therapist tailored much of the treatment verbiage to the patient's much more passionate interests, namely professional football. Of note, in the RCT context session recordings are pulled at random and reviewed to rate therapist adherence, and in this case one of our maintenance sessions for this case was selected for review. Shortly thereafter, a note was received which vigorously encouraged an immediate meeting with the clinical supervisor. This supervisor, Michael J. Kozak, was known for his brilliance as well as his directness, so he got straight to the point: "Martin, it appears that our RA has rated your compliance as a zero for your last maintenance session—perhaps we should review the tape together." Recognizing immediately that this was not actually an invitation, we watched a 45-minute session in which it appeared that the therapist and patient were actively engaged in a very detailed discussion about pro football concepts rather than about relapse prevention per se, which was likely the source of the low adherence rating.

Espousing the need to make the language more flexible to promote engagement and understanding, I narrated over the top of the tape, explaining how the discussion of a football defense's dramatic shift in blitz schemes was a direct result of having successfully blocked that defense's preferred method of "A-gap" blitzes, and was actually relevant in this case: "They've adjusted to the fact that you are blocking that up so well that they're getting no pass rush on you up the middle, so they are now trying to bring pressure off the corner and with the safety on delayed blitzes." Essentially this translated to explain for the patient the shift in OCD symptoms from urges to check repeatedly and wipe down surfaces such as windows when cleaning so that there are no streaks, toward other more novel content such as fear of harm befalling family members and associated efforts to cancel out unwanted thoughts.

Having installed the patient into the role of quarterback, I asked him how he could counteract this adjustment. "I can check out of the play that I called in the huddle and audible to a short pass right behind where the blitzers are coming from."

"Excellent," I answered.

What this meant was that the patient had to design new exposures for the novel content and understand that it was his success at refraining from his typical rituals that likely forced OCD to try other ways to get him to give in, in light of the fact that successful resistance of urges to ritualize is the best way to ultimately reduce the frequency and intensity of obsessions in the long run. After several minutes of essentially translating the football talk back into ERP relapse prevention concepts convergent with our study manual, my exasperated yet ultimately satisfied supervisor proclaimed, "Well, I must commend you for your ... flexibility," after putting the offending adherence rating through the office shredder.

REFERENCES

Aarons, G. A. (2004). Mental health provider attitudes toward adoption of evidence-based practice: The evidence-based practice attitude scale (EBPAS). *Mental Health Services Research, 6*(2), 61–74. https://doi.org/10.1023/B:MHSR.0000024351.12294.65

Aarons, G. A. (2005). Measuring provider attitudes toward evidence-based practice: Consideration of organizational context and individual differences. *Child and Adolescent Psychiatric Clinics, 14*(2), 255–271. https://doi.org/10.1016/j.chc.2004.04.008

Aarons, G. A., Ehrhart, M. G., & Farahnak, L. R. (2014). The implementation leadership scale (ILS): Development of a brief measure of unit level implementation leadership. *Implementation Science, 9*(1), 45. https://doi.org/10.1186/1748-5908-9-45

Abramowitz, J. S. (1996). Variants of exposure and response prevention in the treatment of obsessive compulsive disorder: A meta-analysis. *Behavior Therapy, 27*, 583–600.

Abramowitz, J. S., Foa, E. B., & Franklin, M. E. (2003). Exposure and ritual prevention for obsessive-compulsive disorder: Effects of intensive versus twice-weekly sessions. *Journal of Consulting and Clinical Psychology, 71*, 394–398.

Abramowitz, J. S., Franklin, M. E., & Foa, E. B. (2002). Empirical status of cognitive-behavioral therapy for obsessive compulsive disorder: A meta-analytic review. *Romanian Journal of Cognitive and Behavior Psychotherapies, 2*, 89–104.

Abramowitz, J. S., Franklin, M. E., Zoellner, L. A., & DiBernardo, C. L. (2002). Treatment compliance and outcome in obsessive-compulsive disorder. *Behavior Modification, 26*(4), 447–463.

Abramowitz, J. S., Whiteside, S. P., & Deacon, R. J. (2005). The effectiveness of treatment for pediatric obsessive-compulsive disorder: A meta-analysis. *Behavior Therapy, 36*, 55–63.

Barber, J. P., Sharpless, B. A., Klostermann, S., & McCarthy, K. S. (2007). Assessing intervention competence and its relation to therapy outcome: A selected review derived from the outcome literature. *Professional Psychology: Research and Practice, 38*(5), 493. https://doi.org/10.1037/0735-7028.38.5.493

Beidas, R. S., & Kendall, P. C. (2010). Training therapists in evidence-based prac-
    tice: A critical review of studies from a systems-contextual perspective.
    Clinical Psychology: Science and Practice, 17(1), 1–30. https://doi.org/10.1111/
    j.1468-2850.2009.01187.x

Beidas, R. S., Marcus, S., Aarons, G. A., Hoagwood, K. E., Schoenwald, S., Evans, A. C.,
    Hurford, M. O., Hadley, T., Barg, F. K., Walsh, L. M., Adams, D. R., & Mandell, D.
    S. (2015). Predictors of community therapists' use of therapy techniques in a large
    public mental health system. *JAMA Pediatrics, 169*(4), 374–382. https://doi.org/
    10.1001/jamapediatrics.2014.3736

Benito, K. G., Machan, J., Freeman, J. B., Garcia, A. M., Walther, M., Frank, H., . . .
    Franklin, M. E. (2020). Therapist behavior during exposure tasks predicts habit-
    uation and clinical outcome in three randomized controlled trials for pediatric
    OCD. *Behavior Therapy*, doi:http://dx.doi.org.proxy.library.upenn.edu/10.1016/
    j.beth.2020.07.004.

Craske, M. G., Treanor, M., Conway, C. C., Zbozinek, T., & Vervliet, B. (2014).
    Maximizing exposure therapy: An inhibitory learning approach. *Behaviour Research
    and Therapy, 58*, 10–23. doi:http://dx.doi.org.proxy.library.upenn.edu/10.1016/
    j.brat.2014.04.006

Foa, E. B., Franklin, M. E., & Moser, J. (2002). Context in the clinic: How well do CBT
    and medications work in combination? *Biological Psychiatry, 51*, 989–997.

Foa, E. B., & Kozak, M. J. (1985). Treatment of anxiety disorders: Implications for psy-
    chopathology. In A. H. Tuma & J. D. Maser (Eds.), *Anxiety and the anxiety disorders*
    (pp. 421–452). Erlbaum.

Foa, E. B., & Kozak, M. J. (1986). Emotional processing of fear: Exposure to corrective
    information. *Psychological Bulletin, 99*(1), 20–35.

Foa, E. B., & Kozak, M. J. (1996). Psychological treatment for obsessive-compulsive dis-
    order. In M. R. Mavissakalian & R. F. Prien (Eds.), *Long-term treatments of anxiety
    disorders* (pp. 285–309).) American Psychiatric Association.

Foa, E. B., Liebowitz, M. R., Kozak, M. J., Davies, S. O., Campeas, R., Franklin, M. E.,
    Huppert, J. D., Kjernisted, K., Rowan, V., Schmidt, A. B., Simpson, H. B., & Tu,
    X. (2005). Treatment of obsessive compulsive disorder by exposure and ritual pre-
    vention, clomipramine, and their combination: A randomized, placebo-controlled
    trial. *American Journal of Psychiatry, 162*, 151–161.

Foa, E. B., Steketee, G., Grayson, J. B., Turner, R. M., & Latimer, P. (1984). Deliberate
    exposure and blocking of obsessive-compulsive rituals: Immediate and long-term
    effects. *Behavior Therapy, 15*, 450–472.

Foa, E. B., Yadin, E., & Lichner, T. K. (2012). *Exposure and response (ritual) prevention
    for obsessive-compulsive disorder: Therapist guide* (2nd ed.). Oxford University Press.

Franklin, M. E., Abramowitz, J. S., Kozak, M. J., Levitt, J., & Foa, E. B. (2000). Effectiveness
    of exposure and ritual prevention for obsessive compulsive disorder: Randomized
    compared with non-randomized samples. *Journal of Consulting and Clinical
    Psychology, 68*, 594–602.

Franklin, M. E., Freeman, J. B., & March, J. S. (2019). *Treating OCD in children and
    adolescents: A cognitive-behavioral approach.* The Guilford Press.

Franklin, M., Sapyta, J., Freeman, J., Khanna, M., Compton, S., Almirall, D., Moore, P.,
    Choate-Summers, M., Garcia, A., Edson, A. L., Foa, E. B., & March, J. S. (2011).
    Cognitive behavior therapy augmentation of pharmacotherapy in pediatric

obsessive-compulsive disorder: The Pediatric OCD Treatment Study II (POTS II). *Journal of the American Medical Association, 306*, 1224–1232.

Freeman, J., Sapyta, J., Garcia, A., Compton, S., Khanna, M., Flessner, C., Fitzgerald, D., Mauro, C., Dingfelder, R., Benito, K., Harrison J., Curry, J., Foa, E., March, J., Moore, P., & Franklin, M. (2014). Family-based treatment of early childhood obsessive-compulsive disorder: The pediatric obsessive-compulsive disorder treatment study for young children (POTS jr)—A randomized clinical trial. *JAMA Psychiatry, 71*(6), 689–698.

Garcia, A. M., Sapyta, J. J., Moore, P. S., Freeman, J. B., Franklin, M. E., March, J. S., & Foa, E. B. (2010). Predictors and moderators of treatment outcome in the pediatric obsessive compulsive treatment study (POTS I). *Journal of the American Academy of Child & Adolescent Psychiatry, 49*(10), 1024–1033.

Ginsburg, G. S., Kingery, J. N., Drake, K. L., & Grados, M. A. (2008). Predictors of treatment response in pediatric obsessive-compulsive disorder. *Journal of the American Academy of Child & Adolescent Psychiatry 47*(8), 868–878.

Huppert, J. D., Bufka, L. F., Barlow, D. H., Gorman, J. M., Shear, M. K., & Woods, S. W. (2001). Therapists, therapist variables, and cognitive-behavioral therapy outcome in a multicenter trial for panic disorder. *Journal of Consulting and Clinical Psychology, 69*(5), 747–755.

Jacoby, R. J., & Abramowitz, J. S. (2016). Inhibitory learning approaches to exposure therapy: A critical review and translation to obsessive-compulsive disorder. *Clinical Psychology Review, 49*, 28–40.

Kendall, P. C., & Beidas, R. (2007). Smoothing the trail for dissemination of evidence-based practices for youth: Flexibility within fidelity. *Professional Psychology: Research and Practice, 38*, 13–20.

Kendall, P. C., & Frank, H. (2018). Implementing evidence-based treatment protocols: Flexibility within fidelity. *Clinical Psychology: Science and Practice, 25*, 1–12. doi: 10.1111/cpsp.12271.

Knopp, J., Knowles, S., Bee, P., Lovell, K., & Bower, P. (2013). A systematic review of predictors and moderators of response to psychological therapies in OCD: Do we have enough empirical evidence to target treatment? *Clinical Psychology Review, 33*(8), 1067–1081.

Maher, M. J., Wang, Y., Zuckoff, A., Wall, M. M., Franklin, M., Foa, E. B., & Simpson, H. B. (2012). Predictors of patient adherence to cognitive-behavioral therapy for obsessive-compulsive disorder. *Psychotherapy and Psychosomatics, 81*(2), 124–126.

March, J. S., Franklin, M. E., Leonard, H., Garcia, A., Moore, P., Freeman, J., . . . Foa, E. (2007). Tics moderate the outcome of treatment with medication but not CBT in pediatric OCD. *Biological Psychiatry, 61*, 344–347.

Marks, I. M., Stern, R. S., Mawson, D., Cobb, J., & McDonald, R. (1980). Clomipramine and exposure for obsessive-compulsive rituals: I. *British Journal of Psychiatry, 136*, 1–25.

Miller, W. R., & Mount, K. A. (2001). A small study of training in motivational interviewing: Does one workshop change clinician and client behavior? *Behavioural and Cognitive Psychotherapy, 29*, 457–471.

Miller, W. R., Yahne, C. E., Moyers, T. B., Martinez, J., & Pirritano, M. (2004). A randomized trial of methods to help clinicians learn motivational interviewing.

Journal of Consulting and Clinical Psychology, 72(6), 1050. https://doi.org/10.1037/
0022-006X.72.6.1050

Mowrer, O. H. (1939). A stimulus-response analysis of anxiety and its role as a reinforcing
agent. *Psychological Review, 46*, 553–565.

Mowrer, O. H. (1960). *Learning theory and behavior.* Wiley.

Öst, L., Havnen, A., Hansen, B., & Kvale, G. (2015). Cognitive behavioral treatments
of obsessive-compulsive disorder. A systematic review and meta-analysis of studies
published 1993–2014. *Clinical Psychology Review, 40*, 156–169.

Öst, L., Riise, E. N., Wergeland, G. J., Hansen, B., & Kvale, G. (2016). Cognitive behavioral and pharmacological treatments of OCD in children: A systematic review and
meta-analysis. *Journal of Anxiety Disorders, 43*, 58–69.

Pediatric OCD Treatment Study Team. (2004). Cognitive-behavioral therapy, sertraline,
and their combination for children and adolescents with obsessive-compulsive disorder: The Pediatric OCD Treatment Study (POTS) randomized controlled trial.
Journal of the American Medical Association, 292, 1969–1976.

Peris, T. S., Sugar, C. A., Bergman, L., Chang, S., Langley, A., & Piacentini, J. (2012).
Family factors predict treatment outcome for pediatric obsessive-compulsive disorder. *Journal of Consulting and Clinical Psychology, 80*, 255–263.

Persons, J. B., & Silberschatz, G. (1998). Are results of randomized controlled trials useful
to psychotherapists? *Journal of Consulting and Clinical Psychology, 66*(1), 126–135.

Piacentini, J., Bergman, R. L., Chang, S., Landley, A., Peris, T., Wood, J. J., & McCracken,
J. (2011). Controlled comparison of family cognitive behavioral therapy and
psychoeducation/relaxation training for child obsessive-compulsive disorder.
Journal of the American Academy of Child & Adolescent Psychiatry, 50(11),
1149–1161.

Sanders, M. R., & Turner, K. M. T. (2005). Reflections on the challenges of effective
dissemination of behavioural family intervention: Our experience with the Triple
P–Positive Parenting Program. *Child and Adolescent Mental Health, 10*(4), 158–169.
https://doi.org/10.1111/j.1475-3588.2005.00367.x

Sanders, M., Tully, L., Turner, K., Maher, C., & McAuliffe, C. (2003). Training GPs
in parent consultation skills: An evaluation of training for the Triple P–Positive
Parenting Program. *Australian Family Physician, 32*(9), 763–768.

Schwartz, R. A. (2018). Treating incompleteness in obsessive-compulsive disorder: A meta-analytic review. *Journal of Obsessive-Compulsive and Related
Disorders, 19*, 50–60.

Sholomskas, D. E., Syracuse-Siewert, G., Rounsaville, B. J., Ball, S. A., Nuro, K. F., &
Carroll, K. M. (2005). We don't train in vain: A dissemination trial of three strategies
of training clinicians in cognitive-behavioral therapy. *Journal of Consulting and
Clinical Psychology, 73*(1), 106. https://doi.org/10.1037/0022-006X.73.1.106

Simpson, H. B., Foa, E. B., Liebowitz, M. R., Ledley, D. R., Huppert, J. D., Cahill, S.,
Vermes, D., Schmidt, A. B., Hembree, E., Franklin, M., Campeas, R., Hahn, C. H., &
Petkova, E. (2008). A randomized, controlled trial of cognitive-behavioral therapy
for augmenting pharmacotherapy in obsessive-compulsive disorder. *The American
Journal of Psychiatry, 165*(5), 621–630.

Simpson, H. B., Foa, E. B., Liebowitz, M. R., Huppert, J. D., Cahill, S., Maher, M. J.,
McLean, C. P., Bender, J., Marcus, S. M., Williams, M. T., Weaver, J., Vermes, D.,
Van Meter, P. E., Rodriguez, C. I., Powers, M., Pinto, A., Imms, P., Hahn, C. G., &

Campeas, R. (2013). Cognitive-behavioral therapy *vs* risperidone for augmenting serotonin reuptake inhibitors in obsessive-compulsive disorder: A randomized clinical trial. *JAMA Psychiatry, 70*(11), 1190–1198.

Simpson, H. B., Maher, M., Page, J. R., Gibbons, C. J., Franklin, M. E., & Foa, E. B. (2010). Development of a patient adherence scale for exposure and response prevention therapy. *Behavior Therapy, 41*(1), 30–37.

Simpson, H. B., Maher, M. J., Wang, Y., Bao, Y., Foa, E. B., & Franklin, M. (2011). Patient adherence predicts outcome from cognitive behavioral therapy in obsessive-compulsive disorder. *Journal of Consulting and Clinical Psychology, 79*(2), 247–252.

Simpson, H. B., Marcus, S. M., Zuckoff, A., Franklin, M., & Foa, E. B. (2012). Patient adherence to cognitive-behavioral therapy predicts long-term outcome in obsessive-compulsive disorder. *The Journal of Clinical Psychiatry, 73*(9), 1265–1266.

Simpson, H. B., Zuckoff, A., Page, J. R., Franklin, M. E., & Foa, E. B. (2008). Adding motivational interviewing to exposure and ritual prevention for obsessive-compulsive disorder: An open pilot trial. *Cognitive Behaviour Therapy, 37*(1), 38–49.

Simpson, H. B., Zuckoff, A. M., Maher, M. J., Page, J. R., Franklin, M. E., & Foa, E. B. (2010). Challenges using motivational interviewing as an adjunct to exposure therapy for obsessive-compulsive disorder. *Behaviour Research and Therapy, 48*, 941–948.

Tolin, D. F., & Maltby, N. (2008). Motivating treatment-refusing patients with obsessive-compulsive disorder. In H. Arkowitz, H. A. Westra, W. R. Miller, & S. Rollnick (Eds.), *Motivational interviewing in the treatment of psychological problems* (pp. 85–108). The Guilford Press.

Torp, N. C., Dahl, K., Skarphedinsson, G., Thomsen, P. H., Valderhaug, R., Weidle, B., Holmgren Melin, K., Hybel, K., Becker Nissen, J., Lenhard, F., Wentzel-Larsen, T., Franklin, M. E., & Ivarsson, T. (2015). Effectiveness of cognitive behavior treatment for pediatric obsessive-compulsive disorder: Acute outcomes from the Nordic Long-Term OCD Treatment Study (NORDLOTS). *Behaviour Research and Therapy, 64*, 15–23.

Turner, K. M. T., & Sanders, M. R. (2006). Dissemination of evidence-based parenting and family support strategies: Learning from the Triple P–Positive Parenting Program system approach. *Aggression and Violent Behavior, 11*(2), 176–193. https://doi.org/10.1016/j.avb.2005.07.005

Twohig, M. P., Abramowitz, J. S., Bluett, E. J., Fabricant, L. E., Jacoby, R. J., Morrison, K. L., Reuman, L., & Smith, B. M. (2015). Exposure therapy for OCD from an acceptance and commitment therapy (ACT) framework. *Journal of Obsessive-Compulsive and Related Disorders, 6*, 167–173.

Valderhaug, R., Larsson, B., Gotestam, K. G., & Piacentini, J. (2007). An open clinical trial of cognitive-behaviour therapy in children and adolescents with obsessive-compulsive disorder administered in regular outpatient clinics. *Behaviour Research and Therapy, 45*, 577–589.

Warren, R., & Thomas, J. C. (2001). Cognitive-behavior therapy of obsessive-compulsive disorder in private practice: An effectiveness study. *Journal of Anxiety Disorders, 15*, 277–285.

Westen, D., Novotny, C. M., & Thompson-Brenner, H. (2004). The empirical status of empirically supported psychotherapies: Assumptions, findings, and reporting in controlled clinical trials. *Psychological Bulletin, 130*(4), 631–663.

Wheaton, M. G., Galfalvy, H., Steinman, S. A., Wall, M. M., Foa, E. B., & Simpson, H. B. (2016). Patient adherence and treatment outcome with exposure and response prevention for OCD: Which components of adherence matter and who becomes well? *Behaviour Research and Therapy, 85*, 6–12.

Wheaton, M. G., Rosenfield, D., Foa, E. B., & Simpson, H. B. (2015). Augmenting serotonin reuptake inhibitors in obsessive-compulsive disorder: What moderates improvement? *Journal of Consulting and Clinical Psychology, 83*(5), 926–937.

6

Being Flexible While Maintaining Fidelity for Medical Patients

Patient-Centered and Team-Based Strategies

MIRA REICHMAN, VICTORIA A. GRUNBERG,
JAMES D. DOORLEY, JAFAR BAKHSHAIE,
ETHAN G. LESTER, RYAN A. MACE,
AND ANA-MARIA VRANCEANU ■

INTRODUCTION

For decades, health psychologists have tried to narrow the gap between research and practice. Like behavioral scientists in general, health psychologists tend to prefer the conditions of randomized controlled trials to evaluate interventions. However, translating results from controlled settings to the "real world" of outpatient or inpatient medical clinics and fast-paced intensive care units is a challenge (Glasgow, 2008; Oldenburg & Absetz, 2011; Teachman et al., 2012). The translation of research findings into sustainable changes to health service delivery requires appreciation of both the scientific findings and the complexities of medical populations and settings. Although many health psychology interventions have demonstrated efficacy, and a select few have exhibited effectiveness (Absetz et al., 2009; Ammerman et al., 2002), additional efforts are needed to disseminate and integrate these interventions into practice—efforts that will meaningfully improve the quality of life, emotional functioning, and overall well-being of persons facing the stress of medical illness.

To close this research-practice gap, an important step is to promote the adoption of manual-based and empirically supported health psychology interventions into real-world clinical settings (Kazdin, 2008). Manual-based interventions—in which core evidence-based treatment components are neatly packaged for efficient and consistent delivery—facilitate widespread dissemination and integration of psychological interventions into medical settings. At the same time manual-based interventions are optimal when they take into account the complexities and diversity of medical populations and settings. The fast-paced and unpredictable nature of medical settings may preclude rigid, unvarying delivery of manual-based psychosocial interventions to medical patients. Medical populations are characterized by an interplay between physical and psychosocial issues. These issues direct attention to individual factors to establish a positive therapeutic relationship, enable accessibility of treatment, and triage most pressing patient needs. Enhanced dissemination of manual-based health psychology interventions hinges on evidence-based treatments being implemented with both fidelity and flexibility.

"Flexibility within fidelity" (Kendall, 1998; Kendall et al., 2008; Kendall & Frank, 2018) involves adhering to the core tenets of manual-based treatments while attuning to patient and contextual factors to maximize effectiveness. A balance between flexibility and fidelity is central to evidence-based practice. To find this balance in the delivery of empirically supported treatments (ESTs), clinicians must consider the best available evidence in addition to their own expertise and judgment. For health psychologists, flexibility within fidelity is required to address both the individual patient factors resulting from the dual physical and psychosocial comorbidities that characterize medical populations, and the contextual factors arising from the complexities of medical settings and interdisciplinary medical teams (Mignogna et al., 2018). Flexibility while maintaining fidelity is key in health psychology to enable widespread adoption of ESTs for medical populations.

This chapter presents a model for being flexible while maintaining fidelity for medical populations, addressing flexibility both in the delivery of treatments to patients (i.e., patient-centered flexibility) and in collaborations with multidisciplinary medical teams (i.e., team-based flexibility). We provide examples from our research to illustrate how flexibility within fidelity can be employed for medical patients and offer recommendations to health psychology researchers and providers for exercising thoughtful clinical decision-making in the delivery of evidence-based interventions. Table 6.1 provides a summary of patient-centered and team-based strategies with a focus on application.

A PATIENT-CENTERED AND TEAM-BASED APPROACH TO BEING FLEXIBLE WHILE MAINTAINING FIDELITY

Optimizing Fidelity

Implementing ESTs with fidelity is essential to delivering scientifically informed care and ensuring that patients receive the core treatment components shown to be efficacious in contributing to positive patient outcomes. In health psychology,

Table 6.1. Patient-Centered and Team-Based "Flexibility within Fidelity" Strategies for Medical Populations

Level	Strategy	Context	Flexible Application
Patient-Centered	Motivational interviewing	Addressing barriers to treatment engagement (e.g., stress, substance use, psychiatric comorbidities, neurological illness)	Attune to individual factors that influence patients' readiness, interest, and confidence to engage in treatment (e.g., stigma, physical appearance, culture, values, preferences)
	Education on mental–physical interactions	Medical conditions that have high rates of psychiatric comorbidities (e.g., chronic pain, cancer, diabetes, HIV, obesity, brain injury)	Orient to mind-body connection; emphasize importance of psychological care in long-term physical health; create transdiagnostic conceptualizations
	Treatment planning	Time-limited (e.g., terminal illnesses), fluctuations in health status (e.g., stroke), changes in setting (e.g., care transitions)	Adapt duration (session length and course), frequency (pacing, number of visits), and modality (in-person and remote) of treatment delivery according to stability and chronicity of illness
	Establishing the therapeutic relationship	Initiating treatment, creating a positive group environment	Remain mindful of interactions between group members; discuss session content in a way that facilitates positive patient learning; stay open to relevant topics introduced by patients
	Dyadic and family interventions	High risk for caregiver burden in medical patients, especially degenerative diseases (Alzheimer's) or emergent medical treatment (ICU patients)	Involve family members or caregivers to enhance their well-being and patients' ability to benefit from treatment
	Routine assessments	Expected changes in patients' medical and psychological status (e.g., neurological event, follow-up visit or procedure)	Modify treatment targets based on current emotional distress (e.g., informal 1–10 rating) and interval history

(continued)

Table 6.1. CONTINUED

Level	Strategy	Context	Flexible Application
Team-Based	Staff education	Misunderstandings of psychological care or reluctance to refer patients	Encourage ongoing discussions about roles, services, and appropriate referrals; Add knowledge to the care team on patients' psychiatric/emotional status
	Care coordination	Medical or psychiatric emergencies, deteriorating functioning, missed appointments	Triage issues of higher severity; adapt techniques to target complex comorbidities; adjust timing and delivery of sessions
	Collaborative communication	Documentation in electronic medical records, multidisciplinary rounds	Continuously share psychiatric information with care team; stay vigilant to treatment-interfering comorbidities; engage front-line providers in reinforcing intervention skills
	Needs assessments	Adequately meeting evolving needs of patients and family members	Create open lines of communication with all levels of the team (i.e., front-line to leadership); refine protocols through staff feedback (e.g., referral burden, familiarity with services)
	Patient identification	Presence of psychological risk factors early in medical treatment (e.g., catastrophic thinking about pain), recruitment for clinical research	Create "warm handoff" opportunities; develop a clear understanding of clinic flow; identify barriers to integrating psychological services

high fidelity to ESTs is important given patients' physical comorbidities and providers' aims to enhance patients' mental and physical well-being (Bellg et al., 2004; Compas et al., 1998). Consequently, fidelity can be conceptualized as the necessary framework within which flexibility is exercised. Strategies to optimize fidelity in the delivery of treatment to patients and in collaboration with medical teams serve to strengthen this framework so that clinicians can intentionally and effectively attune to patient and contextual factors.

Patient-Centered Flexibility within Fidelity

High-quality treatment manuals facilitate fidelity in the delivery of treatments to patients through simplicity and clarity in content and structure. Manuals are best when principle-driven, with clear indication of the underlying theoretical framework and the core elements and goals of treatment (Kendall & Frank, 2018). Manuals should include agendas for each session, session goals, and specific activities to meet stated goals (Kendall & Frank, 2018). Supportive aids in manuals, such as decision-making algorithms, help clinicians adapt session content to address and overcome potential patient challenges based on a predetermined set of strategies. Additionally, adherence monitoring through tiered or peer supervision methods strengthens and reinforces fidelity in the delivery of treatment.

Complexities that occur when working with medical populations pose several challenges to fidelity in the implementation of ESTs. First, health psychology providers are often met with resistance, ambivalence, or challenges establishing and maintaining rapport when helping patients process a serious medical diagnosis or change problematic health behaviors. Second, medical patients often present with complex physical and psychiatric comorbidities, which complicate diagnostic assessment and raise questions about which symptoms to target first. Third, the course of acute and chronic medical illness varies in powerful ways across people, which may require deviations from the timeline and session plans of manual-based treatments. Finally, patients who seek treatment in medical or hospital settings often are accompanied by partners, family members, or other caregivers. Therefore, health psychology providers must decide when and how to involve these individuals in treatment. Because the hallmark of good clinical practice is patient-centered care, we argue that unique patient characteristics are the primary driver of flexible deviations in the delivery of manual-based treatments. Below, we outline key considerations for clinicians and clinical researchers for flexibly responding to patient factors in the delivery of manual-based treatments.

FLEXIBLY FACILITATE PATIENT BUY-IN AND ESTABLISH THERAPEUTIC RELATIONSHIP

Patients are referred to health psychologists for many reasons, including stress and difficulties with coping, poor medical treatment adherence, engagement in treatment-interfering behaviors (e.g., substance use), comorbid psychiatric and physical concerns, and end-of-life issues. In any of these instances, referrals may be initiated by primary medical providers following limited discussion with the patient. Health psychologists need to creatively and flexibly use strategies that will build rapport with patients to facilitate willingness and motivation to engage with treatment, usually in a short period of time. Readiness to engage in psychological treatment is particularly important for medical patients (Prochaska, Redding, & Evers, 2015), who may benefit from evidence-based strategies to increase patient buy-in (e.g., motivational interviewing; Lundahl et al., 2013; Miller & Rollnick, 2012). Although some skeptics of ESTs believe manualized treatments inhibit the development of the therapist-patient relationship, research demonstrates that a strong relationship can be built and maintained in the context of manual-based treatments (Creed & Kendall, 2005), even when treatments are brief (Zuroff et al., 2000).

FLEXIBLY TAILOR TREATMENT TO ADDRESS MEDICAL-PSYCHIATRIC COMORBIDITY

Medical populations commonly treated by health psychologists exhibit high rates of psychiatric comorbidity, including patients with chronic pain (Gatchel, 2004), cancer (Knobf, 2007), diabetes (Ducat et al., 2014), HIV (Altice et al., 2010), and obesity (Faith, Matz, & Jorge, 2002). Psychiatric symptoms can exacerbate medical illness, impair physical functioning, and reduce patients' capacity to make health behavior changes. In turn, changes in medical status can precipitate or exacerbate psychopathology. Patients seeking health psychology services for the first time may be unaware of these bidirectional forces. It is important to orient patients to the mind-body connection and set expectations that both psychiatric and medical symptoms may be addressed in tandem through psychosocial intervention. Providers must remain alert to changes in medical and psychiatric needs and use evidence-based skills to flexibly target the most salient symptoms for enhancing health and well-being. Similarly, providers must assess the fluctuating cognitive and mental status of patients with neurological disorders or brain injuries and modify evidence-based skill delivery to meet patients where they are and keep them engaged.

FLEXIBLY ADAPT TIMING AND MODALITY OF TREATMENT IN RESPONSE TO MEDICAL NEEDS

Manual-based treatments may delineate timelines, yet providers may need to tailor these timelines based on the stability and chronicity of patient physical illness. For example, a young, otherwise healthy adult with challenges related to HIV treatment adherence may benefit from a cognitive-behavioral intervention across 10 to 12 weeks (Safren et al., 2009), while a different approach (potentially meaning-centered intervention) and duration of treatment may apply for a patient with terminal cancer (Rosenfeld et al., 2017). Diversity in medical diagnoses, required levels of care, and medical settings impact flexible adaptations to the duration, frequency, and modality of treatment delivery. Interruptions in treatment also should be expected and flexibly accommodated. Fluctuations in patient health status may require hospitalization during treatment, such as an at-risk patient who suffers a stroke or heart attack. These events are both flexibly accommodated and harnessed for their therapeutic value (e.g., highlighting patients' emotions, insights, or motivational shifts that emerge following hospitalization). Providers and clinical researchers also might consider when traditional in-person approaches to treatment delivery may be challenging or suboptimal (e.g., in the intensive care unit [ICU], preceding or following surgery) and when to use virtual versions of treatments to enhance accessibility (Lester et al., 2020; Vranceanu et al., 2019).

FLEXIBLY INVOLVE FAMILY MEMBERS AND CAREGIVERS IN TREATMENT

Partners, family members, and caregivers are routinely present with patients during medical visits and often are involved as allies and facilitators of medical treatment. In contrast, most ESTs in health psychology are designed for individuals. As such, health psychologists may flexibly adapt treatment when family members are present. It is also worth noting that medical patients' family members and caregivers face meaningful stress (Adelman et al., 2014), which is well documented in chronic, degenerative diseases such as Alzheimer's (Etters, Goodall, & Harrison, 2008) and in the context of emergent medical treatment, such as ICU settings (Azoulay et al., 2005; Netzer, 2018). Research suggests that incorporating these significant others into treatments that target health behavior change may be advantageous, particularly when patients and loved ones share health-related risk factors (Carr et al., 2019; Sorkin et al., 2014). A large literature exists on interventions for caregiver burden, and these programs have promise for alleviating distress and enhancing coping among both caregivers and patients (Chung et al., 2009; Segrin et al., 2018). Health psychology providers are faced with situations where flexibility involves including family members and/or caregivers in interventions to enhance family adjustment and facilitate patient buy-in and engagement.

Team-Based Flexibility within Fidelity

The complex physical comorbidities prevalent within medical populations require a multidisciplinary team-based approach. Integrated teams who practice in community clinics, private practices, and inpatient and outpatient hospital settings can include psychologists, physicians, physician assistants, nurse practitioners, registered nurses, physical/occupational/respiratory therapists, social workers, dieticians, and/or pharmacists (Goldstein et al., 2017). Within multidisciplinary teams, providers communicate and collaborate to optimize patients' biopsychosocial outcomes (Hall et al., 2018). Integrated care and interdisciplinary collaborations have been associated with better treatment engagement and improved patient outcomes in psychological care, compared to community-based mental health referrals (Godoy et al., 2017). To our knowledge, very limited research has focused on fidelity and flexibility related to health psychology interventions within the context of multidisciplinary teams and healthcare systems (Cohen et al., 2008; Mignogna et al., 2018).

High fidelity within multidisciplinary team collaborations hinges on clear delineations of professional roles and responsibilities and clear communication regarding the provision of psychological intervention. The team members need to have clear understandings of psychological intervention protocol—treatment plans, goals, and modality—as well as procedures to identify and refer eligible patients (Goldstein et al., 2017). Providing psychoeducation to providers on the evidence underlying psychological skills and their value for medical patients helps service providers maintain fidelity in treatment implementation by enhancing appropriate patient referrals and increasing patient and team engagement in care. Ongoing informal and formal feedback among team members (e.g., through regular meetings) can enhance fidelity by ensuring that providers and patients have the time, support, and resources needed to adhere to treatment protocols (Godoy et al., 2017).

However, given the recent and sometimes precarious integration of psychological services into medical settings, flexibility is key to implementing psychological interventions in collaboration with multidisciplinary teams. First, flexibility allows health psychologists to effectively engage and educate multidisciplinary teams on the utility of psychological intervention for medical patients. Second, health psychology providers must be open to deviations regarding the timing and planned delivery of psychological interventions to medical patients given the fast-paced and unpredictable nature of many medical settings. Finally, health psychology providers must maintain open and frequent communication with multidisciplinary team members to stay appraised of patient status and flexibly adapt treatments in response to changing patient needs. Below, we outline key considerations for clinicians and clinical researchers for flexibly collaborating with multidisciplinary teams in the implementation of psychological interventions.

FLEXIBLY ENGAGE MULTIDISCIPLINARY TEAMS

Health psychologists are challenged when engaging multidisciplinary medical providers with varying levels of knowledge regarding psychological care for medical populations. Despite high levels of psychosocial distress in many medical populations, some medical providers still exhibit misunderstandings regarding psychological care for their patients (Mignogna et al., 2018) and report reluctance to refer patients to psychological service providers (Holopainen et al., 2020). This reluctance in medical providers has been associated with low mental health literacy, lack of understanding and training about integrated care, and/or concern about creating further distress for patients (Holopainen et al., 2020; Vranceanu et al., 2017). Health psychologists who embrace flexibility in their communication and collaboration style can more effectively build interprofessional relationships and encourage ongoing discussions about roles, services, and appropriate referrals for psychological treatments. Additionally, flexibility and openness in interactions with patients enables health psychologists to gather and provide valuable clinical information to other members of patient care teams (e.g., information regarding the psychiatric/emotional status of patients).

FLEXIBLY NAVIGATE UNPREDICTABLE MEDICAL SETTINGS

Flexibility is vital for psychology providers to balance their own treatment goals with patients' needs for medical treatment and the goals of other multidisciplinary team members. Medical settings, especially inpatient hospital settings, can be fast paced and rapidly changing, and often involve emergencies. Adopting a spirit of flexibility for patient goals within team-based care may mean triaging issues of higher severity, adapting techniques to target complex comorbidities, and facilitating communication among patient and team members to adjust care plans (Goldstein et al., 2017). For example, patients who experience medical emergencies will need the immediate attention of medical providers, requiring psychology providers to adapt planned treatment delivery or timing of treatment sessions. Patient attendance also can be a barrier to psychological intervention delivery in outpatient medical settings. Health psychologists can creatively collaborate with other health care professionals to respond flexibly to missed appointments and retain patients in treatment (e.g., maintaining open slots in schedule to accommodate patients who need to reschedule; Godoy et al., 2017).

FLEXIBLY COMMUNICATE WITH TEAMS TO MEET PATIENTS' CHANGING NEEDS

Health psychologists must stay apprised of changing patient needs and adopt strategies to maintain frequent communication with multidisciplinary team members. Openly sharing information with medical providers in addition to the use of electronic medical records provide opportunities for health psychologists to be cognizant of comorbidities that may interfere with treatments and flexibly tailor interventions to the changing needs and status of patients. Additionally, health psychology providers consider when and how to flexibly involve other members of medical treatment teams as facilitators of psychological intervention. For example, nurses, physical therapists, and occupational therapists may spend more time with patients than health psychologists, and thus are well equipped to facilitate and reinforce skills from psychological interventions.

ILLUSTRATIONS OF FLEXIBILITY WHILE MAINTAINING FIDELITY FOR HEALTH PSYCHOLOGY

Several of our evidence-based interventions have used flexibility within fidelity to overcome barriers associated with the provision of psychosocial care to medical patients and on multidisciplinary teams. Our clinical research is based on a mixed method, stage model approach to behavioral intervention development (Onken et al., 2014), which includes prospective studies, qualitative data collection and systematic literature reviews, pilot and feasibility testing, and an iterative intervention development method of refinement. For our interventions, high fidelity is ensured through: (1) clarity and simplicity of core treatment components within manuals, (2) thorough clinician training, (3) provision of manuals to patients as accompaniments and guides to treatment, and (4) peer and tiered supervision. In tandem with this attention to fidelity, our experience demonstrates how interventions can be implemented with flexibility, both in attuning to individual patient factors and in collaborations with multidisciplinary teams. Here we present three interventions as illustrations: Recovering Together for Patients and Caregivers after Acute Neurological Illness, Resiliency for Neurofibromatosis, and the Toolkit for Optimal Recovery after Orthopedic Injury.

Recovering Together for Patients and Caregivers after Acute Neurological Illness

Recovering Together is a six-session, seven-module skills-based resiliency intervention for patients with acute neurological illnesses (ANI; e.g., stroke, traumatic brain injury, hydrocephalus) and their informal caregivers (i.e., family member or friend providing the majority of care; together called "dyads") to prevent chronic emotional distress (i.e., anxiety, depression, and post-traumatic stress; Vranceanu et al., 2020). Recovering Together begins at bedside in the Neuro-ICU shortly after admission, with the first two foundational sessions delivered in-person to both patient and caregiver. After discharge, Recovering Together transitions from in-person to virtual delivery for four additional sessions selected collaboratively from the five possible modules. Recovering Together is a transdiagnostic resiliency program that addresses the comorbidity of depression, anxiety, and post-traumatic stress. The program teaches mindfulness skills (e.g., deep breathing, present focus), coping skills (e.g., dialectics, acceptance, meaning-making), and interpersonal skills (e.g., effective communication, coping with role changes) identified as key drivers of chronic distress in this population (Meyers et al., 2019; Meyers, McCurley et al., 2020; Meyers, Presciutti et al., 2020; Shaffer et al., 2016a; Shaffer et al., 2016b). Recovering Together was iteratively developed and optimized with feedback from patients, caregivers, and medical teams (Bannon et al., 2020; McCurley et al., 2019; Meyers, McCurley, et al., 2020). The last iteration of Recovering Together demonstrates feasibility and acceptability, as well as efficacy in improving depression, anxiety, and post-traumatic stress in both patients and caregivers (Vranceanu et al., 2020).

Patient-Centered Flexibility within Fidelity for Recovering Together

Flexibly facilitate patient buy-in and establish therapeutic relationship.   ANIs often present critical junctures when patients and families are asked to make life-altering and time sensitive decisions for their current and future care with little preparation or support. The complex nature of this juncture can present in the form of unwillingness to commence psychosocial treatment in tandem with biomedical treatment while in the ICU, or resistance to psychosocial treatment based on perceived lack of relevance to the dyad's specific ANI. To engage dyads, psychologists attune to the presenting resistance and clearly communicate the rationale for treatment, specifically the fact that emotional distress is a common experience for both patients and caregivers after ANIs, regardless of the type and timing of the injury (Netzer, 2018). Clear explanation of this rationale as well as giving the dyad time to consider the treatment often results in dyads' willingness to address emotional needs in tandem with biomedical needs, beginning in the ICU. Support from the medical team is key in ensuring that patients understand psychological care as an important aspect of their health care, with strong implications for long-term recovery.

Flexibly tailor treatment to address medical-psychiatric comorbidity. ANIs are heterogeneous in terms of medical diagnoses, clinical presentation, psychiatric profile, and social context. The modular design of the Recovering Together manual allows clinicians and dyads to select skills that are most relevant for each dyad's needs, while also tailoring the skills of the intervention to dyad-specific scenarios. Additionally, patients' medical and psychological status and needs can change drastically over the course of treatment. This could occur in the form of a new neurological event, a disappointing or frightening follow-up visit or procedure, and problems with rehabilitation protocols. It is also common that dyadic treatment goals and priorities change once outside the immediate intensive care setting due to factors such as a greater familiarity with functional limitations and changing social support, resources, and roles. To attune to changing needs, clinicians delivering Recovering Together assess weekly emotional distress (informally; rating scale 1 to 10) and take an interval history of the most recent psychosocial stressors experienced since the last visit. Based on this information, clinicians flexibly modify treatment delivery to the dyad's most relevant needs.

Flexibly adapt timing and modality of treatment to medical needs. Recovering Together features a flexible treatment delivery modality (i.e., in-person sessions in the ICU and sessions over live video after ICU discharge) to increase treatment accessibility. Dyads can join videoconferencing sessions using laptops, tablets, or smartphones, and from separate devices if they are not physically together. We strive to adhere to the treatment plan with weekly sessions postdischarge, but some missed appointments are unavoidable as dyads juggle hectic schedules, role reversals, and adjustments to new responsibilities. We accommodate by promptly rescheduling and/or delivering two sessions consecutively in the following week. We observed that these flexible approaches helped to eliminate barriers, increase access to care, and provide continuity of care to the dyad throughout ANI recovery.

Flexibly involve family members and caregivers in treatment. As a dyadic treatment, Recovering Together includes both patients and primary caregivers, and targets emotional distress in both partners. Primary caregivers who participate in Recovering Together with patients include spouses, romantic partners, children, parents, and siblings. This approach is supported by prior research, which shows that caregivers have similar levels of emotional distress to patients, and that patients' and caregivers' risk and resiliency factors are interdependent (Meyers et al., 2019; Meyers, McCurley, et al., 2020; Meyers, Presciutti, et al., 2020; Shaffer et al., 2016a; Shaffer et al., 2016b). Psychologists build rapport with both members of the dyad, and the treatment goal is improvement of dyadic emotional distress with patients and caregivers as equal participants.

TEAM-BASED FLEXIBILITY WITHIN FIDELITY FOR RECOVERING TOGETHER

Flexibly engage multidisciplinary teams. Multidisciplinary work is essential in an effective clinical research initiative in the high-stress, busy Neuro-ICU setting. During the Recovering Together trial, our work benefitted from several years of building relationships with members of the multidisciplinary care team, particularly the critical care nurses, who became indispensable partners in this research. Weekly team meetings, case conferences, and focus groups allowed us to iteratively incorporate feedback from the medical team into the intervention and procedures. In turn, the medical team became invested in this work and helped to make referrals, identify caregivers, schedule appointments at a time when patients were able to participate, and act as liaisons with families. Recovering Together clinicians and research coordinators provided the broader multidisciplinary team with useful information that benefitted the patient and family care. Clinicians and research coordinators summarized clinically relevant observations (e.g., depression, anxiety, or interpersonal dynamics) gathered during baseline assessments and treatment sessions to nurses and other members of the care team to support effective communications with dyads and better delivery of care.

Flexibly navigate unpredictable medical settings. A psychosocial intervention in an acute setting such as the Neuro-ICU can sometimes be confused as a "competing priority" for time and resources, and psychologists are wise to adopt a flexible attitude to navigate the fast-paced and unpredictable setting. Clinicians and research coordinators for Recovering Together routinely attended nursing rounds to familiarize themselves with the unit, current admissions, medical diagnoses, medical treatments, and referrals made to various specialties. By coordinating effectively and flexibly with the multidisciplinary team (including intensivists, occupational and physical therapists, and social workers), we were able to develop and sustain a strong, familiar, and collaborative workflow.

Flexibly communicate with teams to meet patients' changing needs. The Recovering Together team benefitted from regular and frequent check-ins and open lines of communication with the care team, bedside nurses, and Neuro-ICU leadership. During monthly nursing meetings, we took a "pulse" of whether, based on nurses' perspectives, Recovering Together was meeting patient and family needs and integrating within the Neuro-ICU workflow. We gathered monthly feedback from nurses related to burden of referrals, familiarity with the program, and perceived benefits of the program. With this data, we were able to refine recruitment protocols over time to ensure that we were meeting the needs of the team while also maintaining fidelity to our treatment protocol.

Resiliency for Neurofibromatosis

Resiliency for Neurofibromatosis (NF) is an eight-session, group-based, virtual resiliency intervention for patients with Neurofibromatoses (i.e., neurological conditions that cause benign tumors to grow on the nervous system) to improve ability to cope with NF symptoms and stress, as well as physical and psychological quality of life (Lester et al., 2020; Vranceanu et al., 2016). The Resiliency for NF intervention was iteratively adapted from the Relaxation Response Resiliency Program (Park et al., 2013), which was based on feedback from patients and developed for both adults (eight weeks, 90-minute sessions) and adolescents (eight weeks, 45-minute sessions). The programs teach relaxation response skills (e.g., deep breathing, body scan), cognitive behavioral skills (e.g., adaptive thinking), and positive psychology skills (e.g., gratitude, social support) tailored to population needs and cognitive/learning disabilities frequent in this population. The adapted programs demonstrated feasibility and preliminary efficacy (Funes et al., 2019; Lester et al., 2020; Vranceanu et al., 2016), with full efficacy trials ongoing (Reichman et al., 2020; Vranceanu et al., 2018).

PATIENT-CENTERED FLEXIBILITY WITHIN FIDELITY FOR RESILIENCY FOR NEUROFIBROMATOSIS

Flexibly facilitate patient buy-in and establish therapeutic relationship. Given the group-based format of Resiliency for NF (with typically four to eight patients in each group), psychologists are challenged not only to establish rapport with individual patients, but to cultivate positive and therapeutic group relationships. Few components of treatment delivery require flexibility more than cultivation of group camaraderie. When delivering Resiliency for NF, clinicians are wise to be mindful of interactions between group members in order to deliver and discuss session content in a way that facilitates positive patient learning. Group interaction is a valuable part of the psychosocial interventions for rare medical illnesses, given that it helps normalize patients' experiences. Remaining flexible to novel topics introduced by patients can facilitate positive outcomes and group camaraderie.

Flexibly tailor treatment to address medical–psychiatric comorbidity. Neurofibromatosis has a diverse set of clinical presentations; therefore, flexibility in treatment delivery is essential to ensure accessibility and relevance of treatment for individual patients. NF patients exhibit differences in cognitive limitations and learning disabilities, symptom presentations (e.g., idiopathic pain, self-consciousness due to appearance), and home cultures. Clinicians flexibly adapt the delivery of skills to promote the greatest engagement by group members (e.g., allow patients with appearance concerns due to tumors to turn cameras off; frequently assess comprehension in younger adolescents with learning disabilities). Sometimes, individual patients present a more pressing need for specific resiliency skills based on personal stressors and symptoms, and clinicians may decide to emphasize certain skills within or across sessions, if it is beneficial to the group.

Flexibly adapt timing and modality of treatment in response to medical needs. Resiliency for NF uses live video for treatment delivery to promote accessibility of the intervention and enable participation from geographically diverse patients. We schedule group sessions based on patient availability to accommodate patients who work full-time and are from multiple time zones (e.g., schedule evening sessions). For our adolescent and NF2-deaf interventions, we use other adaptations such as weekend scheduling and captioning services. When participants miss weekly group sessions, we accommodate with individual make-up sessions. Although we cannot recreate the actual group experience or cover the materials in the same level of detail, clinicians deliver useful individual make-up sessions, summarizing session content and simulating group participation by recalling contributions unique to the group session from other participants.

TEAM-BASED FLEXIBILITY WITHIN FIDELITY FOR RESILIENCY FOR
NEUROFIBROMATOSIS
Flexibly engage multidisciplinary teams. Strong collaborations with multidisciplinary care teams for patients with NF are essential to successful implementation of Resiliency for NF. In particular, referrals from well-known NF clinics and
providers can serve as an endorsement for our programs, given that patients tend
to trust providers treating their medical ailments, especially when they are rare.
In forming relationships with referring medical providers, it is important to emphasize the way in which we are able to provide a needed service for their patients.
For example, NF providers at our hospital noted that patients were experiencing
high levels of stress and reduced quality of life; however, there were no specialists
to whom they could refer patients. In this way, Resiliency for NF was seen as
useful to our multidisciplinary collaborators. Additionally, we flexibly engage in
community events and patient forums to present on psychosocial factors related
to NF and to engage participants as study champions. Because implementation
of the program is the larger goal, we also collaborate with the Children's Tumor
Foundation, the largest NF nonprofit organization, which will support our efforts
of implementing the intervention and work with us to develop a training program
for potential clinicians.

The Toolkit for Optimal Recovery after Orthopedic Injury

The Toolkit for Optimal Recovery after Orthopedic Injury (TOR) is a four-
session, live video, mind-body program for patients with acute musculoskeletal
injuries (e.g., fractures, dislocations) to prevent chronic pain and disability. TOR
is informed by the fear avoidance model (Vlaeyen et al, 2012), which explains
how pain anxiety and catastrophic thinking about pain can cause patients to avoid
activity and give rise to symptom persistence and chronic disability. Accordingly,
TOR is specifically designed for patients who endorse high pain anxiety and catastrophic thinking about pain, established risk factors for persistent pain and disability (Vranceanu et al., 2014). The program teaches mindfulness and relaxation
skills (e.g., breath awareness, body scan), cognitive behavioral skills (e.g., adaptive
thinking, activity pacing), and acceptance and commitment therapy skills (e.g.,
value-based goals). The program is delivered one to two months after orthopedic
injury when all activity restrictions are removed. TOR has demonstrated excellent
feasibility and acceptability, and was associated with sustained improvement in
pain, disability, emotional distress, and treatment targets (Vranceanu et al., 2019).

PATIENT-CENTERED FLEXIBILITY WITHIN FIDELITY FOR TOOLKIT FOR
OPTIMAL RECOVERY AFTER ORTHOPEDIC INJURY
**Flexibly facilitate patient buy-in and establish therapeutic relation-
ship.** Rapport building with patients is an essential aspect of TOR because
patients are referred by their orthopedic treatment team, and TOR often serves
as patients' first point of contact with mental health care. We have observed that

warm hand-off referrals from orthopedic surgeons, in which surgeons personally connect patients with members of the research team, maximize patient willingness to engage in treatment (Vranceanu et al., 2019). In delivery of the first TOR session, clinicians target stigma related to mental health services and enhance patient motivation to participate by providing comprehensive psychoeducation on treatment rationale and goals. Clinicians can enhance patient buy-in by (a) normalizing the experience of pain after injury and (b) moving patients away from the mind-body dichotomy by discussing how all pain sensations originate in the brain. Clinicians ensure patients understand that while TOR is psychosocial in nature, the intervention is designed to ultimately prevent patients' having persistent pain and disability.

Flexibly tailor treatment to address medical–psychiatric comorbidity. The Toolkit for Optimal Recovery after Orthopedic Injury is designed to target (a) pain anxiety and (b) catastrophic thinking about pain after acute orthopedic injury. However, patients present with diverse types and severities of orthopedic injuries as well as psychological symptoms (e.g., depression, post-traumatic stress; Nota et al., 2015; Vranceanu et al., 2014; Vranceanu, Barsky, & Ring, 2009). In delivering TOR, clinicians attune to patients' symptom presentations and the differing impacts patients experience as a result of their injuries. For example, a lower extremity injury might impact a young avid runner differently from an older, mostly sedentary person. In aiming to break down myths and challenge negative cognitions about pain, TOR requires clinicians to attune to patients' beliefs and thoughts about their injury. TOR excludes patients with impaired cognitive function, but sudden changes in medical and psychiatric condition are possible given patients' recent histories of injuries, and clinicians pay attention to changing patient status when flexibly adjusting the pacing of treatment.

Flexibly adapt timing and modality of treatment in response to medical needs. The Toolkit for Optimal Recovery after Orthopedic Injury uses a live-video delivery model for all four sessions to maximize accessibility of the intervention and enable higher flexibility regarding the timing of treatment. We have found live-video delivery to be particularly important for orthopedic patients given the stigma associated with mental health services within orthopedic populations.

TEAM-BASED FLEXIBILITY WITHIN FIDELITY FOR TOOLKIT FOR OPTIMAL RECOVERY AFTER ORTHOPEDIC INJURY

Flexibly engage multidisciplinary teams. Implementation of TOR requires close collaboration with orthopedic care teams who treat patients during the acute phase after orthopedic injuries to identify patients exhibiting pain anxiety and catastrophic thinking about pain. Biomedical approaches tend to be prioritized over biopsychosocial approaches across most medical settings, and our prior work has shown that orthopedic surgeons in particular are neutral to psychosocial factors in their patients, and struggle with how to communicate with patients regarding psychosocial issues when they do notice them (Vranceanu et al., 2017). Understanding the nuanced barriers and facilitators to incorporating psychosocial care can lead to the creation of targeted educational materials based on data, which can support surgeons and orthopedic staff in making referrals. Ensuring buy-in from surgeons hinges on helping them understand how addressing psychosocial factors in their patients can benefit their orthopedic practice through increased patient satisfaction as well as decreased risk of medical complications and repeat surgeries.

Flexibly navigate unpredictable medical settings.   Orthopedic providers may perceive a "lack of time" to discuss psychosocial issues within their clinic, which is another barrier to integration of psychological care. This was the case with several surgeons in our pilot randomized controlled trial (RCT). We found it helpful to develop an understanding of the clinical flow when establishing relationships with all care providers. Clinicians and research coordinators adopted various strategies to facilitate patient recruitment, including approaching patients while they waited to see orthopedic surgeons and asking orthopedic surgeons to introduce patients to the study team. Flexibility helped us integrate within the streamlined clinical flow of orthopedic practices.

RECOMMENDATIONS FOR CLINICAL DECISION-MAKING IN FLEXIBLE TREATMENT DELIVERY

Differentiating between Flexibility and Nonadherence

To attune to patient and contextual factors in active medical settings without jeopardizing the delivery of scientifically informed care, health psychologists are encouraged to recognize the difference between a flexible application of a manual while preserving fidelity versus fidelity-inconsistent modification (i.e., nonadherence). Various considerations can help psychologists distinguish between flexibility and nonadherence (Kendall et al., 2008). Flexible delivery of ESTs requires that clinicians deliver all essential skills for each session, meet all stated session goals, and enact flexible deviations from the manual only in ways that adhere to the overarching conceptual framework of the EST. Nonadherence occurs in circumstances in which essential treatment skills are not delivered, session goals are not met, skills outside the manual are introduced, supportive therapy is offered in place of skill-delivery, or alternative conceptual frameworks are used that are inconsistent with the EST.

Determining When Nonadherence May Be Acceptable

Despite the importance of preserving fidelity, there may be times when nonadherence to ESTs is needed to preserve the safety and well-being of medical patients (Kendall et al., 2008). In research, nonadherence impacts the evaluation of the intervention and needs to be considered in data analyses. In practice, adherence to ESTs may not be appropriate for patients experiencing severe worsening psychiatric symptoms or acute medical crises. When patients present with severe worsening psychiatric symptoms (e.g., delusional thinking), clinicians have to weigh the degree to which discontinuation of treatment is in the best interest of the patient. For example, a diabetic patient with increasingly severe depression who develops suicidal ideation and plans might need an increase in the dosage of her weekly interventions or possible removal from the protocol. Additionally, a crisis that is not directly related to the originally targeted problem may constitute a reason for nonadherence. For example, a recent diagnosis of late-stage cancer and concomitant post-traumatic stress symptoms in a patient being treated for irritable bowel syndrome (IBS) might justify no longer adhering to the IBS-related protocol.

Several factors related to a medical patient's presentation and engagement with treatment may dictate nonadherence. Nonadherence may be the result when the patient's understanding or cognitive engagement with the materials is severely lacking, for example during a self-management intervention for a poststroke patient with a cognitive impairment that prevents the uptake of the psychoeducational materials. Nonadherence may also be justified when there is a lack of data to support the EST for the specific medical population. For example, a pain-focused intervention for orthopedic patients suffering from emotional distress may not yet be tested with patients with self-injurious thoughts or behaviors (SITBs). Adopting another treatment approach entirely may be appropriate.

A Framework for Flexibility-Related Decision-Making

We suggest a step-by-step set of decision-making rules for applying flexibility in the provision of psychosocial interventions for medical patients. The model is adapted from the general decision-making model for the provision of psychosocial interventions proposed by Miller and colleagues (2020). We focus on modifications that constitute "planned adaptations" in this decision-making algorithm as opposed to unintentional deviations from manuals.

Step 1. Clinicians should determine whether the goal of the adaptation is justified based on clinical, stakeholder, or empirical data. The clinician should find and examine any relevant evidence that supports the need for modifications related to the presenting medical–psychiatric comorbidity. Further, it is always important for the clinician to take into account factors such as therapist knowledge, patient characteristics, potential predictors and moderators of outcomes, and evidence of generalizability before considering modifications (Kendall & Frank, 2018).

Step 2. Next, the "function" of the EST for the particular medical patient needs to be identified to decide whether the adaptation is needed. As an example, for an intervention that aims to improve diabetes outcomes, a module on medication adherence may be essential for some individuals or populations but unnecessary for others.

Step 3. The next important consideration is related to the potential negative impact of the adaptation on outcomes. Is there any evidence that the clinician can apply adaptations without impacting the adherence to the protocol (i.e., flexibility while preserving fidelity)? Does time allow for pilot testing such a hypothesis? Any potential negative impact of adaptations under consideration is a red flag for their application and requires close analysis of the costs and benefits by the clinician and medical team.

Step 4. The last step includes conducting the adaptations while gauging their success using proper constructs, with considerations for the stakeholders' satisfaction and acceptance of potential reduction in efficacy. An example might include conducting focus groups among the professional healthcare providers of a physical activity program for older adults to test feasibility, acceptability, and appropriateness of the applied adaptations (Moore et al., 2014).

CONCLUSION

As the biopsychosocial model for medicine gains scientific support, popularity, and prevalence, health psychologists and other mental health practitioners are more commonplace in medical settings (e.g., community health clinics, inpatient intensive care units). To further integrate psychologists and other mental health professionals into medical settings and to disseminate evidence-based psychological treatments for medical patients, both fidelity and flexibility must be prioritized. We presented here a novel approach for being flexible while maintaining fidelity; namely, an approach for health psychologists in which flexibility is enacted to enable patient-centered care and clinician attunement to individual patient factors, as well as to enable effective collaboration with multidisciplinary teams in medical settings.

REFERENCES

Absetz, P., Oldenburg, B., Hankonen, N., Valve, R., Heinonen, H., Nissinen, A., Fogelholm, M., Talja, M., Uutela, A. (2009). Type 2 diabetes prevention in the real world: three-year results of the GOAL lifestyle implementation trial. *Diabetes Care, 32*(8), 1418–1420.

Adelman, R. D., Tmanova, L. L., Delgado, D., Dion, S., & Lachs, M. S. (2014). Caregiver burden: A clinical review. *JAMA, 311*(10), 1052–1060.

Altice, F. L., Kamarulzaman, A., Soriano, V. V., Schechter, M., & Friedland, G. H. (2010). Treatment of medical, psychiatric, and substance-use comorbidities in people infected with HIV who use drugs. *The Lancet, 376*(9738), 367–387.

Ammerman, A. S., Lindquist, C. H., Lohr, K. N., & Hersey, J. (2002). The efficacy of be-havioral interventions to modify dietary fat and fruit and vegetable intake: A review of the evidence. *Preventive Medicine, 35*(1), 25–41.

Azoulay, E., Pochard, F., Kentish-Barnes, N., Chevret, S., Aboab, J., Adrie, C., Annane, D., Bleichner, G., Bollaert, P. E., Darmon, M., Fassier, T., Galliot, R., Garrouste-Orgeas, M., Goulenok, C., Goldgran-Toledano, D., Hayon, J., Jourdain, M., Kaidomar, M., Laplace, C., Larché, J., Liotier, J., Papazian, L., Poisson, C., Reignier, J., Saidi, F., & Schlemmer, B.; FAMIREA Study Group. (2005). Risk of post-traumatic stress symptoms in family members of intensive care unit patients. *American Journal of Respiratory and Critical Care Medicine, 171*(9), 987–994. doi:10.1164/rccm.200409-1295OC. Epub 2005 Jan 21. PMID: 15665319.

Bannon, S., Lester, E., Gates, M., Rosand, J., & Vranceanu, A-M. (2020). Recovering Together: Building resiliency in dyads of stroke patients and their caregivers at risk for chronic emotional distress: A feasibility RCT. *Pilot and Feasibility Study, 25*(6),75.

Bellg, A. J., Borrelli, B., Resnick, B., Hecht, J., Minicucci, D. S., Ory, M., Ogedegbe, G., Orwig, D., Ernst, D., & Czajkowski, S.; Treatment Fidelity Workgroup of the NIH Behavior Change Consortium. (2004). Enhancing treatment fidelity in health beha-vior change studies: Best practices and recommendations from the NIH Behavior Change Consortium. *Health Psychology, 23*(5), 443–451. doi:10.1037/0278-6133.23.5.443. PMID: 15367063.

Carr, R. M., Prestwich, A., Kwasnicka, D., Thøgersen-Ntoumani, C., Gucciardi, D. F., Quested, E., Hall, L. H., & Ntoumanis, N. (2019). Dyadic interventions to promote physical activity and reduce sedentary behaviour: Systematic re-view and meta-analysis. *Health Psychology Review, 13*(1), 91–109. doi:10.1080/17437199.2018.1532312. Epub 2018 Oct 14. PMID: 30284501.

Chung, M. L., Moser, D. K., Lennie, T. A., & Rayens, M. K. (2009). The effects of depres-sive symptoms and anxiety on quality of life in patients with heart failure and their spouses: Testing dyadic dynamics using Actor–Partner Interdependence Model. *Journal of Psychosomatic Research, 67*(1), 29–35.

Cohen, D. J., Crabtree, B. F., Etz, R. S., Balasubramanian, B. A., Donahue, K. E., Leviton, L. C., Clark, E. C., Isaacson, N. F., Stange, K. C., & Green, L. W. (2008). Fidelity versus flexibility: Translating evidence-based research into practice. *American Journal of Preventive Medicine, 35*(5), S381–S389.

Compas, B. E., Haaga, D. A., Keefe, F. J., Leitenberg, H., & Williams, D. A. (1998). Sampling of empirically supported psychological treatments from health psy-chology: Smoking, chronic pain, cancer, and bulimia nervosa. *Journal of Consulting and Clinical Psychology, 66*(1), 89.

Creed, T. A., & Kendall, P. C. (2005). Therapist alliance-building behavior within a cognitive-behavioral treatment for anxiety in youth. *Journal of Consulting and Clinical Psychology, 73*(3), 498.

Ducat, L., Philipson, L. H., & Anderson, B. J. (2014). The mental health comorbidities of diabetes. *JAMA, 312*(7), 691–692.

Etters, L., Goodall, D., & Harrison, B. E. (2008). Caregiver burden among dementia pa-tient caregivers: A review of the literature. *Journal of the American Academy of Nurse Practitioners, 20*(8), 423–428.

Faith, M. S., Matz, P. E., & Jorge, M. A. (2002). Obesity–depression associations in the population. *Journal of Psychosomatic Research, 53*(4), 935–942.

Funes, C. J., Mace, R. A., Macklin, E. A., Plotkin, S. R., Jordan, J. T., & Vranceanu, A-M. (2019). First report of quality of life in adults with neurofibromatosis 2 who are deafened or have significant hearing loss: Results of a live-video randomized control trial. *Journal of Neuro-oncology, 143*(3), 505–513.

Gatchel, R. J. (2004). Comorbidity of chronic pain and mental health disorders: The biopsychosocial perspective. *American Psychologist, 59*(8), 795.

Glasgow, R. (2008). What types of evidence are most needed to advance behavioral medicine? *Annals of Behavioral Medicine, 35*(1), 19–25.

Godoy, L., Long, M., Marschall, D., Hodgkinson, S., Bokor, B., Rhodes, H., Crumpton, H., Weissman, M., & Beers, L. (2017). Behavioral health integration in health care settings: Lessons learned from a pediatric hospital primary care system. *Journal of Clinical Psychology in Medical Settings, 24*(3–4), 245–258.

Goldstein, C. M., Gathright, E. C., & Garcia, S. (2017). Relationship between depression and medication adherence in cardiovascular disease: The perfect challenge for the integrated care team. *Patient Preference and Adherence, 11*, 547.

Hall, M., Bifano, S. M., Leibel, L., Golding, L. S., & Tsai, S. L. (2018). The elephant in the room: The need for increased integrative therapies in conventional medical settings. *Children, 5*(11), 154.

Holopainen, R., Simpson, P., Piirainen, A., Karppinen, J., Schütze, R., Smith, A., O'Sullivan, P., & Kent, P. (2020). Physiotherapists' perceptions of learning and implementing a biopsychosocial intervention to treat musculoskeletal pain conditions: A systematic review and metasynthesis of qualitative studies. *Pain, 161*(6), 1150–1168.

Kazdin, A. E. (2008). Evidence-based treatment and practice: New opportunities to bridge clinical research and practice, enhance the knowledge base, and improve patient care. *American Psychologist, 63*, 146–159.

Kendall, P. C. (1998). Empirically supported psychological therapies. *Journal of Consulting and Clinical Psychology, 66*(1), 3.

Kendall, P. C., & Frank, H. E. (2018). Implementing evidence-based treatment protocols: Flexibility within fidelity. *Clinical Psychology: Science and Practice, 25*(4), e12271.

Kendall, P., Gosch, E., Furr, J. M., & Sood, E. (2008). Flexibility within fidelity. *Journal of the American Academy of Child and Adolescent Psychiatry. 47*(9), 987–993.

Knobf, M. T. (2007). Psychosocial responses in breast cancer survivors. *Seminars in Oncology Nursing, 23*(1), 71–83.

Lester, E., DiStefano, S., Mace, R., Macklin, E., Plotkin, S., & Vranceanu, A-M. (2020). Virtual mind-body treatment for geographically diverse youth with neurofibromatosis: A pilot randomized controlled trial. *General Hospital Psychiatry, 62*, 72–78.

Lundahl, B., Moleni, T., Burke, B. L., Butters, R., Tollefson, D., Butler, C., & Rollnick, S. (2013). Motivational interviewing in medical care settings: A systematic review and meta-analysis of randomized controlled trials. *Patient Education and Counseling, 93*(2), 157–168.

McCurley, J. L., Funes, C. J., Zale, E. L., Lin, A., Jacobo, M., Jacobs, J., Salgueiro, D., Tehan, T., Rosand, J., & Vranceanu, A-M. (2019). Preventing chronic emotional distress in stroke survivors and their informal caregivers. *Neurocritical Care, 30*(3), 581–589.

Meyers, E., Lin, A., Lester, E., Shaffer, K., Rosand, J., & Vranceanu, A-M. (2019). Baseline resilience and depression symptoms predict trajectory of depression in dyads of patients and their informal caregivers following discharge from the Neuro-ICU. *General Hospital Psychiatry, 62*, 87–92.

Meyers, E., McCurley, J., Lester, E., Jacobo, M., Rosand, J., & Vranceanu, A-M. (2020). Building resiliency in dyads of patients admitted to the Neuroscience Intensive Care Unit and their family caregivers: Lessons learned from William and Laura. *Cognitive and Behavioral Practice, 27*(3), 321–335.

Meyers, E., Presciutti, A., Shaffer, K. M., Gates, M., Lin, A., Rosand, J., & Vranceanu, A-M. (2020). The impact of resilience factors and anxiety during hospital admission on longitudinal anxiety among dyads of neurocritical care patients without major cognitive impairment and their family caregivers. *Neurocritical Care, 33*(2), 468–478.

Mignogna, J., Martin, L. A., Harik, J., Hundt, N. E., Kauth, M., Maik, A. D., Morocco, K., Benzer, J., & Cully, J. (2018). "I had to somehow still be flexible": Exploring adaptations during implementation of brief cognitive behavioral therapy in primary care. *Implementation Science, 13*, 76.

Miller C. J., Wiltsey-Stirman, S., Baumann, A. A. (2020). Iterative Decision-Making for Evaluation of Adaptations (IDEA): A decision tree for balancing adaptation, fidelity, and intervention impact. *Journal of Community Psychology, 48*(4), 1163–1177.

Miller, W. R., & Rollnick, S. (2012). *Motivational interviewing: Helping people change.* Guilford Press.

Moore, J. E., Mascarenhas, A., Marquez, C., Almaawiy, U., Chan, W. H., D'Souza, J., Liu, B., Straus, S. E., & MOVE ON Team. (2014). Mapping barriers and intervention activities to behaviour change theory for Mobilization of Vulnerable Elders in Ontario (MOVE ON), a multi-site implementation intervention in acute care hospitals. *Implementation Science, 9*(1), 160. https://doi.org/10.1186/s13012-014-0160-6

Netzer, G. (Ed.) (2018). *Families in the intensive care unit: A guide to understanding, engaging, and supporting at the bedside.* Springer. https://doi.org/10.1007/978-3-319-94337-4

Nota, S. P., Bot, A. G., Ring, D., & Kloen, P. (2015). Disability and depression after orthopaedic trauma. *Injury, 46*(2), 207–212.

Oldenburg, B., & Absetz, P. (2011). Lost in translation: Overcoming the barriers to global implementation and exchange of behavioral medicine evidence. *Translational Behavioral Medicine, 1*(2), 252–255.

Onken, L. S., Carroll, K. M., Shoham, V., Cuthbert, B. N., & Riddle, M. (2014). Reenvisioning clinical science: Unifying the discipline to improve the public health. *Clinical Psychology Science, 2*(1), 22–34.

Park, E. R., Traeger, L., Vranceanu, A.-M., Scult, M., Lerner, J. A., Benson, H., Denninger, J., & Fricchione, G. L. (2013). The development of a patient-centered program based on the relaxation response: The Relaxation Response Resiliency Program (3RP). *Psychosomatics, 54*(2), 165–174. https://doi.org/10.1016/j.psym.2012.09.001

Prochaska, J. O., Redding, C. A., & Evers, K. E. (2015). The transtheoretical model and stages of change. In K. Glanz, B. K. Rimer, & K. "V." Viswanath (Eds.), *Health behavior: Theory, research, and practice* (pp. 125–148). Jossey-Bass/Wiley.

Reichman, M., Riklin, E., Macklin, E., & Vranceanu, A-M. (2020). Virtual mind-body treatment for adolescents with neurofibromatosis: Study protocol for a single-blind randomized controlled trial. *Contemporary Clinical Trials, 95*, 106078.

Rosenfeld, B., Saracino, R., Tobias, K., Masterson, M., Pessin, H., Applebaum, A., Brescia, R., & Breitbart, W. (2017). Adapting meaning-centered psychotherapy for the palliative care setting: Results of a pilot study. *Palliative Medicine, 31*(2), 140–146.

Safren, S. A., O'cleirigh, C., Tan, J. Y., Raminani, S. R., Reilly, L. C., Otto, M. W., & Mayer, K. H. (2009). A randomized controlled trial of cognitive behavioral therapy for adherence and depression (CBT-AD) in HIV-infected individuals. *Health Psychology, 28*(1), 1.

Segrin, C., Badger, T. A., Sikorskii, A., Crane, T. E., & Pace, T. W. (2018). A dyadic analysis of stress processes in Latinas with breast cancer and their family caregivers. *Psycho-oncology, 27*(3), 838–846.

Shaffer, K. M., Riklin, E., Jacobs, J. M., Rosand, J., & Vranceanu, A-M. (2016a). Mindfulness and coping are inversely related to psychiatric symptoms in patients and informal caregivers in the neuroscience ICU: Implications for clinical care. *Critical Care Medicine, 44*(11), 2028–2036.

Shaffer, K. M., Riklin, E., Jacobs, J. M., Rosand, J., & Vranceanu, A-M. (2016b). Psychosocial resiliency is associated with lower emotional distress among dyads of patients and their informal caregivers in the neuroscience intensive care unit. *Journal of Critical Care, 36*, 154–159.

Sorkin, D. H., Mavandadi, S., Rook, K. S., Biegler, K. A., Kilgore, D., Dow, E., & Ngo-Metzger, Q. (2014). Dyadic collaboration in shared health behavior change: The effects of a randomized trial to test a lifestyle intervention for high-risk Latinas. *Health Psychology, 33*(6), 566.

Teachman, B. A., Drabick, D. A., Hershenberg, R., Vivian, D., Wolfe, B. E., & Goldfried, M. R. (2012). Bridging the gap between clinical research and clinical practice: Introduction to the special section. *Psychotherapy, 49*(2), 97.

Vlaeyen, J. W. S., & Linton, S. J. (2012). Fear-avoidance model of chronic musculoskeletal pain: 12 years on. *Pain, 153*(6), 1144.

Vranceanu, A-M., Bachoura, A., Weening, A., Vrahas, M., Smith, R. M., & Ring, D. (2014). Psychological factors predict disability and pain intensity after skeletal trauma. *The Journal of Bone and Joint Surgery. American volume, 96*(3), e20.

Vranceanu, A-M., Bannon, S. M., Mace, R., Lester, E. G., Meyers, E., Gates, M., Popok, P., Lin, A., Salgueiro, S., Tehan, T., Macklin, E., & Rosand, J. Feasibility and efficacy of a resiliency intervention on chronic emotional distress among survivor-caregiver dyads admitted to the Neuroscience Intensive Care Unit: A pilot randomized controlled trial. (2020). *JAMA Network Open, 3*(10).

Vranceanu, A-M., Barsky, A., & Ring, D. (2009). Psychosocial aspects of disabling musculoskeletal pain. *The Journal of Bone and Joint Surgery, 91*(8), 2014–2018.

Vranceanu, A-M., Beks, R. B., Guitton, T. G., Janssen, S. J., & Ring, D. (2017). How do orthopaedic surgeons address psychological aspects of illness? *The Archives of Bone and Joint Surgery, 5*(1), 2–9.

Vranceanu, A-M., Jacobs, C., Lin, A., Greenberg, J., Funes, C. J., Harris, M. B., Heng, M. M., Macklin, E. A., & Ring, D. (2019). Results of a feasibility randomized controlled trial (RCT) of the Toolkit for Optimal Recovery (TOR): A live video program to prevent chronic pain in at-risk adults with orthopedic injuries. *Pilot and Feasibility Studies, 5*(1), 30. doi:10.1186/s40814-019-0416-7. PMID: 30820341; PMCID: PMC6381627.

Vranceanu, A-M., Riklin, E., Merker, V. L., Macklin, E. A., Park, E. R., & Plotkin, S. R. (2016). Mind-body therapy via videoconferencing in patients with neurofibromatosis: An RCT. *Neurology, 87*(8), 806–814.

Vranceanu, A-M., Zale, E. L., Funes, C. J., Macklin, E. A., McCurley, J., Park, E. R., Jordan, J. T., Lin, A, & Plotkin, S. R. (2018). Mind-Body treatment for international English-speaking adults with neurofibromatosis via live videoconferencing: Protocol for a single-blind randomized controlled trial. *JMIR Research Protocols, 7*(10), e11008. doi:10.2196/11008. PMID: 30355560; PMCID: PMC6231775.

Zuroff, D. C., Blatt, S. J., Sotsky, S. M., Krupnick, J. L., Martin, D. J., Sanislow III, C. A., & Simmens, S. (2000). Relation of therapeutic alliance and perfectionism to outcome in brief outpatient treatment of depression. *Journal of Consulting and Clinical Psychology, 68*(1), 114.

7

Goodness of Fit

Flexing Manualized Treatment for Hoarding Disorder

SUZANNE OTTE, CHRISTIANA BRATIOTIS,
AND GAIL STEKETEE ∎

FEATURES OF HOARDING DISORDER

Frost and Hartl described "compulsive hoarding" in 1996, identifying the main elements that are central to the current diagnosis of hoarding disorder (HD) per the *Diagnostic and Statistical Manual of Mental Disorders, Fifth Edition* (DSM-5; see Box 7.1 for diagnostic criteria; American Psychiatric Association, 2013). Frost and Hartl described three main elements: (1) excessive acquiring and failure to discard a large number of possessions, often items that seem useless or of little value to others; (2) cluttered living spaces that are not accessible for ordinary activities; and (3) significant distress or impairment in functioning because of the hoarding. The items saved by people with HD are similar to those kept by most people without HD—clothing, magazines, papers, books, supplies, kitchen items, toys, and decorative objects. Occasionally, people with HD save unusual items such as trash, old food, or even their own body products. People with and without HD also save objects for similar reasons—emotional attachment, usefulness, and/ or attractiveness (Frost, Steketee, Tolin, Sinopoly, & Ruby, 2015). About 80% to 90% of people who hoard acquire their items excessively by buying or finding free objects, and sometimes by stealing, although this is rare (Frost, Rosenfield, Steketee, & Tolin, 2013). What distinguishes hoarding from ordinary object collecting and ownership is the extreme difficulty people who hoard experience when trying to part with possessions they own. Discarding items is especially difficult when strong feelings arise, such as guilt about waste and anxiety about needing the item in future, supported by beliefs that objects have meaning, value, and utility. This leads them to save too many items that accumulate as clutter, the byproduct of excessive acquiring and saving. Thus, although clutter is a defining

Box 7.1.

SUMMARY OF THE DSM-5 DIAGNOSTIC FEATURES OF HOARDING DISORDER

- Persistent difficulty discarding or parting with possessions, regardless of their value;
- Difficulty discarding due to a perceived need to save items and/or distress about discarding them;
- Accumulation of many possessions that clutter the active living areas of the home so rooms cannot be used as intended. In some cases, living areas have little clutter because other people intervene (e.g., family members, authority figures);
- Hoarding symptoms cause significant distress or impairment in social, occupational, or other areas of functioning, including difficulty maintaining a safe environment;
- Hoarding symptoms are not caused by other medical conditions (e.g., brain injury) and are not better accounted for by other mental disorders such as major depression, obsessive-compulsive disorder, or dementia.

Specifiers:

Excessive Acquisition—difficulty discarding is accompanied by frequent acquiring
Insight—degree of recognition that hoarding is a problem:

- good or fair—recognizes that hoarding behavior is problematic
- poor—mostly convinced hoarding behavior is not problematic
- absent/delusional—completely convinced hoarding behavior is not problematic despite contrary evidence

*See APA, 2013.

---

feature of hoarding, it is merely a consequence of excessive acquisition and saving, and of the disorganization evident in nearly all hoarded homes. In such homes, similar items are not grouped together, leading to difficulty finding important papers and objects that must be repurchased. The organizing problem stems from cognitive processing traits common among those who hoard, including difficulty categorizing objects, sustaining attention, and making decisions (Frost & Hartl, 1996; Woody, Kellman-McFarlane, & Welsted, 2014).

A diagnosis of hoarding disorder requires at least moderate clutter in the living areas of the home that impairs functioning (APA, 2013). Often, furniture and floors are piled with jumbled papers and objects so they cannot be used without extensive clearing. In severe cases, people with HD have difficulty cooking, cleaning, using bathrooms, and sleeping in their beds because of the clutter. People with HD experience distress when attempting to let go of or avoid acquiring possessions, and many find their behavior distressing but feel unable to resolve the problem. Often, family members, neighbors, and friends of those with HD are also distressed and may be an impetus for seeking treatment.

Based on careful clinical observations, Frost and Hartl (1996) proposed a model for understanding hoarding (see also Steketee & Frost, 2003), articulating the relationship among behavioral, cognitive, and emotional features (see Figure 7.1). Their model identified genetic, familial, and personal vulnerability factors that may play a role in onset, along with information processing problems (e.g., attention deficit, problems with organizing and/or decision-making) that reflect executive functioning challenges. These vulnerabilities appear to influence a person's beliefs about their possessions (e.g., object meaning, value, utility, need),

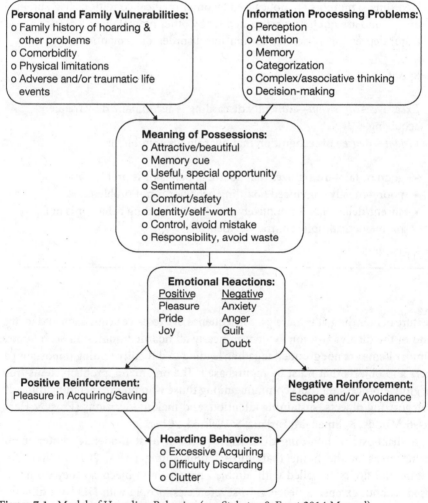

Figure 7.1. Model of Hoarding Behavior (see Steketee & Frost 2014 Manual)

which in turn generate positive and negative emotions that reinforce acquiring and saving behaviors and result in difficulty discarding. Positive emotions can include pleasure in acquiring a new item or finding a possession amidst the clutter, and negative emotions include anxiety and/or guilt when deciding whether to discard an object. This model has guided the development of Steketee and Frost's (2014) manual for treating hoarding disorder.

TREATMENTS AND IMPACT ON HOARDING DISORDER SYMPTOMS

Cognitive and behavioral treatments (CBT) have shown benefits for HD, although intervention strategies that improve outcomes are still needed. Treatment includes the following elements: case formulation based on the model for HD, motivational enhancement including establishing goals and values, skills training for sorting and organizing, practice (exposure) not acquiring, and practice decision-making and discarding. Early pilot studies indicated that clinical trainees can deliver CBT effectively using a preliminary manual and that clients with moderate-to-severe HD and various comorbid problems benefitted from the treatment (e.g., Hartl & Frost, 1999; Steketee, Frost, Wincze, Greene, & Douglass, 2000; Turner, Steketee, & Nauth, 2010). The treatment manual was refined based on initial work (Tolin, Frost, & Steketee, 2007a) and a waitlist-controlled research evaluation (Steketee, Frost, Tolin, Rasmussen, & Brown, 2010), resulting in the current CBT manual by Steketee & Frost (2014).

In the initial open trial by Tolin and colleagues (2007a), 10 women who met criteria for HD were treated with 26 sessions of individual CBT delivered over six to nine months, with home visits spaced approximately monthly. Overall hoarding severity, difficulty discarding, and acquisition reduced by 25% to 37%, and clutter improved 31%. Using a modified treatment manual, the controlled trial (Steketee et al., 2010) found that 12 weeks of individual CBT for HD (n = 23) was much more successful than 12 weeks of waitlist (n = 23). CBT produced significantly more reduction in hoarding symptoms (15% to 27% vs. 2% to 11% for waitlisted participants). Among 37 clients who completed 26 sessions of CBT over a period of 9 to 12 months, the reductions in hoarding symptoms ranged from 27% to 39%.

Approximately 75% of participants were rated "much" or "very much" improved (71% for therapist ratings and 81% for self-ratings). Only 10% of participants discontinued treatment. A follow-up study of 31 of the 37 completers (Muroff, Steketee, Frost, & Tolin, 2014) indicated that nearly all had maintained their gains up to 12 months after CBT. The rates of those showing much or very much improved were generally stable at approximately 70% (62% for clinician ratings and 79% for self-ratings). Higher initial hoarding severity, perfectionism, social anxiety, and male gender were associated with worse outcome, but only greater perfectionism and male gender were significant when initial hoarding severity was controlled.

Group CBT (GCBT) offers a potentially more cost-effective therapy option that may also reduce social isolation and improve motivation for some clients with HD. The first group treatment yielded modest benefits for six participating clients (Steketee, Frost, Wincze, Green, & Douglass, 2000), most of whom were men with primary hoarding problems and comorbid major depression and/or social phobia. This group had 10 weekly two-hour sessions followed by five twice monthly sessions plus in-home clinician visits between group sessions. Modest benefits were evident for acquisition and problematic beliefs, while clutter improved slightly. Three participants who received additional sessions improved 28% on their HD symptoms after one year.

Muroff and colleagues (2009) tested group CBT for a larger sample of 32 mainly white middle-aged women with HD as a primary problem; 75% also reported comorbid depression. Groups of 5-8five to eight people met for 16 two-hour weekly sessions, with one group meeting for 20 weeks. The social work and psychology coleaders also provided two home visits. GCBT led to a 14% reduction in HD symptoms and modest benefits for depression and social isolation for the 27 completers after five people dropped out of the study.

This feasibility study was followed by another GCBT evaluation that omitted home-based sessions in order to test group treatment suitable for community mental health settings (Gilliam et al., 2011). Five therapy groups averaging nine members met for 90 minutes for 16 or 20 sessions. Among the mainly white middle-aged women who participated, one third discontinued treatment, leaving 30 who completed GCBT. Clinically significant improvement in HD symptoms occurred for 31% of these clients, who also improved on anxiety, depression, and quality-of-life measures.

Muroff, Steketee, Bratiotis, and Ross (2012) compared GCBT to a control condition in which participants read *Buried in Treasures* (Tolin, Frost, & Steketee, 2007b), a self-help book based on the CBT model. The 38 mainly white women clients were assigned randomly to GCBT with extra home assistance (n = 11), GCBT with limited home assistance (n = 14), or individual bibliotherapy with no clinical assistance (n = 13). All groups met for 20 weekly sessions plus four 90-minute clinician home visits. Only one person dropped out. Improvement rates after treatment were 30% for GCBT with extra home visits, 23% for standard GCBT, and 9% for bibliotherapy. Both group methods were significantly better than reading the self-help book but did not differ from each other. Additional home visits improved clutter a little more (34%–35%) than did standard treatment (24%–30%), and these outcomes were similar to those achieved by individual treatment. In summary, 20 sessions of group CBT for hoarding are effective for HD, and in-home assistance might provide additional benefit.

A meta-analysis examined the comparative benefits of various forms of CBT for HD on hoarding symptoms and on functional impairment as well as potential moderators of treatment response (Tolin, Frost, Steketee, & Muroff, 2015). Findings from 12 studies with a total sample of 232 people indicated a large effect of CBT on HD symptom severity. The strongest effects occurred for difficulty discarding, followed by clutter and acquiring. Functional impairment improved moderately. Most studies reported reliable changes on HD symptoms, but the rates of clinically significant change were lower, ranging from 24% to 43%, indicating that after treatment most clients' scores were closer to the clinical range than to the normal range for hoarding symptoms. Factors associated with better clinical outcomes were being female, younger, receiving more CBT sessions, and more home visits. These treatment studies suggest that CBT developed specifically for HD is promising but there is room for improvement.

HOARDING DISORDER THERAPY COMPONENTS AND IMPLEMENTATION

Manualized CBT for hoarding problems includes elements based on Frost and Hartl's model of HD. During assessment and case formulation therapists help clients build their own individual model to understand their behavior. Motivational enhancement strategies that include goal setting and treatment planning are used throughout treatment whenever clients seem reluctant or ambivalent. Hoarding-specific therapy elements include organizing, problem-solving, and decision-making skills training; practice not acquiring and discarding; and modifying beliefs about possessions. These components often are intermingled so that skills are learned and beliefs are examined during nonacquisition and discarding practice sessions. In the sections to follow we give descriptions of these components and ways to flex them to fit clients' symptoms and immediate needs.

FLEXIBILITY OF THE ESSENTIAL THERAPY COMPONENTS

As noted, people who hoard often experience co-occurring mental and physical health conditions, psychosocial problems, and fluctuating levels of insight that complicate their hoarding disorder. This necessitates a flexible approach to treatment from the outset, because no standard method offers effective treatment for the range of people who experience HD. To plan a successful intervention, it is helpful to consider mental health comorbidities, to match early phases of treatment to clients' insight and values, to order the components of treatment to the symptoms, and to manage challenges as they arise during therapy.

Early treatment phases: The complex features of HD require flexible delivery of treatment components. Flexibility begins at the outset of the clinical relationship, with a shared understanding of the client's view of their hoarding problem and an initial conceptualization of the situation. This determines where treatment begins, both within the client's living space *and* in the intervention sequence. Readiness for change varies considerably from person to person, so providing therapy with flexibility, and with creativity, is a must. Steketee and Frost's (2014) manual, *Treatment for Hoarding Disorder*, presents a modular approach that accommodates shifting client needs and reprioritization of clinical focus based on factors such as inconsistent motivation and the immediate need to clear living space due to an impending housing inspection. The manual supports clinical practice by helping therapists meet clients wherever they are in their HD experience.

Responding to clients' needs: Careful consideration of unique client needs and soliciting input throughout the assessment and case formulation process is essential to establishing the client-clinician relationship at the core of this treatment. Some clients may hold presumptions about the therapist's role as an expert. We recommend a conversation to reiterate the collaborative nature of treatment, emphasizing that consistent input from *both* therapist and client is welcomed and expected. A flexible strategy is appropriate based on the readiness of the client to begin work and in consideration of existing comorbidities and complex life circumstances. For example, a client who is highly motivated to engage in the work might benefit from "diving in" to practical exercises that pinpoint their challenges related to sorting, discarding, and resisting acquiring (Steketee & Frost, 2014, p. 94). However, clients who express ambivalence may require a slower introduction. Allocating time to help clients identify treatment strategies that fit their specific clutter challenges is an important step in the therapeutic process.

Order of components: Flexibility is inherent in CBT for HD, so that modules for working on organizing skills, as well as beliefs about hoarding, acquisition, and discarding may be reordered as needed. For example, clients who experience problems with acquiring items may benefit from front-loading treatment with non-acquisition-related treatment, including education, discussion of acquisition-related values and goals, and practice exercises to curb additional clutter. For clients whose acquisition is quite limited, that module can be shifted to the latter part of treatment. In the same vein, those who have great difficulty figuring out how to organize objects may need to concentrate on this work early in the program. Clinicians and clients work together to decide the order and modify it as needed.

Dealing with complications: The HD clinical population includes people with major depressive disorder (MDD, more than 50%) and anxiety disorders, most commonly social phobia (about 30%), generalized anxiety disorder (GAD, about 30%), and to a lesser extent obsessive compulsive disorder (OCD, 17%; Frost, Steketee, & Tolin, 2011). Additionally, among hoarding participants in research studies, attention deficit problems occurred in nearly 30% and hyperactivity was evident in over 15% (Frost et al., 2011; see also Sheppard et al., 2010). Research suggests that PTSD is diagnosed less often (about 6%), yet it presents a challenging barrier to intervention when hoarding behavior is directly linked to the traumatic event (Bratiotis, Schmalisch, & Steketee, 2011; Frost et al., 2011).

Some clients with hoarding may suffer from psychotic conditions or dementia, though this appears to be rare among hoarding clients who receive mental health services, including older adults. Some clients present with personality disorders (PD) or personality features such as dependent, obsessive compulsive (OCPD) and paranoid personalities that can complicate the relationship with the therapist. Perfectionism and rigidity sometimes occur in the context of OCPD and can slow the intervention process (Bratiotis et al., 2011), leading clinicians to be flexible in the timing of applying the modules as they help clients focus on their goals. For example, when clients resist a decision to discard an item because it is somehow incomplete (missing a part; not clean enough), clinicians can include cognitive strategies to help clients reflect on their previously stated values and goals for the future and inquire whether completeness helps advance those goals. How might they be able to tolerate the discomfort they feel when something does not feel complete?

Physical health problems including obesity and chronic medical concerns are also a significant factor for those who hoard. In a study that examined the health status of people with hoarding behavior, 63.6% met diagnostic criteria for at least one chronic or severe condition, including hypertension, arthritis, high cholesterol, arthritis, lung problems (asthma and emphysema), autoimmune disorders, and stomach or bladder troubles (Tolin, Frost, Steketee, Gray, & Fitch, 2008). These impairments and related discomforts can impair sustained attention, focused decision-making, and the physical effort needed for clients to engage in the process of decluttering. Flexible accommodations to these problems can take various forms, such as assistance with hauling items for those who cannot lift or move heavy things, prioritizing the organizing of paperwork to resolve late bill payments for clients with financial management challenges, or initiating landlord communication to extend housing for clients in danger of eviction. Mental health comorbidities might require clinicians to help clients design activity schedules to alleviate their depressive symptoms and improve motivation to work on clutter. Introducing the perfectionism continuum, a cognitive therapy strategy, can help identify the advantages of being less perfectionistic in order to reduce anxiety (Steketee & Frost, 2014, p. 177). These actionable steps integrate flexibility into the treatment approach to HD.

STANDARD ASSESSMENT METHODS AND BRIEF ALTERNATIVES

Observing clutter: Gaining an understanding of HD requires careful assessment at the outset of treatment that includes direct observation of clutter severity. This is accomplished by one or more meetings at the therapist's office and ideally one or more visits to the client's home. An in-office meeting provides uninterrupted and comfortable space in which clients may be less distracted by the clutter that surrounds them at home and less anxious without a visitor in their home. If a home visit is feasible, therapists benefit from personally experiencing the living space where the physical clutter exists. A flexible timeline and approach to assessing clutter may be required if the client's circumstances are particularly complex and/or their level of ambivalence is high. Direct home observation can be particularly challenging given the stigma surrounding hoarding disorder, the shame that often accompanies it, and the social isolation clients experience due to not having visitors in their home for long periods. In such situations, a home visit can be replaced by a request for photos of each room. Alternatively, a virtual visit to the home via web technology can be used as noted further on in this chapter.

In a similar vein, it is not unusual for clinicians to modify treatment plans as the clinical conceptualization becomes clearer and alternative strategies seem useful. Clients who are homebound due to health problems and/or unable to travel to meet in-person require modified treatment planning to exchange in-office visits for at-home or online sessions. Client and therapist comfort with technology will require time to adapt when using virtual platforms for sessions. A therapist may be called upon to step outside their clinical role to help clients secure Internet access or training to facilitate online meetings.

Measuring hoarding symptoms and severity: As described in Steketee and Frost's CBT manual for hoarding, an initial step toward the comprehensive understanding of a client's hoarding problem is to conduct a Hoarding Interview (see Appendix in Steketee & Frost, 2014) that includes questions about the client's symptoms of hoarding, their degree of impairment, safety concerns, and their general life situation. The interview questions can be asked in any sequence that seems to fit the circumstances in order to create an idiographic conceptual model of the client's hoarding symptoms. The interview can be conducted in the office, at home, or remotely online. Although the ideal option is an in-home visit, the essential goal is for clinicians to understand the client's rationale for acquiring and keeping items, and how objects are organized and stored. When in-home or virtual visits are not feasible, photos can substitute for direct observation and help foster questions to build the client's model.

Standardized assessments help determine the type, volume, and hazards of clutter in clients' homes. Clinicians can select the measures that seem most useful for each client and will help measure progress during treatment. The self- and assessor-rated Hoarding Rating Scale (HRS; Tolin, Frost, & Steketee, 2010) contains five questions about the defining features of hoarding, including clutter, difficulty discarding, acquisition, distress, and interference; it identifies clinically significant hoarding. The self-rated Saving Inventory–Revised (SI-R; Frost, Steketee, & Grisham, 2004) measures the severity of acquisition (compulsive buying and acquiring free items), clutter volume and associated problems, and difficulty discarding.

The Clutter Image Rating (CIR; Frost, Steketee, Tolin, & Renaud, 2008) contains a series of nine photos of a living room, a kitchen, and a bedroom showing progressively greater levels of clutter. Clients and clinicians, as well as family members or service providers who have visited the home choose the photo that best mirrors the volume of the clutter in each room. Because clutter diminishes more slowly than the acquisition and difficulty discarding that are assessed on the HRS and SI-R, clinicians should remind clients to take heart from their progress on specific areas they have worked on rather than focusing on the amount of clutter in the home as a whole; rooms often look worse before they look better as progress is made.

Two additional standardized questionnaires can be completed at home, in the clinician's office, or online. The Saving Cognitions Inventory (SCI; Steketee,

Frost, & Kyrios, 2003) assesses clients' beliefs and attitudes when discarding, including their emotional attachment to objects, beliefs about items as memory aids, responsibility to avoid wasting objects, and the need to control belongings. Activities of Daily Living for Hoarding (ADL-H; Frost, Hristova, Steketee, & Tolin, 2013) investigates the level of interference caused by clutter for clients' ability to complete ordinary activities such as meal preparation, bathing, and dressing. These two tools are helpful in guiding treatment toward thoughts and beliefs of special significance, as well as problems with ordinary activities that may be special motivators for clients. Overall, these several assessment instruments support the therapist's working case conceptualization and guide the development of a client-centric treatment plan.

CASE FORMULATION AND TREATMENT PLANNING

Essential treatment guide: Providing clients with the manual's general description titled, "What is hoarding?" is a helpful first step in ensuring clients' understanding of HD, including what hoarding is and isn't, as well as the role of information processing problems in thinking about possessions. After clients complete their assessments, the therapist shares a summary of the findings, which is used to develop an individualized hoarding model and to plan treatment.

Client observation and developing a personal hoarding model: Constructing a model of the hoarding problem is a helpful way to encourage collaboration between the client and the therapist, who uses open-ended questions and objective statements to convey and verify observations. Building upon findings from the hoarding interview, clinicians flesh out each client's personal hoarding model as depicted in Figure 7.1. This includes the personal and family vulnerabilities (comorbid problems, adverse life events), information processing problems (attention, perception, memory), meaning/value of possessions (uniqueness, avoidance of waste, comfort/safety, etc.), positive and negative emotional reactions, learning processes through positive and negative reinforcement, and effects on hoarding behaviors. Responses to these questions help clients work collaboratively with their clinicians to understand their hoarding behavior by building a historical and current model of how they think, feel, and behave toward objects in their lives. Building the model deepens their understanding of what contributes to their hoarding behavior and opens pathways to changing behavior.

Clinicians are best when they are flexible in reformulating the hoarding model and subsequent treatment plans when unexpected events arise for clients. Examples include health problems that limit mobility, current major depression, housing status that is threatened by home safety concerns, and ambivalence about reducing clutter that necessitates the reconsideration of treatment timing. Changing course to respond to disruption fits within the manualized approach to HD and requires initiative and timely problem solving by both therapist and client to maintain progress.

Imagining a difference: To better understand motivation for treatment, visualization exercises encourage clients to imagine their home in both a cluttered and uncluttered state while capturing their discomfort and other emotional responses and their thoughts about the space in both conditions. Therapists can flex this approach by using photos of the home to help clients who have difficulty articulating their reactions, and by asking a client to describe their ideal home layout and décor. Clients who have difficulty maintaining motivation to resist acquiring objects and remove clutter can benefit from viewing "before" pictures of their home as a visual reminder of progress during treatment. Spending additional time to explain treatment steps and how they connect to the hoarding model may help increase client confidence, improve readiness for change, and establish a clear vision of steps ahead.

ENHANCING MOTIVATION

Family versus personal goals: Many people with HD live alone (Samuels et al., 2008), whereas others live with or are closely connected to family and friends. Depending on the role of family and friends, clinicians will need to be flexible in determining how the client's personal treatment goals are influenced by the interpersonal dynamics. For example, some clients' depression and defensiveness stem from prolonged conflicts with family members that have reduced their motivation to resolve the problem. One client shared a painful consequence of her hoarding, saying, "I'm not allowed to see my grandkids because my son thinks my home is unhealthy and I'm too lazy to clean up after myself." In such a case, the therapist can suggest that being able to spend time with grandchildren be included among her treatment goals.

In some cases, challenging family dynamics necessitate that therapists devote treatment time to examining how these shape clients' ability to make progress in reducing clutter. Less commonly, family and friends with whom clients have generally good relationships can serve as personal motivators and helping hands for resisting acquisition, skill-building, and removing clutter the client discards during treatment. Thus, just as adversarial relationships must be acknowledged, the presence of positive influencers can shape treatment goals and how treatment components are delivered. Above all, it is critical that therapists empower and encourage clients to create *their* own personal goals.

External pressure: Motivation to address a hoarding problem can be influenced by factors outside of self or immediate family, including internalized stigma about hoarding, pressure from the housing authority, health department, and/or protective services when vulnerable children or older adults live in the home. In cases where community service organizations are involved, clinicians will want to keep client motivation at the forefront of their work in order to meet mandated deadlines to meet mandated requirements. For example, when a homeowner or renter is in violation of housing codes, external pressure from authorities—including the local fire department, board of health, or building inspectors—will require immediate improvements in order show a good faith effort to address the problem and to comply with relevant codes (Bratiotis et al., 2011). Preserving housing and proving that the home is a safe place for their children are important motivators for reducing clutter and learning to maintain a safe and sanitary home environment.

Matching motivational strategies to therapist style: Motivational interviewing (MI) theory (Miller & Rollnick, 2013) provides a helpful context to examine low client motivation. Therapists ask a series of questions and summarize clients' statements to help them clarify the pros and cons of change, develop confidence in their ability to change, and increase the discrepancy between the disadvantages and advantages of proceeding with treatment. They do this while avoiding any effort to convince clients that they "should" change their hoarding behavior. Open-ended questions, reflective listening, and affirming language reflects support and respect for the client. At the same time, therapists using MI methods need to be aware of their own therapeutic style to develop their ability to be authentically nonjudgmental, affirming, reflective, respectfully curious, and clear communicators. These traits will inevitably support effective treatment delivery.

Goal reminders: The use of MI offers a flexible client experience by assuming that motivation and commitment to change can be enhanced and that clients must articulate their *own* reasons for change (Miller & Rollnick, 2013, pp. 72–73). This depends on therapists' commitment to maintaining a working partnership with clients, focusing on clients' ambivalence, asking evocative questions to discover motivations to change, eliciting clients' talk about change, and developing action plans to bring about the change (Miller & Rollnick, p. 73). As one client shared, "After a lifetime of others walking all over my decisions, I feel like I'm finally in control of my future and can get to work on my home to make it the way *I* want it to be."

Practice success enhances motivation: Motivation grows through the successful application of new skills and knowledge related to hoarding. To encourage a consistent practice routine, the therapist may encourage the client to:

1. Schedule specific work times
2. Link homework time to other routine activities that serve as reminders
3. Ask someone to be present at home or in acquisition settings during practice
4. Play pleasant music during homework sessions
5. Find ways to interrupt self-defeating thoughts, and
6. Monitor homework completion (time spent, where and when).

Additional options include a brief phone call between therapist and client to check in before and after homework as a reminder to continue practice between sessions. When clients seem reluctant, additional flexibility is available from a range of methods to boost motivation. This includes emphasizing client self-determination, asking for their wisdom about how to proceed, asking clients about previously stated goals, and exploring the pros and cons of hoarding to acknowledge both positive and negative aspects of the problem (Steketee & Frost, 2014).

Supporting and sustaining motivation: Based on our experiences, maintaining motivation throughout CBT for HD demands more consistent effort than for many clinical problems. This requires the clinician to recognize the need to shift focus from applying CBT strategies to using MI whenever ambivalence is evident in verbal or behavioral actions. At such times, therapists can dedicate a portion of a clinical session to MI to elucidate the client's ambivalence about proceeding with therapy methods and to revisit their confidence that change is beneficial and possible through their own efforts. This interruption of CBT to focus on motivation helps reignite clients' efforts to implement CBT strategies. When clients express concern that they are being "difficult," clinicians can reiterate how hard it is to combat a lifelong problem and can normalize the client's ambivalence and pattern of "two steps forward, one step back," which often characterizes progress in treating HD. *Motivational Interviewing and CBT: Combining Strategies for Maximum Effectiveness* (Naar & Safren, 2017) is a useful resource for clinicians to understand how integration of MI and CBT can improve treatment outcomes rather than applying each approach independently.

REDUCING ACQUISITION

Easy gains or not? Some clients are reluctant to acknowledge or are simply unaware that their acquisition habits have played a significant role in cluttering their homes. "I just loved to collect sports memorabilia," explained one person, "but when I was tripping over a pile of baseball cards that I had paid good money for, I finally looked up and really saw the mess I was in. I needed to do something." For others, acquiring is less of a challenge, enabling the client to reduce acquiring quickly so sorting, organizing, and discarding work can begin concurrently (Steketee & Frost, 2014, p. 108). When a client's acquisition behavior continues to add to their clutter and disorganization, the treatment plan flexes to focus first on acquisition in order to stem the incoming tide of objects and facilitate learning of organizing and discarding skills.

Use of acquiring questions to change attitudes: Excessive acquiring, the inability to suppress ongoing urges to do so, and the positive emotions stemming from buying or finding new items reinforce problems with acquisition. Clients benefit from learning to tolerate and resist urges to acquire via several flexible approaches that include:

1. Identifying activities (e.g., cooking, watching a film) to replace the pleasure of acquisition and to alleviate distress,
2. Choosing questions that work for clients' specific acquiring situations, such as asking about the benefits of buying new clothes when the wardrobe is large or searching for model train parts when there is no place to put them,
3. Examining the client's "need" versus "want" for an item, followed by questions to evaluate the desire to acquire (Steketee & Frost, 2014, p. 121).

Practice hierarchies: Not acquiring is reinforced through a hierarchical approach in which clients practice easier tasks and progress to more difficult ones (Steketee & Frost, 2014). The acquiring situations are ranked based on client discomfort. For example, reading an advertisement for a favorite store is likely to elicit less discomfort (= 10 out of 100) than seeing a final sale item in that store (= 90 out of 100). Developing a list of acquiring scenarios with the client can be used to plan real-time acquisition practice with gradual increases in discomfort. For example, if a client experiences strong urges to buy and great discomfort in a particular store, the clinician may plan to accompany the client on an experiential shopping trip to that location. The trip may begin with driving past the store, followed by the client entering and browsing around the store without making a purchase. Exposure to gradual increases in discomfort during this practice shopping trip will help clients to decide what triggers they can tolerate while resisting the urge to acquire. Practicing nonacquisition requires clients to identify locations, types of goods, and related variables that trigger acquiring, allowing a flexible approach that targets clients' specific vulnerabilities to acquisition.

Practicing behavioral change: As clients practice acquiring fewer items, they benefit from establishing personal rules for their own acquisition. For example, the rules may require that the client (1) does not own a similar item already, (2) pays cash (not credit), and (3) has space to store the item without compromising progress in decluttering. For instance, a client might decide that "If I can't think of a specific place to put it or how to use it, I don't need it." Rules and modifications can be suggested by clinicians as items in the client's living space are cleared and organized, but only clients should make the decisions. Clinicians can accompany clients for nonshopping trips to help them use coping skills taught during therapy (e.g., questions for acquiring, advantages/disadvantages of acquiring) in settings that provide current challenges (Steketee & Frost, 2014, p. 114).

Because the discomfort experienced by clients during acquiring exposures varies, therapists are best when they are flexible in suiting the circumstances by first identifying faulty thinking that reinforces acquisition behavior. After identifying automatic thoughts, the therapist can:

1. Apply Socratic questioning to examine the meaning and evidence for the need to acquire,
2. Use the Downward Arrow cognitive technique to clarify thoughts and beliefs,
3. Discuss alternative thoughts,
4. Estimate the probability of benefits gained from acquiring the item, and/or
5. Determine the importance of the item by examining the degree of need versus want.

For example, one client who wanted to purchase a consignment shop item said, "I've *never* seen vintage earrings like these before . . . they match my eye color and they're on sale! If I miss out on this, I'll regret it *forever.*" Given the catastrophic thinking about lifelong regret, the clinician began by examining and testing the client's faulty thinking, beginning with an estimation of the probability of her feared outcome. Clients with acquisition problems will require repeated exposures before integrating work on organizing, sorting, and discarding.

SKILLS TRAINING

Organizing: Guiding clients while upholding their goals and priorities: An essential part of HD treatment is teaching the skills necessary for clients to reduce clutter, maintain space, and manage hoarding vulnerabilities. Skills training should be guided by clients' wishes. Clinicians can begin the conversation about organizational goals based on the case formulation that identified skills gaps that contribute to hoarding. Collaborating on a list of goals and relevant skill-building opportunities requires a thoughtful approach that suits the client's needs. For example, clients who struggle to make discarding decisions, picking up items and putting them down somewhere else, are likely to benefit from putting the "OHIO" rule (Only Handle It Once—no more than twice) on their list of treatment goals. Other possibilities include creating categories for "keep" items, deciding on a discarding plan for unwanted things, and learning to problem solve situational challenges, such as feeling overwhelmed.

Categorizing unwanted and wanted items: It's not unusual for clients to create too many categories while sorting (Wincze, Steketee, & Frost, 2007) and to voice uncertainty about when or where to put belongings. Creating categories for *unwanted* items first can help clients make early progress in clutter reduction. Here are points of flexibility to consider:

1. Difficulty categorizing—Ask where (what room) the item would be easy to find and store (closet, drawer, shelf);
2. Working at the therapist's office—Bring a bag of randomly selected items from home to practice sorting in order to mirror an at-home experience;
3. Nonhousehold items—Suggest a specialty retail website (i.e., cookware, collectibles) for inspiring categorizing ideas. Several retailers specializing in organizing also post online tips for categorizing.

Sorting and removing unwanted and wanted items: "Pick the low hanging fruit" is good advice for clients to gain momentum at the beginning of the sorting process as removing unwanted items creates space and confidence. When clients are concerned about wastefulness, planning to recycle items may increase their willingness to let go. Collaborative efforts to identify donation sites, coordinate trash disposal, and select items to sell can be helpful. For wanted items, therapists may need to be flexible in their approach by (1) rolling up their sleeves to actively haul, lift, and move things; (2) using cognitive strategies to help clients who fear making wrong choices; and (3) reminding clients (and family members) that spaces often look worse initially (for a brief time) as items are temporarily shuffled until permanent storage solutions are found. Additional guidance is available in *Treatment for Hoarding Disorder* (Steketee & Frost, 2014).

Problem solving—When? How? Problem solving is a difficult skill for many HD clients to learn, and also a pivotal one. Common problem types that arise for clients include reluctance to begin sorting, running out of time to complete tasks, and being unsure of where to move items because space is lacking. Problem-solving steps often are presented at the outset of treatment because they are so commonly needed during the treatment process (Steketee & Frost, 2014, p. 127). Opportunities to flex the problem-solving approach include:

1. Planning a check-in via e-mail or phone after completing a challenging part of treatment,
2. Generating as many solutions to a problem as possible using creative thinking without judging whether the ideas are feasible or practical,
3. Anticipating motivational and practical problems and deciding on a response,
4. Encouraging the client to write down successful solutions for future use when similar challenges arise.

Working with attentional problems: Sustaining attention on repetitive chores such as organizing and sorting is difficult or impossible for many HD clients (Hartl, Duffany, Allen, Steketee, & Frost, 2005). Therapists who are unfamiliar with ADHD are advised to seek additional information to assist clients with these symptoms—one comprehensive source of information is *Mastering Your Adult ADHD* (Safren, Sprich, Otto, & Perlman, 2005). Strategies to encourage focused attention include:

1. Measuring attention span while gradually increasing practice time so clients can understand and extend their working capacity;
2. Creating structure in clients' lives by utilizing calendars, task lists, and routines;
3. Asking clients to create a priority list, choose a goal at the beginning of each session, and practice breaking down the goal or project into manageable steps.

We suggest that therapists be mindful of distractions posed by clients, such as extended storytelling about an item or focusing on negative emotions about other problems (Steketee & Frost, 2014, pp. 130–131). Taking steps to limit the visual field while sorting helps focus attention on one designated area at a time. Some clients engage in small distracting tasks because of their attention difficulties and/or to avoid discomfort during decluttering. Therapists can anticipate these potential interruptions and engage clients in problem solving to avoid these problems.

Maintaining new systems: As clients practice new skills and gain confidence, they must develop new routines to maintain their gains and prevent the re-emergence of clutter. A former client shared her advice: "I post my new rules above my kitchen sink so that I'm reminded about what I need to do to keep my home in good shape." Such a list might include putting away new items immediately, returning items to their original location right after use, and doing dishes/mail sorting at an appointed time each day. Therapists might focus on more challenging areas for clients and spend additional time problem solving to generate workable solutions. We recommend dedicating two or more sessions to skill-building, understanding that not every skill-building method will be needed by all clients. We suggest working on the skills that are most productive for clients while letting others go if they seem less useful.

PRACTICING DECISION-MAKING—WHAT TO KEEP AND WHAT TO DISCARD

Behavioral experiments and longer practice sessions: Decision-making is a central and required component of HD treatment, given that discarding decisions are essential to reducing clutter. Engaging in behavioral experiments (BEs) is helpful to clients who experience a high level of discomfort and believe a dire outcome will result if they discard an item. Therapists can apply BEs when they believe their client would benefit from testing their thinking to change HD beliefs and behavior patterns. We suggest imagining discarding before actually doing it when clients fear harmful outcomes. This approach also may be useful for clients who have unrealistic fears about losing possessions, information, or needing to keep objects in sight (Steketee & Frost, 2014).

   Managing strong emotions when discomfort habituates slowly: Clients' discomfort (anxiety, guilt, sadness) about discarding lessens with practice. Therapists can take the opportunity to remind clients that some discomfort is part of making progress and that sometimes they will progress faster and other times more slowly. If discomfort persists, therapists can dedicate more time to decision-making exercises, repeating practice exposures, incorporating additional MI methods, and emphasizing client progress for encouragement. The extension of practice time helps clients habituate to decluttering, better tolerate discomfort, and learn skills to navigate the process.

   Firm or fluid approach? Throughout HD treatment, therapists are called upon to help clients identify and pursue their goals. Choosing between a firm or fluid style is somewhat subjective, based upon the observations and experience of the therapist. We suggest that a firmer approach be taken when increased exposure to discomfort seems to support resilience and habituation, when an urgent safety issue or housing deadline must be addressed through decluttering, and when clients have not fully engaged in treatment (e.g., avoiding homework). In such cases, clinicians can emphasize parts of the treatment protocol while limiting or eliminating others. For example, for a client who seems overwhelmed by efforts to clear clutter, the therapist can spend more time discussing feelings and helping structure the tasks to increase clarity and simplicity. Therapists can also brainstorm ideas about a helper or coach who visits the home to provide a supportive and calming presence as the client works independently on sorting and discarding. Sometimes comorbidity that interferes with functioning (e.g., major depression) requires separate evaluation and a possible treatment detour from initial plans for HD symptoms.

Decision-making helpers? "Coaches aren't only for sports," a client recently reminded us as she shared her experiences while working with a clutter coach during HD treatment. As clients work with therapists for limited time periods, we've found it helpful to encourage those who will benefit from additional structure and motivation to work with a coach. These can include professional organizers and life coaches, as well as trusted family members or friends who are patient, calm, and consistent. We recommend that clinicians talk with their clients about the role of a coach, and if the client expresses interest, consider who might best serve in that role. Additional guidelines for coaches may be found in *Treatment for Hoarding Disorder* (Steketee & Frost, 2014, pp. 233–235).

CHANGING BELIEFS

Improving observations of internal processes: We have met many clients whose decision-making is limited by errors in their thinking. The inclination to use emotional reasoning rather than logic, to label self or others negatively, or to jump to conclusions about negative outcomes while lacking supportive facts are hallmarks of problematic thinking styles. Cognitive therapy (CT) strategies can help clients be more observant of their self-talk and underlying beliefs about acquiring, organizing, and discarding and evaluate the accuracy of those beliefs about the objects and themselves. Clients need time to learn and practice cognitive strategies. If decisions to discard after using CT methods remain slow, therapists can assess whether ambivalence is present and use motivational methods accordingly (Steketee & Frost, 2014, p. 160).

Thought-listing versus therapist-guided cognitive modifications: Thought Listing (TL) is a simple exercise aimed to help clients observe their attachment to possessions by documenting their initial distress if they were to discard it and then talk aloud or write down their thoughts. Clients aren't required to throw the item away, but if they do, they are asked to notice and record their distress over the next few minutes to better understand how they feel after discarding. TL increases exposure to the uncomfortable task of decision-making while avoiding pressure on clients who often "talk themselves into" discarding. When clients do decide to keep the item, they gain practice in sorting and organizing (Steketee & Frost, 2014, pp. 146–148).

Cognitive therapy strategies are designed to help clients assess the accuracy of their beliefs and promote rational alternatives that fit the facts (Steketee & Frost, 2014, p. 163). Clients are encouraged to take various perspectives on their hoarding problems during sorting and decision-making (Steketee & Frost, 2014, pp. 159–160). Because research suggests that clients generally make more decisions to discard items when asked to list their thoughts than when asked questions designed to modify their thinking, clinicians are advised not to use cognitive challenges prematurely when thought listing may suffice (Frost, Ong, Steketee, & Tolin, 2016). Therapists can decide whether to apply CT methods based on the client's response.

Melding cognitive strategies with skills training and practice sessions: Cognitive strategies can be selected to fit clients' needs as they are interwoven into skills training for decision-making and sorting/discarding practice. For example, a client who is reluctant to part with a stack of dated magazines and voices a plan to read them "later" may benefit from the "Valuing Time" exercise. This exercise asks the client to think about how they'd prefer to spend their time given their goals and values versus feeling obligated to attend to their belongings. Questions such as "Are there other parts of your life you'd be missing by reading all of these magazines?" may help the client consider how they are valuing their possessions and what they may be giving up (Steketee & Frost, 2014, p. 179).

Selecting cognitive strategies to fit therapist and client: Therapists are advised to become familiar with the range of CT methods to select those that seem most appropriate as clients verbalize their thoughts and beliefs during practice sessions. There is considerable flexibility in the CT approach and a range of options, depending on presenting symptoms and treatment objectives. For example, clients with strong emotional and/or somatic anxiety responses often benefit from completing a thought record (TR) to establish the connections between triggering events (discarding, acquiring) and their thoughts, emotions, and behaviors, followed by alterative ideas that strengthen their resilience. The Downward Arrow exercise helps clients clarify strong beliefs about objects as well as core beliefs that impede progress. Problems completing homework might benefit from discussion of the perfection continuum (when these problems stem from holding high performance standards) and/or metaphors and stories that enable clients to take another perspective on their goals and abilities (Steketee & Frost, 2014, pp. 163–179). A number of other CT interventions described in the manual may prove useful, and clinicians should select those that are well received by clients and effective in reducing their hoarding symptoms.

ARE CLEANOUTS EVER HELPFUL?

The delivery of CBT for HD rests on the assumption of systematic and flexible implementation of manualized treatment modules in a stepwise progression that accounts for client skill and tolerance. Clients should be full participants in the intervention process. In some instances, however, severe clutter and associated threats to the health and safety of the home, occupants, and nearby neighbors necessitate immediate intervention, supplanting the step-by-step approach to clutter reduction that typically accompanies skill development across the course of treatment.

Evaluations of the use of cleanouts is scant. In fact, this term often is used without precision to represent a range of interventions. The most common use refers to nonvoluntary immediate removal of most (if not all) possessions from the home, carried out with little to no involvement or control from the client. Such drastic cleanouts are presumed to result in recidivism because clients do not learn new skills, although this has not been adequately studied (see Steketee & Frost, 2014). Risk to vulnerable and protected populations (e.g., children, older adults) and/or the community typically necessitates legally mandated removal of clutter and correction of structural problems in the home (e.g., wiring, exit openings) assisted by community agencies such as fire departments, housing inspection, and protective services. Not surprisingly, forced cleanouts are usually experienced as traumatic events. When they are necessary due to mandated reporting for clinicians, clinical treatment must be altered, and sometimes halted temporarily, to accommodate the client's emotional and pragmatic needs.

On the other hand, a carefully planned intensive cleanout of the home can be a treatment goal for clients with heavily hoarded homes who are motivated to remove a large quantity of objects. These cleanouts, if supportive and well-executed, can be flexibly implemented, usually at middle to later stages of treatment. Clients appear to benefit most when they have learned the skills of decision-making, problem-solving, and organizing, and when they have practiced sorting and discarding sufficiently that they can meaningfully direct the intervention themselves. This means that clients can articulate rules for what types of items to keep, what types to discard, and where these should go. Therapist role, timing and duration, as well as involvement of family and/or friends are important considerations when planning a cleanout intervention that will take place over several days as part of the treatment program. Client characteristics such as age, ability, and financial resources, as well as home circumstances (e.g., logistics of object removal, local town or community assistance) inform clinical decisions.

FLEXIBILITY WITHIN FIDELITY FOR GROUP HOARDING DISORDER TREATMENTS

Meeting the needs of a dispersed population during a pandemic: In 2018, an online version of a *Buried in Treasures* support group was piloted, followed by two CBT treatment groups (Muroff & Otte, 2019). The decision to conduct these groups was initially inspired by requests from clients for a virtual experience, sometimes for convenience due to long commutes and sometimes to accommodate those with mobility and transportation challenges who could not otherwise join. After nearly two years of practice with online group facilitation, online assistance became the only option in early 2020 when the COVID-19 pandemic quarantine eliminated the possibility of in-person groups. This web-based clinical work is ongoing amidst research efforts dedicated to improving its efficacy. For such groups, we recommend a conversation between therapist and clients prior to the first virtual group meeting to review group expectations and norms, confirm that connectivity device and Internet service are functional, and to answer any questions. That is, although in-person office group sessions have some initial requirements (prescreening of client, need to arrive on time at a specified location), online sessions necessitate considerable pretreatment coordination and client guidance.

Flexing HD intervention to telehealth delivery: Clinicians are encouraged to take care to transfer the components of support groups and treatment groups to an online modality. For example, an online chat box substitutes for writing on a whiteboard during an in-person group. Whereas a quiet meeting space for an in-person group ensures a consistent atmosphere for all members, the atmosphere of virtual meetings depends on all group members finding a private space to login. Practicing nonacquisition during an experiential shopping trip shifts from a retail store to an online shopping excursion as clients share their screen with group participants to give a real-time view of items in their cart (Muroff & Otte, 2020). The considerable stress created by quarantine has further isolated some clients who are already physically and socially distanced. This can amplify comorbid conditions such as depression and anxiety, making intervention efforts more complex as time is needed to process difficult emotions.

As we have noted throughout this chapter, we hope that continued creative thinking and flexibility within the clinical community will enable us to deliver effective HD intervention to those who need it.

REFERENCES

American Psychiatric Association, DSM-5 Task Force. (2013). *Diagnostic and statistical manual of mental disorders: DSM-5™* (5th ed.). American Psychiatric Publishing, Inc. https://doi.org/10.1176/appi.books.9780890425596

Bratiotis, C., Schmalisch, C. S., Steketee, G. (2011). *The hoarding handbook: A guide for human service professionals.* Oxford University Press.

Frost R. O. & Hartl, T. L. (1996). A cognitive-behavioral model of compulsive hoarding. *Behaviour Research and Therapy, 34,* 341–350. https://doi.org/10.1016/0005-7967(95)00071-2

Frost, R. O., Hristova, V., Steketee, G., & Tolin, D. F. (2013). Activities of daily living scale in hoarding disorder. *Journal of Obsessive-Compulsive and Related Disorders, 2*(2), 85–90. https://doi.org/10.1016/j.jocrd.2012.12.004

Frost, R. O., Ong, C., Steketee, G., & Tolin, D. F. (2016). Behavioral and emotional consequences of thought listing versus cognitive restructuring during discarding decisions in hoarding disorder. *Behaviour Research and Therapy, 85,* 13–22. https://doi.org/10.1016/j.brat.2016.08.003

Frost, R. O., Rosenfield, E., Steketee, G., & Tolin, D. F. (2013). An examination of excessive acquisition in hoarding disorder. *Journal of Obsessive-Compulsive and Related Disorders, 2*(3), 338–345. https://doi.org/10.1016/j.jocrd.2013.06.001

Frost, R. O., Steketee, G., & Grisham, J. (2004) Measurement of compulsive hoarding: Saving inventory-revised. *Behaviour Research and Therapy, 42*(10), 1163–1182. https://doi.org/10.1016/j.brat.2003.07.006

Frost, R. O., Steketee, G., & Tolin, D. F. (2011). Comorbidity in hoarding disorder. *Depression and Anxiety, 28*(10), 876–884. https://doi.org/10.1002/da.20861

Frost, R. O., Steketee, G., Tolin, D. F., & Renaud, S. (2008). Development and validation of the clutter image rating. *Journal of Psychopathology and Behavioral Assessment, 30*(3), 193–203. https://doi.org/10.1007/s10862-007-9068-7

Frost, R. O., Steketee, G., Tolin, D. F., Sinopoli, N., & Ruby, D. (2015). Motives for acquiring and saving in hoarding disorder, OCD, and community controls. *Journal of Obsessive-Compulsive and Related Disorders, 4*, 54–59. https://doi.org/10.1016/j.jocrd.2014.12.006

Gilliam, C. M., Norberg, M. M., Villavicencio, A., Morrison, S., Hannan, S., & Tolin, D. F. (2011). Group cognitive-behavioral therapy for hoarding disorder: An open trial. *Behaviour Research and Therapy, 49*(11), 802–807. https://doi.org/10.1016/j.brat.2011.08.008

Hartl, T. L., Duffany, S. R., Allen, G. J., Steketee, G., & Frost, R. O. (2005). Relationships among compulsive hoarding, trauma, and attention-deficit hyperactivity disorder. *Behaviour Research and Therapy, 43*(2), 269–276. https://doi.org/10.1016/j.brat.2004.02.002

Hartl, T. L., & Frost, R. O. (1999). Cognitive-behavioral treatment of compulsive hoarding: A multiple baseline experimental case study. *Behaviour Research and Therapy, 37*(5), 451–461. https://doi.org/10.1016/S0005-7967(98)00130-2

Kendall, P. C., & Frank, H. E. (2018). Implementing evidence-based treatment protocols: Flexibility within fidelity. *Clinical Psychology: Science and Practice, 25*(4), 1–12. https://doi.org/10.1111/cpsp.12271

Miller, W. R., & Rollnick, S. (2013). *Motivational interviewing: Helping people change* (3rd ed.). Guilford Press.

Muroff, J., & Otte, S. (2019). Innovations in CBT treatment for hoarding: Transcending office walls. *Journal of Obsessive-Compulsive and Related Disorders, 23*, 100471. https://doi.org/10.1016/j.jocrd.2019.100471

Muroff, J., Steketee, G., Bratiotis, C., & Ross, A. (2012). Group cognitive and behavioral therapy and bibliotherapy for hoarding: A pilot trial. *Depression and Anxiety, 29*(7), 597–604. https://doi.org/10.1002/da.21923

Muroff, J., Steketee, G., Frost, R. O., & Tolin, D. F. (2014). Cognitive behavioral therapy for hoarding disorder: Follow-up findings and predictors of outcome. *Depression and Anxiety, 31*(12), 964–971. https://doi.org/10.1002/da.22222

Muroff, J., Steketee, G., Rasmussen, J., Gibson, A., Bratiotis, C., & Sorrentino, C. (2009). Group cognitive behavioral treatment for compulsive hoarding: A preliminary trial. *Depression and Anxiety, 26*(7), 634–640. https://doi.org/10.1002/da.20591

Naar, S., & Safren, S. A. (2017). *Motivational Interviewing and CBT: Combining strategies for maximum effectiveness*. Guilford Press.

Safren, S. A., Sprich, S., Otto, M. W., & Perlman, C. (2005). *Mastering your adult ADHD: A cognitive-behavioral treatment program therapist guide*. Oxford University Press. https://doi.org/10.1093/med:psych/9780195188196.001.0001

Samuels, J. F., Bienvenu, O. J., Grados, M. A., Cullen, B., Riddle, M. A., Liang, K.-Y., Eaton, W. W., & Nestadt, G. (2008). Prevalence and correlates of hoarding behavior in a community-based sample. *Behaviour Research and Therapy, 46*(7), 836–844. https://doi.org/10.1016/j.brat.2008.04.004

Sheppard, B., Chavira, D., Azzam, A., Grados, M. A., Umaña, P., Garrido, H., & Mathews, C. A. (2010). ADHD prevalence and association with hoarding behaviors in childhood-onset OCD. *Depression and Anxiety, 27*(7), 667–674. http://doi.org/10.1002/da.20691

Steketee, G., & Frost, R. O. (2003). Compulsive hoarding: Current status of the research. *Clinical Psychology Review, 23,* 905–927. https://doi.org/10.1016/j.cpr.2003.08.002

Steketee, G., & Frost, R. O. (2014). *Treatment for hoarding disorder: Therapist guide* (2nd ed.). Oxford University Press. https://doi.org/10.1093/med:psych/9780199334964.001.0001

Steketee, G., Frost, R. O., & Kyrios, M. (2003). Cognitive aspects of compulsive hoarding. *Cognitive Therapy and Research, 27*(4), 463–479. https://doi.org/10.1023/A:1025428631552

Steketee, G., Frost, R. O., Tolin, D. F., Rasmussen, J., & Brown, T. A. (2010). Waitlist-controlled trial of cognitive behavior therapy for hoarding disorder. *Depression and Anxiety, 27*(5), 476–484. https://doi.org/10.1002/da.20673

Steketee, G., Frost, R. O., Wincze, J., Greene, K. A. I., & Douglass, H. (2000). Group and individual treatment of compulsive hoarding: A pilot study. *Behavioural and Cognitive Psychotherapy, 28*(3), 259–268. https://doi.org/10.1017/S1352465800003064

Tolin, D. F., Frost, R. O., & Steketee, G. (2007a). An open trial of cognitive-behavioral therapy for compulsive hoarding. *Behaviour Research and Therapy, 45*(7), 1461–1470. https://doi.org/10.1016/j.brat.2007.01.001

Tolin, D. F., Frost, R. O., & Steketee, G. (2007b). *Buried in treasures: Help for compulsive hoarding.* Oxford University Press. https://doi.org/10.1093/med:psych/9780199329250.001.0001

Tolin, D. F., Frost, R. O., & Steketee, G. (2010). A brief interview for assessing compulsive hoarding: The Hoarding Rating Scale-Interview. *Psychiatry Research, 178*(1), 147–152. https://doi.org/10.1016/j.psychres.2009.05.001

Tolin, D. F., Frost, R. O., Steketee, G., Gray, K. D., & Fitch, K. E. (2008). The economic and social burden of compulsive hoarding. *Psychiatry* Research, *160*(2), 200–211. https://doi.org/10.1016/j.psychres.2007.08.008

Tolin, D. F., Frost, R. O., Steketee, G., & Muroff, J. (2015). Cognitive behavioral therapy for hoarding disorder: A meta-analysis. *Depression and Anxiety, 32*(3), 158–166. https://doi.org/10.1002/da.22327

Turner, K., Steketee, G., & Nauth, L. (2010). Treating elders with compulsive hoarding: A pilot program. *Cognitive and Behavioral Practice, 17*(4), 449–457. https://doi.org/10.1016/j.cbpra.2010.04.001

Wincze, J. P., Steketee, G., & Frost, R. O. (2007). Categorization in compulsive hoarding. *Behaviour Research and Therapy, 45*(1), 63–72. https://doi.org/10.1016/j.brat.2006.01.012

Woody, S. R., Kellman-McFarlane, K., & Welsted, A. (2014). Review of cognitive performance in hoarding disorder. *Clinical Psychology Review, 34*(4), 324–336. https://doi.org/10.1016/j.cpr.2014.04.002

8

Treatment of Chronic Pain

Importance of Flexibility and Fidelity

JOHN D. OTIS ■

INTRODUCTION

Chronic pain is one of the most frequent reasons that people seek medical care. Pain conditions affect at least 116 million U.S. adults at a cost of $560–$635 billion annually in direct medical treatment costs and lost productivity due to pain (Institute of Medicine, 2011; Gaskin & Richards, 2012). Common types of chronic pain conditions include low back pain, knee pain, headache, arthritis, multiple sclerosis, fibromyalgia, and shingles. Our understanding of the factors that contribute to the experience of chronic pain has meaningfully evolved over the past 30 years, and we are now aware of how biological, psychological, and social factors contribute to and impact the experience of pain. This understanding has helped to shape the development of interventions designed to help patients cope more effectively with pain. Cognitive behavioral therapy (CBT) is considered the "gold-standard" psychological treatment approach for chronic pain. CBT for chronic pain focuses on identifying and changing negative thoughts and behaviors that contribute to and maintain the experience of pain, as well as teaching ways of safely reintroducing enjoyable activities into patients' lives. The essential components of CBT for chronic pain include behavioral activation, psychoeducation on pain, relaxation training, challenging negative thinking, time-based activity scheduling, and sleep hygiene. All of these components are included to decrease patients' avoidance of activity and reintroduce a healthy, more active lifestyle (Otis, 2007a; 2007b). A substantial literature exists documenting the efficacy of CBT for a variety of chronic pain conditions including osteoarthritis, chronic back and neck pain (Linton & Ryberg, 2001), diabetic neuropathic pain (Otis et al., 2013), and tension headache (Holroyd et al., 2001). In a meta-analysis of 22 randomized controlled trials of psychological treatments for chronic low-back pain, cognitive-behavioral and self-regulatory treatments specifically were found to be efficacious (Hoffman, Papas, Chatkoff, & Kerns, 2007).

There are components of treatment for chronic pain that are "vital" or "core" components, and the delivery of each should be tailored to the needs of the patient. Other components are considered "optional" and chosen based on patient characteristics and other factors. In the following chapter, we first present the core components of CBT for pain, along with suggestions as to how these components might be flexibly tailored based on patient needs. Next, we review optional treatment components, as well as factors that should be considered when tailoring treatment to patients. Consistent with the call for "flexibility within fidelity" (Kendall & Beidas, 2007; Kendall & Frank, 2018), it is essential that manual-based treatments for pain be implemented flexibly, while also maintaining fidelity to the essential elements of treatment. Therapist flexibility has been found to increase patient-therapist rapport, patient engagement in the treatment process, and adherence to treatment recommendations.

ESSENTIAL COMPONENTS OF PAIN TREATMENT REQUIRED TO MAINTAIN FIDELITY

Behavioral Activation

Patients with chronic pain often report that the experience of pain has interfered with their ability to engage in regular daily functioning and other activities that they once found enjoyable. As a result, one of the first objectives when engaging a patient in CBT for pain is to work collaboratively with the patient to create a set of overall goals. Therapy goals are best when designed to decrease the patient's avoidance of activity and reintroduce a healthy and more active lifestyle, but they also should be flexibly tailored to each patient. Developing goals and working toward them in small steps from the very first session of therapy is important because successful goal completion demonstrates to the patient that change is possible, increases the patient's perceptions of self-efficacy, and communicates to the patient that CBT is an active treatment that will require participation. When developing behavioral treatment goals, tailoring the goals to the interests and physical abilities of each patient is a priority. For example, while some patients may choose goals that involve a high level of physical functioning such as walking, playing sports, or going to the gym, other patients may have physical disabilities that limit their ability to perform many activities. It also may be the case that a patient can identify an activity that they once found enjoyable; however, they are no longer able to perform the activity because of pain or other issues. In these cases, therapists work with the patient to select goals that are realistic and consistent with their abilities. These types of situations can be used as opportunities for the patient to consider alternative ways of engaging in enjoyable activities. For example, a patient may not be able to jog like they once could, but they could go for a walk around the block or perform yoga and stretches in order to keep in shape. Goals are best when behavioral and quantifiable rather than vague or general such as "experiencing less pain" or "having a better outlook on life." The wise therapist collaborates with the patient to develop goals in areas where the patient can reasonably expect change over the course of therapy. Goals do not have to focus on exercise; rather, goals can include performing valued activities such as working on a puzzle, reading, or spending more time with a partner. Goals should be flexible so that if a goal is achieved before the end of treatment it can be updated or replaced by another goal. Once overall therapy goals are created, the therapist can incorporate small goals at the end of each therapy session that help the patient take small steps toward achieving them. For example, if a patient has set an overall therapy goal of swimming five days a week by the end of the treatment program, they could begin by setting the goal of swimming once a week and gradually increasing the number of times swimming with each visit to the therapist.

Psychoeducation on Pain

The first session of CBT for pain includes education designed to inform the patient about our current understanding of pain. Providing education increases the patient's understanding and confidence in talking about pain, increases feelings of self-efficacy related to pain, and encourages patients to take a more active role in treatment. When speaking with a patient about their experience of chronic pain it is often helpful to discuss the "Cycle of Pain," which includes Pain, Distress, and Disability. This cycle can be drawn on a sheet of paper or presented on a computer screen if a therapist is conducting sessions by telehealth. A key point when presenting this cycle is to provide an opportunity for the patient to describe the specific types of thoughts they have experienced in response to pain, and the ways in which pain has interfered in their daily life. In this way, the explanation of the cycle of pain can be tailored to the experience of each patient, and can serve to validate the patient's experience of pain. The review provides a rationale for the patient as to why CBT will be specifically targeting thoughts and behaviors that are contributing to their experience of pain.

In addition to providing information on the cycle of pain, the early session provides education on the adaptive nature of pain, the various types of nerve fibers that transmit pain, and how the transmission of pain signals work in the body. Presenting the Gate Control Theory (Melzack & Wall, 1965) can be particularly useful because it describes the important role of psychological factors in the experience of pain. Therapists can vary the complexity of the biological information shared about pain transmission to the level of interest of each patient. For example, although a basic understanding of the pain theory may be sufficient for some patients, other patients with higher levels of interests in science, mechanics, engineering, and biology may request more information on the biological processes involved.

Relaxation Training

There are a number of reasons why relaxation training is often one of the first skills taught to patients with chronic pain. First, relaxation training is a tangible skill, which can often be easily learned, and the benefits of relaxation can be recognized by patients within a short period of time. This early success can provide a patient a greater sense of control over something that was previously believed to be beyond control, and thus can reinforce therapy participation. This is particularly important given that research has shown that beliefs about self-efficacy and control are associated with reductions in distress and disability (French, Holroyd, Pinell, Malinoski, O'Donnell, & Hill, 2000; Ahlstrand, Vaz, Falkmer, Thyberg, & Bjork, 2017), and can mediate the effects of CBT on chronic pain (Turner, Holtzman, & Mancl, 2007). Second, learning to relax can help the patient to notice and release stress and muscle tension that may be contributing to the experience of pain. Third, the practice of taking time to "slow the mind" and notice thoughts will pave the way for the practice and development of cognitive skills (i.e., cognitive restructuring, stress and anger management, sleep hygiene) in subsequent sessions of therapy. Relaxation can be taught in a number of ways, including Diaphragmatic Breathing, Progressive Muscle Relation (PMR), and Visual Imagery. Diaphragmatic Breathing is a core component in meditation, yoga, Tai Chi, and mindfulness-based practices that focuses on the breath and teaches people to clear the mind and release stress and tension in the body. Diaphragmatic breathing involves taking slow deep inhalations and exhalations by contracting the diaphragm, expanding the belly, and pulling air into the lungs. Studies have found that breathing practice can be an effective nonpharmacological intervention that can result in reduced anxiety (Brown & Gerberg, 2005) and workplace burnout (Salyers et al., 2011). Research data suggest that they also can have positive health effects including reductions in oxidative stress (Martarelli, Cocchioni, Scuri, & Pompei, 2011) and decreases in cortisol (Ma et al., 2017). Progressive Muscle Relaxation (PMR) is another technique that can be helpful for learning to notice and release muscle tension. PMR is a widely used relaxation strategy that can help people achieve a deep state of relaxation by alternating the tensing and relaxing of muscle groups. Studies have found that PMR can have many positive health effects including immunoenhancement (Pawlow & Jones, 2005) and significant decreases of stress in the workplace (Sundram, Dahlui, & Chinna, 2016). PMR is particularly helpful for patients who experience muscle tension that contributes to pain. Visual Imagery is a technique that helps the patient create a relaxing image that they can use to relax and reduce stress. Visual Imagery has been shown to be an effective treatment component for pain related to arthritis (Baird & Sands, 2004), fibromyalgia (Hadhazy, Ezzo, Creamer, & Berman, 2000), and other chronic pain conditions (Akerman & Turkoski, 2000). The visually relaxing image that the patient uses should be tailored to the patient by receiving input from the patient. For example, some patients might find the beach to be relaxing, whereas others might find imagining themselves camping outside under the stars to be relaxing. The particular images used do not matter, what matters is that the patient is taught how to use relaxing images to reduce stress. Although it does not matter which technique a patient prefers to use (breathing practice, visual imagery, or PMR), patients are given the opportunity to decide and therapists should praise all efforts to learn any of the strategies presented. Therapists may be tempted to reduce time spent teaching relaxation techniques if a patient seems initially resistant to learning (e.g., Patient: "I tried this and it doesn't work"), reports prior experience with one or more relaxation strategies (e.g., Patient: "Oh, I learned all about this with another therapist"), or if there are other seemingly "more important" targets for intervention identified in the assessment. Given the variability that can occur in the therapeutic setting, however, it is important to review and practice each of the strategies with the patient to ensure that the patient's training with the skill is consistent with evidence-based practices.

Challenging Negative Thinking

Cognitive skill training is a core component of all CBT programs, and given the relationship between thoughts and the experience of pain, it is particularly important when working with patients who have chronic pain. When teaching this skill, it is important to begin by providing the patient with education on the role of thoughts in the experience of emotions and pain. Patients are often well-aware of this connection and can give examples of when an increase in pain contributed to an increase in feelings of stress, anxiety, anger, or other emotions. Conversely, patients also will be able to give examples of when strong negative emotions contributed to an increase in their pain. This dialogue is important because it provides an opportunity for the therapist to validate the patient's connection between pain and emotions, and it also provides a rationale for learning to examine thoughts that are contributing to pain. Therapy begins with the patient being taught how to develop an awareness of categories of automatic thoughts called cognitive errors. One particular type of cognitive error called "catastrophizing," which may be thought of as an irrationally negative or exaggerated response to anticipated or actual pain, has long been considered a maladaptive coping strategy and has been proposed to be a key factor in the transition from acute to chronic pain (Niederstrasser, Slepian, Mankovsky-Arnold, Lariviere, Vlaeyen, & Sullivan, 2014; Vlaeyen & Linton, 2000). Research has found strong relationships between catastrophizing and outcomes including pain severity, pain interference, disability, depression, reduced social support, and increased suicidal ideation (Sullivan et al., 2001; Edwards, Bingham, Bathon, & Haythornthwaite, 2006; Edwards, Smith, Kudel, & Haythornthwaite, 2006). The relationship between pain catastrophizing and clinical outcomes also has been found in pediatric chronic pain samples (Miller, Meints, & Hirsh, 2018). For these reasons, it can be helpful to address the role of catastrophizing with the patient directly and to place greater emphasis on addressing these types of thoughts when conducting CBT for pain.

For patients with chronic pain, some particularly common automatic thoughts may include: "I'm going to be this way forever," "I'm worthless," or "I did this to myself." In CBT for pain, patients are taught to notice the connections among thoughts, feelings, behaviors, and pain. They are then taught to use cognitive restructuring to recognize automatic thoughts that give rise to negative emotions, to evaluate thoughts by gathering evidence for and against the thought, and then to replace negative thoughts with more adaptive thoughts that are based on the evidence. When attempting to teach patients to examine their own thoughts, it's important to keep in mind that many different types of patient-level issues can make it more challenging for patients to engage in cognitive tasks. For example, physical traumas that have resulted in concussions or traumatic brain injuries can make it difficult for patients to engage in higher-level cognitive processing. For patients with post-traumatic stress disorder (PTSD), the idea of closely examining one's thoughts may be particularly frightening and could result in avoidance of homework or a focus on trauma-related thoughts rather than pain. Further, there may be patients who are experiencing neurological deficits associated with a disease process, such as Alzheimer's disease, who may find it challenging to think about their thoughts, but who could still benefit from learning pain management skills. In these cases, therapists adapt the treatment approach by altering the manner in which the content is provided (e.g., create simplified forms and tailor them to the level of the patient) and focusing on ways to make learning more behavioral and concrete.

Time-Based Activity Scheduling

Time-based activity pacing is a behavioral strategy in which patients learn to balance being active with resting in order to accomplish daily activities without overdoing it and experiencing increased pain. Pacing is a key treatment component used by physical therapists when treating patients with chronic pain (Beissner et al., 2009; Wallman, Morton, Goodman, Grove, & Guilfoyle, 2004). Pacing is an important skill to learn because patients who have pain, but who are accustomed to leading an active life, tend to push themselves to get things done even when they are in pain. This can result in a pain flare-up afterward, which reduces function and productivity. Time-based activity pacing is a process in which physical activity breaks are based on time intervals, not on how much of the job is completed. For example, a patient is asked to identify a job that they frequently do that can result in increased pain. The patient is asked to estimate how long she can perform the job before her pain increases (active time) and how long she will need to rest before becoming active again (rest time). This active–rest schedule is then used when completing the entire project. Although different jobs will require different active–rest cycles, using a time-based activity pacing strategy will reduce time spent recovering from pain flare-ups due to overactivity and will actually result in a higher level of productive functioning.

In spite of the benefits of pacing, it can be challenging to implement for some active patients. Slogans such as "No pain–No gain" and "Pain is weakness leaving the body" have contributed to the perception that pacing oneself is somehow demonstrating a sign of physical weakness. For example, pacing can be difficult for U.S. military veterans who have been trained to continue with a task until it is completed, and who still identify with that way of approaching all activities. For these patients, it is often helpful to use examples that demonstrate how pacing can actually maximize performance in the long run, such as when runners are racing in a marathon or when athletes are playing a professional sport and need to last the entire game. Activity pacing can be challenging for individuals who are not accustomed to slowing down and taking breaks, as well as for those who tend to lose track of time while they are performing computer work that requires concentration. For these individuals, activity pacing can be introduced by setting the goal of having them take small breaks away from their computer at regular time intervals where they stretch and relax tense muscles. Other individuals may not like pacing and taking breaks because they would rather keep busy than provide an opportunity for their mind to wander to uncomfortable and unpleasant thoughts. For these individuals, this provides an opportunity to discuss the role of avoidance of thoughts and the benefits of using the time to practice relaxation strategies and cognitive restructuring.

Sleep Hygiene

Sleep problems are common among patients with chronic pain (Finan & Smith, 2013). Approximately 20% of the people living with chronic pain report at least one symptom of insomnia compared to only 7.4% in those without chronic pain (Ohayon, 2005). Research indicates that these two conditions can interact with each other (Raymond, Nielsen, Lavigne, Manzini, & Choiniere, 2001), with one meta-analysis finding that pain was consistently associated with greater sleep disturbance, reduced sleep duration and sleep quality, increased time taken to fall asleep, poor day-time function, and greater sleep dissatisfaction and distress (Kelly, Blake, Power, O'keeffe, & Fullen, 2011). Some research suggests dopamine may be a neurobiological factor associated with symptoms of insomnia and pain; however, the exact nature of the associations has yet to be elucidated (Finan & Smith, 2013).

Cognitive Behavioral Therapy for Insomnia (CBT-I) is considered the gold-standard psychological treatment for insomnia and includes instructions such as sleep restriction, stimulus control, relaxation, and thought restructuring (Trauer, Qian, Doyle, Rajaratnam, & Cunnington, 2015). Prior to teaching CBT-I skills, however, it's important to conduct a thorough sleep assessment to determine the factors that may be contributing to the sleep issue. For example, people with pain often report difficulty falling asleep, frequent nighttime awakenings due to pain, or pain associated with certain sleep positions. Some sleep disorders, however, may be unrelated to pain, such as in the case of obstructive sleep apnea, or may be the result of medication side effects. Difficulty with sleep also may be caused by psychological conditions such as anxiety, depression, or PTSD. A combination of factors may be contributing to sleep difficulties, but by conducting a sleep assessment and considering all possible comorbidities that may be contributing to the problem, therapists can create a sleep intervention that is tailored to the needs of the patient with pain.

FLEXIBLE, CLIENT-FOCUSED IMPLEMENTATION

Optional Treatment Components to Consider When Flexibly Tailoring Treatment to Patients

ANGER MANAGEMENT

Anger is not uncommon in patients who have chronic pain (Okifuji, Turk, & Curran, 1999), and research supports an association between anger and pain intensity (Gaskin, Green, Robinson, & Geisser, 1992), unpleasantness (Wade, Price, Hamer, Schwartz, & Hart, 1990), and emotional distress (Duckro, Chibnall, & Tomazic, 1995). In many cases, patients who report experiencing anger can benefit from developing an awareness of anger triggers, learning to modify internal responses through relaxation or cognitive restructuring, and practicing responding in constructive ways. When considering teaching anger management, however, it's important to assess for the source of a patient's anger. For some patients, the experience of anger may be related to frustrations with a significant other or not feeling listened to by medical providers when discussing their pain. In these cases, helping the patient to develop skills for communicating their needs to the provider or the partner can be helpful. Frequent anger may suggest the presence of issues such as PTSD or substance use.

STRESS MANAGEMENT

Patients often report that in times of stress their pain can seem more intense, and conversely, when they are in pain their tolerance for minor annoyances is lowered. Stress occurs when an individual perceives that their coping resources are being overwhelmed, and this can cause physiological changes within the body as well as interfere with health-related behaviors that can be used for stress reduction, such as sleep, diet, and exercise. Given the strong evidence linking stress and pain (Abdallah & Geha, 2017), many patients with pain can benefit from learning techniques to identify and adapt to internal and external sources of stress. It's important for therapists to consider the source of stress that a patient is experiencing. For example, some sources of stress may be temporary (e.g., a transition to a new job) and other perceived sources of stress may be considered long-term (e.g., a cancer diagnosis) and may require a different set of coping skills. Therapists help patients learn techniques for approaching controllable problems with problem-solving techniques and uncontrollable problems with emotion-focused techniques. By having a repertoire of coping skills, patients will be equipped to deal with a variety of stressors that might have an impact on their pain and their emotional functioning.

Pleasant Activity Scheduling

Often times when patients are experiencing chronic pain they respond by reducing pleasant activities. Although some patients stop pleasant activities altogether, others might reduce the frequency at which they engage in activities they once found enjoyable, and both scenarios can have negative impacts on everyday life. Without intervention, this response to pain can contribute to depressed mood and disability. The goal when teaching pleasant activity scheduling is to identify pleasant and reinforcing activities that patients can introduce into their lives. Even if some activities are no longer possible due to an injury or pain, the therapist and patient can brainstorm new activities or alternate ways to perform activities the patient once enjoyed. Therapists can consider consulting with a patient's physician or physical therapist to determine the extent to which a patient can engage in certain activities. By doing so, therapists and patients can be "on the same page" when it comes to selecting activities that patients can safely reintroduce into their lives. Activity scheduling is a core component in the evidence-based treatment of depression and a substantial literature exists demonstrating the positive effects of scheduling social and pleasant activities on depressed mood (Lewinsohn & Atwood, 1969; Cuijpers, van Straten, & Warmerdam, 2007). As is the case with the other treatment components, however, it is important that pleasant activities are tailored to each patient's individual hobbies and interests.

Optional Treatment Format Variations to Consider When Flexibly Tailoring Treatment to Patients

Telehealth Delivered Treatment

Patients with chronic pain and comorbid physical health conditions (e.g., cardiac conditions, spinal cord injuries, kidney failure) often encounter physical, financial, and logistical barriers that interfere with mobility and the availability of transportation to appointments. In addition, patients also may have limited geographic access to therapists with specialized training in CBT for pain. One method for overcoming these barriers is the use of Internet-based telehealth sessions to deliver CBT for pain management. A number of simple modifications can be made to ensure that the essential elements of CBT for pain can be delivered effectively. One of the first modifications that can be completed by the therapist is to convert CBT treatment manual content to an electronic format. Separating the electronic content by session will facilitate sharing of information between the patient and therapist. For example, a fillable version (e.g., MS Word or pdf file) of a cognitive restructuring worksheet can be shared during the video session and completed collaboratively. After the session, the therapist can send the completed form to the patient to serve as an example of how to complete the assignment. Similarly, homework assignments completed by the patient can be securely sent to the therapist after completion so that they are ready to review prior to the session. Telehealth methods have the advantage of increasing patients' access to evidence-based care. This format of treatment might not be preferable for all patients, but many of them might appreciate the convenience of telehealth, namely, the opportunity to remain at home and save money on transportation costs, and thus, might prefer the telehealth modality of treatment. Again, the delivery method of treatment could be tailored to suit the needs of the patient.

GROUP VERSUS INDIVIDUAL FORMAT

Cognitive Behavioral Therapy for pain management can be delivered in either group or individual formats, both of which have potential benefits and challenges. There are a number of advantages to conducting a pain management group. First, a group approach can allow one or more therapists to help several patients simultaneously; as a result this approach is more resource efficient even when co-therapists are involved in the delivery of CBT. Second, group treatment provides an opportunity for patients to learn effective coping skills from other group members. Third, interacting with others in a group may provide opportunities for patients to develop a social support network that will provide added benefits well beyond the end of therapy.

In other situations, individual therapy will be the treatment approach of choice. For example, patients may request individual therapy if they feel uncomfortable sharing personal information with a group, or if they feel threatened by groups due to a history of trauma. Individual therapy allows a therapist to devote more time to addressing the specific issues and challenges reported by the patient, to tailor the treatment to the specific needs of the patient, and to engage in patient-specific problem solving and goal setting. Because sessions only need to be scheduled for one person rather than an entire group, individual therapy offers more flexibility in the timing of sessions.

Patient-Centered Variables to Consider When Flexibly Tailoring Treatment to Patients

The presence of chronic pain can negatively impact every aspect of a person's life. As a result, it is not uncommon for individuals with chronic pain to experience mental health issues such as anxiety, depression, or traumatic stress. Regardless of whether these conditions were precipitated or exacerbated by the development of pain, the interaction between pain and other mental health comorbidities can impact symptom presentation and treatment engagement. This should be considered by the clinician when developing a treatment plan.

ANXIETY AND DEPRESSION

Given the impact that chronic pain can have on all aspects of a person's life, it is not uncommon to find high rates of comorbidity between pain and emotional disorders such as anxiety and depression. Rates of anxiety are reported to be as high as 45% in pain populations (Kroenke et al., 2013). Anxiety and fear play an important role in the experience of pain, with one study finding that for patients with low-back pain, anxiety accounted for 32% of the disability and 14% of the severity of the pain (Staerkle et al., 2004). Studies have found depression prevalence rates ranging from 30% to 54% in chronic pain samples (Banks & Kerns, 1996; Elliott, Renier, & Palcher, 2003), and depression is associated with more frequent pain complaints and impairment (Bair, Robinson, Katon, & Kroenke, 2003). The presence of anxiety and depression can complicate the delivery of many elements of CBT, including goal setting, activity engagement, challenging negative thinking, and motivation to participate. For example, patients with pain and anxiety may catastrophize and worry about the meaning of pain (i.e., pain is a sign of damage being done) or avoid activities that have the potential to cause pain. Similarly, patients who have depressed mood may report understanding the benefits of goal setting but feel unable to make goals or take the first step toward achieving those goals. For individuals who report anxiety and depression, it is often helpful to provide reassurance that you believe their pain is "real," but explicitly make the connection that their engagement in worry thoughts about pain is actually contributing to the experience of pain. To accomplish this, it may be helpful in the psychoeducation phase of treatment to introduce the Cognitive-Behavioral Fear–Avoidance Model of chronic pain (Vlaeyen & Linton, 2000) to explain how fear and avoidance play a role in the transition from acute pain to the development of chronic pain. Other modifications may include cognitive restructuring exercises focused on challenging thoughts that are generating anxiety. For patients who are depressed, a greater emphasis can be placed on the use of motivational interviewing in order to help the patient develop intrinsic motivation for engaging in desired behaviors.

POST-TRAUMATIC STRESS DISORDER

Chronic pain may be caused by normal degenerative changes that occur over a lifetime—the onset of pain also can be associated with traumatic injuries caused by motor vehicle accidents or engagement in military combat. Studies estimate that between 20% and 34% of patients referred for the treatment of chronic pain have significant PTSD symptomatology or are diagnosed with PTSD (Geisser, Roth, Bachman, & Ekert, 1996; Asmundson, Norton, Allerdings, Norton, & Larson, 1998). Importantly, research indicates that individuals with comorbid chronic pain and PTSD report greater pain, PTSD symptoms, depression, anxiety, disability, and opioid use than those with only one of these conditions (Asmundson, Wright, & Stein, 2004; Sullivan et al., 2009; Jenewein, Wittmann, Moergeli, Creutzig, & Schnyder, 2009; Outcalt et al., 2015). When working with a patient who has pain and PTSD, clinicians may notice avoidance behaviors, anger issues, or themes related to trauma being expressed while attempting to conduct restructuring exercises. Rather than ignoring the presence of trauma, it is often helpful to acknowledge the interaction between pain and PTSD early in therapy.

Setting Variables

Therapists who have been trained to deliver CBT for pain will need to flexibly apply this treatment approach depending on the settings in which they are working. Therapists who work in an individual outpatient or group-based practice setting can offer CBT for pain as one of several evidence-based treatments. When practicing in this type of setting, however, it will be important for therapists to obtain a release of information from patients in order to coordinate care with the patient's other health providers and ensure that CBT treatment goals are consistent with other recommendations. For example, by communicating with a patient's neurologist a therapist may be able to reinforce the physician's suggestion that the experience of pain is not a sign of increased pathology and that engaging in a walking program is of great physical benefit to the patient. Therapists trained in CBT also will have the opportunity to join multidisciplinary pain management programs that include disciplines such as occupational therapy, physical therapy, nursing, psychiatry, neurology, and rheumatology. In these types of programs, providers work together in a coordinated manner to provide care that is integrated and tailored to the needs of the patient. Given the high prevalence of pain complaints in the primary care setting, therapists who are integrated into primary care will have an opportunity to deliver pain management skills to a broad sample of the population. Primary care appointments are typically spaced apart in time, so therapists may need to carefully select elements of treatment that will yield the greatest benefit for their patients. Additional opportunities will exist for therapists to practice in specialty programs such as surgical centers, facial pain clinics, dental clinics, burn units, or orthopedic surgical centers, because skills learned in CBT for pain will help patients in these programs achieve reduced pain and disability, and more fully participate in treatment interventions. Therapists also will have the opportunity to assist patients in developing pain management skills in the inpatient setting. The selection of CBT skills should match the needs of the individual, because patients may be experiencing a combination of acute pain due to a medical procedure or injury and chronic pain sensations from an existing painful medical condition. For example, pain management skills will be very different for a patient who has experienced knee replacement surgery as opposed to a patient with a spinal cord injury who is also on a ventilator. Other patients may be engaged in rehabilitative services, such as physical or occupational therapy, that require regular participation in order to maximize functional gains. Regardless of the setting, therapists communicate with all providers involved in a patient's pain care to ensure that the patient is receiving a consistent message across providers, and in the process they deliver a coordinated overall plan for the patient's recovery.

SUMMARY AND CONCLUSIONS

Chronic pain is one of the most prevalent disorders to affect adults, and warrants treatment to help reduce its associated impairment and negative effects on everyday life. Fortunately, CBT for chronic pain has been developed that can complement or in many cases even replace pharmacological interventions for pain. Manual-based CBT for chronic pain offers many benefits; patients who receive the "core" treatment ingredients (fidelity) tend to experience significant improvements in their pain severity and level of disability, and also show improved mood and everyday functioning. Like other manual-based and evidence-based treatments, however, this intervention is best when patient-centered. By flexibly tailoring the delivery of each of the core treatment components, and by carefully choosing optional treatment components based on a patient's individual needs, patients can achieve maximal benefit. Fortunately, empirical research on pain guides therapists on how to appropriately tailor treatment to various subpopulations of patients with pain. Research is needed, however, to help determine the various setting factors, treatment format considerations, individual characteristics, and therapist factors that might influence outcomes.

REFERENCES

Abdallah, C. G., & Geha, P. (2017). Chronic pain and chronic stress: Two sides of the same coin? Chronic Stress (Thousand Oaks, Calif.).

Ahlstrand, I., Vaz, S., Falkmer, T., Thyberg, I., & Bjork, M. (2017). Self-efficacy and pain acceptance as mediators of the relationship between pain and performance of valued life activities in women and men with rheumatoid arthritis. *Clinical Rehabilitation, 31*, 824–834.

Akerman, C. J., & Turkoski, B. (2000). Using guided imagery to reduce pain and anxiety. *Home Healthcare Nurse: The Journal for the Home Care and Hospital Professional, 18*, 524–530.

Asmundson, G., J. G., Norton, G., Allerdings, M., Norton, P., & Larsen, D. (1998). Post-traumatic stress disorder and work-related injury. *Journal of Anxiety Disorders, 12*, 57–69.

Asmundson, G. J. G., Wright, K. D., & Stein, M. B. (2004). Pain and PTSD symptoms in female veterans. *European Journal of Pain, 8*(4), 345–350.

Bair, M. J., Robinson, R. L., Katon, W., & Kroenke, K. (2003). Depression and pain comorbidity: A literature review. *Archives of Internal Medicine, 163*, 2433–2445.

Baird, C. L., & Sands, L. (2004). A pilot study of the effectiveness of guided imagery with progressive muscle relaxation to reduce chronic pain and mobility difficulties of osteoarthritis. *Pain Management Nursing, 5*(3) 97–104.

Banks, S. M., & Kerns, R. D. (1996). Explaining high rates of depression in chronic pain: A diathesis-stress framework. *Psychological Bulletin, 119*, 95–110.

Beissner, K., Henderson C. R., Papaleontiou, M., Olkhovskaya, Y., Wigglesworth, J., & Reid, M. C. (2009). Physical therapists' use of cognitive-behavioral therapy for older adults with chronic pain: A nationwide survey. *Physical Therapy, 89*(9), 456–469.

Brown, R. P., & Gerbarg, P. L. (2005). Sudarshan Kriya Yogic breathing in the treatment of stress, anxiety, and depression. Part II—clinical applications and guidelines. *Journal of Alternative and Complementary Medicine, 11*(4), 711–717.

Cuijpers, P., van Straten, A., & Warmerdam, L. (2007). Behavioral activation treatments of depression: A meta-analysis. *Clinical Psychology Review, 27*(3), 318–326.

Duckro, P. N., Chibnall, J. T., & Tomazic, T. J. (1995). Anger, depression, and disability: A path analysis of relationships in a sample of chronic posttraumatic headache patients. *Headache, 35,* 7–9.

Edwards, R. R., Bingham, C. O., III, Bathon, J., & Haythornthwaite, J. A. (2006). Catastrophizing and pain in arthritis, fibromyalgia and other rheumatic disease. *Arthritis Rheum, 55,* 325–332.

Edwards, R. R., Smith, M. T., Kudel, I., & Haythornthwaite, J. (2006). Pain-related catastrophizing as a risk factor for suicidal ideation in chronic pain. *Pain, 126(1–3),* 272–279.

Elliott, T. E., Renier, C. M., & Palcher, J. A. (2003). Chronic pain, depression, and quality of life: Correlations and predictive value of the SF-36. *Pain Medicine, 4(4),* 331–339.

Finan, P. H., & Smith, M. T. (2013). The comorbidity of insomnia, chronic pain, and depression: Dopamine as a putative mechanism. *Sleep Medicine Reviews, 17*(3), 173–183.

French, D. J., Holroyd, K. A., Pinell, C., Malinoski, P. T., O'Donnell, F., & Hill, K. R. (2000). Perceived self-efficacy and headache-related disability *Headache, 40,* 647–656.

Gaskin, D. J., & Richard, P. (2012). The economic costs of pain in the United States. *The Journal of Pain, 13*(8), 715–724.

Gaskin. M. E., Greene, A. F., Robinson, M. E., & Geisser, M. E. (1992). Negative affect and the experience of chronic pain. *Journal of Psychosomatic Research, 36,* 707–713.

Geisser, M. E., Roth, R. S., Bachman, J. E., & Eckert, T. A. (1996). The relationship between symptoms of post-traumatic stress disorder and pain, affective disturbance and disability among patients with accident and non-accident related pain. *Pain, 66,* 207–214.

Hadhazy, V. A., Ezzo, J., Creamer, P., & Berman, B. M. (2000). Mind–body therapies for the treatment of fibromyalgia: A systematic review. *Journal of Rheumatology, 227,* 2911–2918.

Hoffman, B. M., Papas, R. K., Chatkoff, D. K., & Kerns, R. D. (2007). Meta-analysis of psychological interventions for chronic low-back pain. *Health Psychology, 26*(1), 1–9.

Holroyd, K. A., O'Donnell, F. J., Stensland, M., Lipchik, G. L., Cordingley, G. E., & Carlson, B. (2001). Management of chronic tension-type headache with tricyclic antidepressant medication, stress-management therapy, and their combination: A randomized controlled trial. *JAMA, 285,* 2208–2215.

Institute of Medicine. (2011). *Relieving pain in America: A blueprint for transforming prevention, care, education, and research.* Washington, DC: National Academies Press.

Jenewein, J., Wittmann, L., Moergeli, H., Creutzig, J., & Schnyder, U. (2009). Mutual influence of posttraumatic stress disorder symptoms and chronic pain among injured accident survivors: A longitudinal study. *Journal of Traumatic Stress, 22,* 540–548.

Kelly, G. A., Blake, C., Power, C. K., O'keeffe, D., & Fullen, B. M. (2011). The association between chronic low back pain and sleep: A systematic review. *Clinical Journal of Pain, 27*(2), 169–181.

Kendall, P. C., & Beidas, R. (2007). Smoothing the trail for dissemination of evidence-based practices for youth: Flexibility within fidelity. *Professional Psychology: Research and Practice, 38,* 13–20.

Kendall, P. C., & Frank, H. (2018). Implementing evidence-based treatment protocols: Flexibility within fidelity. *Clinical Psychology: Science and Practice, 25*, 1–12. doi: 10.1111/cpsp.12271.

Kroenke, K., Outcalt, S., Krebs, E., Bair, M. J., Wu, J., Chumbler, N., & Yu, Z. (2013). Association between anxiety, health-related quality of life and functional impairment in primary care patients with chronic pain. *General Hospital Psychiatry, 35*(4), 359–365.

Lewinsohn, P. M., & Atwood, G. E. (1969). Depression: A clinical-research approach. *Psychotherapy: Theory, Research & Practice, 6*(3), 166.

Linton, S. J., & Ryberg, M. (2001). A cognitive-behavioral group intervention as prevention for persistent neck and back pain in a non-patient population: A randomized controlled trial. *Pain, 90*, 83–90.

Ma, X., Yue, Z. Q., Gong, Z. Q., Zhang, H., Duan, N. Y., Shi, Y. T., Wei, G. X., & Li, Y. F. (2017). The effect of diaphragmatic breathing on attention, negative affect and stress in healthy adults. *Frontiers in Psychology, 8*, 874.

Martarelli, D., Cocchioni, M., Scuri, S., & Pompei, P. (2011). Diaphragmatic breathing reduces exercise-induced oxidative stress. *Evidence-based Complementary and Alternative Medicine*, eCAM, 932430. https://doi.org/10.1093/ecam/nep169

Melzack, R., & Wall, P. D. (1965). Pain mechanisms: A new theory. *Science, 150*(3699), 971–979.

Miller, M. M., Meints, S. M., & Hirsh, A. T. (2018). Catastrophizing, pain, and functional outcomes for children with chronic pain: A meta-analytic review. *Pain, 159*(12), 2442–2460.

Niederstrasser, N. G., Slepian, P. M., Mankovsky-Arnold, T., Lariviere, C., Vlaeyen, J. W., & Sullivan, M. J. (2014). An experimental approach to examining psychological contributions to multisite musculoskeletal pain. *Journal of Pain, 15*, 1156–1165.

Ohayon, M. M., (2005). Relationship between chronic painful physical condition and insomnia. *Journal of Psychiatric Research, 39*(2), 151–159.

Okifuji, A., Turk, D. C., & Curran, S. L. (1999). Anger in chronic pain: Investigations of anger targets and intensity. *Journal of Psychosomatic Research, 47*(1), 1–12.

Otis, J. D. (2007a). *Managing chronic pain: A Cognitive-Behavioral Therapy approach, therapist guide*. Treatments that Work Series, Oxford University Press.

Otis, J. D. (2007b). *Managing chronic pain: A Cognitive-Behavioral Therapy approach, patient workbook*. Treatments that Work Series, Oxford University Press.

Otis, J. D., Sanderson, K., Hardway, C., Pincus, M., Tun, C., & Soumekh, S. (2013). A randomized controlled pilot study of a Cognitive Behavioral Therapy approach for painful diabetic peripheral neuropathy. *Journal of Pain, 14*(5), 475–482.

Outcalt, S. D., Kroenke, K., Krebs, E. E. Chumbler, N. R., Wu, J., & Bair, M. J. (2015). Chronic pain and comorbid mental health conditions: Independent associations of posttraumatic stress disorder and depression with pain, disability, and quality of life. *Journal of Behavioral Medicine, 38*, 535–543.

Pawlow, L. A., & Jones, G. E. (2005). The impact of abbreviated progressive muscle relaxation on salivary cortisol and salivary immunoglobulin A (sIgA). *Applied Psychophysiology and Biofeedback, 30*(4), 375–387.

Raymond, I., Nielsen, T., Lavigne, G., Manzini, C., & Choiniere, M. (2001). Quality of sleep and its daily relationship to pain intensity in hospitalized adult burn patients. *Pain, 92*, 381–388.

Salyers, M. P., Hudson, C., Morse, G., Rollins, A. L., Monroe-Devita, M., Wilson, C., & Freeland, L. (2011). BREATHE: A pilot study of a one-day retreat to reduce burnout among mental health professionals. *Psychiatric Services, 62*(2), 214–217.

Staerkle, R., Mannion, A. F., Elfering, A., Junge, A., Semmer, N. K., Jacobshagen, N., Grob, D., Dvorak, J., & Boos, N. (2004). Longitudinal validation of the fear-avoidance beliefs questionnaire (FABQ) in a Swiss-German sample of low back pain patients. *European Spine Journal, 13*(4), 332–340.

Sullivan, M. J. L., Thibault, P., Simmonds, M. J., Milioto, M., Cantin, A. P., & Velly, A. M. (2009). Pain, perceived injustice and the persistence of post-traumatic stress symptoms during the course of rehabilitation for whiplash injuries. *Pain, 145*(3), 325–331.

Sullivan, M. J. L., Thorn, B., Haythornthwaite, J. A., Keefe, F. J., Martin, M., Bradley, L. A., & Lefebvre, J. C. (2001). Theoretical perspectives on the relation between catastrophizing and pain. *Clinical Journal of Pain, 17*, 52–64.

Sundram, B. M., Dahlui, M., & Chinna, K. (2016). Effectiveness of progressive muscle relaxation therapy as a worksite health promotion program in the automobile assembly line. *Industrial Health, 54*(3), 204–214.

Trauer, J. M., Qian, M. Y., Doyle, J. S., Rajaratnam, S. M., & Cunnington, D. (2015). Cognitive Behavioral Therapy for chronic insomnia: A systematic review and meta-analysis. *Annals of Internal Medicine, 163*(3), 191–204.

Turner, J., Holtzman, S., & Mancl, L. (2007). Mediators, moderators, and predictors of therapeutic change in cognitive-behavioral therapy for chronic pain. *Pain, 127*, 276–286.

Vlaeyen, J. W., & Linton, S. J. (2000). Fear-avoidance and its consequences in chronic musculoskeletal pain: A state of the art. *Pain, 85*(3), 317–332.

Vlaeyen, J. W., & Linton, S. J. (2000). Fear-avoidance and its consequences in chronic musculoskeletal pain: A state of the art. *Pain, 85*(3), 317–332.

Wade, J. B., Price, D. D., Hamer, R. M., Schwartz, D. M., & Hart, R. P. (1990). An emotional component analysis of chronic pain. *Pain, 40*, 303–310.

Wallman, K. E, Morton, A. R., Goodman, C., Grove, R., & Guilfoyle, A. M. (2004). Randomised controlled trial of graded exercise in chronic fatigue syndrome. *Medical Journal of Australia, 180*(9), 444–448.

9

Flexible Applications of Family-Based Therapy for Youth with Bipolar Spectrum Disorders

HALEY M. BRICKMAN AND MARY A. FRISTAD ■

AUTHOR NOTE

Haley M. Brickman: ⓘ Mary A. Fristad: ⓘ
Bipolar Spectrum Disorders (BPSD), which include bipolar disorder type 1 (BD1), bipolar disorder type 2 (BD2), cyclothymic disorder (CYC), and other specified bipolar and related disorders (OSBARD), are persistent, often debilitating conditions that affect approximately 3.9% of youth internationally, while BD1, or "classic" BD, has an average prevalence of 0.6% (Van Meter et al., 2020). BD1 requires one or more episodes of mania, while BD2 requires one or more episodes each of hypomania plus depression. CYC refers to hypomania and subthreshold depressive symptoms that are persistent for a year or longer (two years for adults), while OSBARD refers to a combination of impairing manic and depressive symptoms that do not meet criteria for BD1, BD2, or CYC. Diagnostic criteria are identical for youth and adults, although demonstrations of symptoms will differ across age groups (e.g., poor judgment for a nine-year-old might involve giving away all prized video games whereas an adult might run up a large credit card bill). Pediatric BPSD is associated with meaningful impairment and reduced quality of life (Freeman et al., 2009) as well as high rates of hospitalization and suicidality (Hauser et al., 2013). Although it is likely that a primary cause of BPSD is at least partially genetic, with twin studies providing evidence that it is one of the most heritable of all mental health disorders (79%–83%; Kieseppa et al., 2004), research suggests that its course and prognosis is heavily influenced by environmental and psychosocial factors (Johnson et al., 2017).

With increased understanding of the prevalence and impairment associated with childhood BPSD, the need for evidence-based psychosocial interventions has become increasingly apparent. Early symptom onset appears to be associated with a worse course of the disorder (Birmaher et al., 2014; Estrada-Prat et al., 2019); thus, early intervention is crucial for improving both short- and long-term outcomes. This association may be, in part, attributable to the fact that those with adult-onset BPSD experience fewer impairments over the course of development and have had the opportunity to develop coping skills, social support, and vocational/occupational training necessary for effective functioning. Providing early intervention to assist in acquisition of these skills, then, is likely to improve course and prognosis of the disorder, decreasing frequency and severity of episodes (Youngstrom & Algorta, 2014). Additionally, given the high heritability rate in childhood-onset BPSD (Faraone et al., 2003), early intervention has the potential to benefit the entire family, which, in turn, is likely to improve the course of the disorder (Sullivan et al., 2012).

The following sections introduce well-established manual-based interventions for youth with BPSD. Their shared core components and ways in which these components have been applied flexibly and effectively across settings, populations, and contexts are highlighted. In short, the core components are key to treatment fidelity, but they can be applied with flexibility (Kendall & Beidas, 2007; Kendall & Frank, 2018). One such intervention, Multi-Family Psychoeducational Psychotherapy (MF-PEP; Fristad et al., 2003), is then discussed in detail to illustrate flexible implementation of this intervention.

PSYCHOSOCIAL INTERVENTIONS FOR YOUTH WITH BIPOLAR SPECTRUM DISORDERS

Multiple randomized clinical trials (RCTs) have demonstrated efficacy of three manualized treatments for treating youth with Bipolar Spectrum Disorders (BPSD), in conjunction with pharmacotherapy. All three incorporate family psychoeducation and skill building, indicating they can be considered a well-established *class* of interventions. These interventions include family-focused treatment for adolescents (FFT-A; Miklowitz et al., 2008; 2011; 2013), child- and family-focused CBT (CFF-CBT; Pavuluri et al., 2004; West et al., 2007; 2009; 2014), and psychoeducational psychotherapy (PEP: Fristad, 2006; Fristad et al., 2009; 2015). Of note, there is also growing evidence for dialectical behavior therapy (DBT; Goldstein et al., 2015) and interpersonal and social rhythm therapy (IPSRT; Goldstein et al., 2018; Hlastala et al., 2010) for adolescents with BPSD.

Family Focused Therapy for Adolescents (FFT-A). FFT-A (Miklowitz et al., 2004) was adapted for 12- to 17-year-olds from a well-established treatment for adults with BPSD (i.e., family-focused treatment, FFT). Informed by research linking expressed emotion (EE; i.e., the amount of criticism, hostility, or emotional over involvement exhibited by family members) with poor outcomes for individuals with BPSDs, a main focus of FFT-A includes providing psychoeducation and skills to affected adolescents and their families, with over-arching goals being to encourage family members to develop a common understanding of the disorder, decrease EE levels in the family, and provide psychoeducation and skill building regarding symptom management, coping strategies, mood charting, and prevention planning. Three phases of treatment (psychoeducation, communication enhancement training, and problem-solving skills training) are provided to adolescents, parents, and siblings over the course of up to 21 sessions.

Numerous randomized controlled trials (RCTs) have demonstrated FFT-A's efficacy in improving outcomes. A 46% improvement in manic symptoms (Miklowitz, et al., 2004), faster recovery from depressive symptoms, more time in remission, and a more favorable 2-year symptom trajectory (Miklowitz et al., 2008) have been reported. Adolescents who receive FFT-A also exhibit increased stabilization of manic symptoms (Miklowitz et al., 2014) and report an improved quality of life (O'Donnell et al., 2017). FFT-A is also beneficial for those at high risk for developing BPSD (Miklowitz et al., 2011; 2013; 2020). Finally, FFT-A produces beneficial effects for families; increased cohesion has been reported to persist two years following intervention (O'Donnell et al., 2020).

Child- and Family-Focused Cognitive Behavioral Therapy (CFF-CBT). CFF-CBT (Pavuluri et al., 2004; West et al., 2007; 2009; 2014) is designed for youth ages 5 to 17 years and their parents. CFF-CBT includes 12 sessions, with additional booster sessions available for maintenance. CFF-CBT skills are represented by the acronym RAINBOW: **R**outine; **A**ffect regulation; **I** can do it; **N**o negative thoughts/live in the **N**ow; **B**e a good friend/**B**alanced lifestyle; **O**h, how can we solve it?; and **W**ays to get support.

Open trials and an RCT of CCF-CBT have demonstrated significant improvements in depressive and manic symptoms as well as comorbid symptoms of ADHD, aggression, and psychosis, and global functioning in youth with BPSD (Pavuluri et al., 2004; West et al., 2007; 2009; 2014). In addition, an open trial of a multifamily adaptation of CFF-CBT with children ages 6 to 12 years provided evidence for improvements in parental stress as a result of treatment, which was associated with children's increased prosocial behaviors (West et al., 2009).

Psychoeducational Psychotherapy (PEP). PEP (Fristad et al., 1998) was originally designed for children ages 8 to 12 years with depressive and bipolar spectrum disorders but was later modified for adolescents (Fristad et al., 2018). PEP includes multifamily group (MF-PEP) and individual-family formats (IF-PEP; Fristad et al., 2006).

Randomized controlled trials of both MF-PEP and IF-PEP have supported their efficacy in decreasing mood symptom severity up to 18 months following the intervention (Fristad, 2006; Fristad et al., 2003; 2009). Impact on family functioning includes improved family interactions and increased perceived social support from parents up to six months following intervention (Fristad et al., 2003), and decreased EE within the family (Fristad, 2006). In addition, a recent longitudinal follow-up study of IF-PEP combined with omega-3 fatty acid supplementation indicated parent- and self-reported improved coping and emotion regulation skills in youth that lasted two to five years following the intervention (Fristad et al., 2021).

PREDICTORS OF DIFFERENTIAL OUTCOMES

A limited number of studies have examined predictors and moderators of treatment outcomes, and findings are mixed for the role of baseline mood severity, comorbidities, parental depression, expressed emotion, and socioeconomic status (Roley-Roberts & Fristad, 2020). Two studies indicate that sex, age, race, baseline mania, and suicidal ideation/nonsuicidal self-injury do *not* moderate outcomes. There is some suggestion that greater baseline child and family impairment, including high levels of family conflict and untreated ADHD, is associated with greater improvement following treatment (Macpherson et al., 2014; Miklowitz et al., 2009;2013; O'Donnell et al., 2020; Sullivan et al., 2012; Weintraub et al., 2019).

CORE COMPONENTS

FFT-A, CFF-CBT, and PEP are all manual-based and family-based interventions that begin with psychoeducation and shift to skill building later in treatment. Each has a foundation in CBT, attends to family systems issues, and focuses on communication and problem solving. All are intended to be implemented in conjunction with pharmacotherapy; psychoeducation includes information on medication management and adherence. Although the protocols, specific activities, and methods of delivery vary somewhat between particular interventions, each exerts its treatment effects through the application of similar core components, evidencing the inherent ability for this class of interventions to be flexibly applied to meet the needs of families.

Family Focused. Research has long acknowledged the struggles that families of individuals with BPSD face, as well as the importance of including families in treatment. In each intervention described above, family members play an integral part. They are included in both psychoeducation and skills building. The theoretical basis for including families in treatment is based on the bidirectional impact of family environment on symptoms and treatment outcomes in individuals with BPSD. Interventions that improve family environment may produce beneficial effects on symptoms, course, and outcome of BPSD, and improvement in symptoms can lead to improved family functioning. Thus, a major goal of these treatments is to improve individual coping and family environment, which necessitates working with family members as well as the affected individual.

Studies have consistently identified that families of children and adolescents with BPSD exhibit increased levels of conflict, control, and EE, as well as decreased levels of cohesion and expressiveness (see Stapp et al., 2020 for review). This increased rate of impairment in families with BPSD is particularly detrimental because of the profound effects of family environment on the rate, course, and progression of BPSD. For example, negative family environments characterized by high degrees of conflict and hostility have been found to exacer- bate symptoms, and in some cases prolong the course of disorder in adolescents with BPSD (Sullivan et al., 2012). Improved family functioning following FFT-A leads to decreased symptomology in adolescents with BPSD (Sullivan et al., 2012). Families of youth with BPSD exhibit decreased levels of expressiveness (i.e., "extent to which family members are encouraged to express their feelings openly"; Moos & Moos, 1994) compared to unaffected families (Vance et al., 2008), which is neg- atively correlated with depressive symptoms in children (Nussbaum et al., 2017).

Given that it is not uncommon for multiple family members to experience mood disorders (Faraone et al., 2003), an added benefit of including family members in treatment may include improved parental functioning or willingness to seek treatment, which may occur through increased awareness of symptoms, knowledge of coping strategies, using newly learned skills, and increased social support (particularly in treatments delivered in a group of families).

Psychoeducation. Psychoeducation is provided at treatment onset and continues throughout all sessions. Information about etiology, course, prognosis, and treatment of mood disorders, including access to treatment, resources, edu- cational services, and other supports, is provided. Family members are equipped with information and strategies on how to manage symptoms, prevent re- lapse, and provide a supportive environment for the affected individual. A key takeaway is that both the youth and their family members play a role in man- aging the disorder, and parents are encouraged to become advocates and active members of their child's treatment team. Research supports a strong emphasis on psychoeducation, which, when combined with pharmacotherapy, has consistently been found to contribute to better short- and long-term outcomes in individuals with BPSD (Miklowitz, 2008).

Skill Building. Specific treatment modules address family problem solving and communication, the primary goal of which is to increase the frequency of posi- tive interactions and decrease the amount of EE in families. Communication and problem solving are central components of interpersonal relationships and family functioning; deficits in these areas may contribute to the impaired family envi- ronment reported in families with children with BPSD (Belardinelli et al., 2008). Because communication styles and problem-solving techniques can be learned and adjusted with coaching and practice, targeting these areas is often an effective way to improve family functioning and, consequently, treatment outcomes.

FLEXIBILITY

A critical aspect of these treatments is to tailor sessions to deliver core treat- ment components in a developmentally appropriate way, such that the interven- tion is appropriate for younger children as well as adolescents. In fact, FFT-A itself represents a developmental adaptation of an adult-focused treatment, and

CFF-CBT was created as an adaptation of FFT-A to be applied with a younger age range. PEP was initially designed for 8- to 12-year-olds and later adapted for adolescents. These interventions have been successfully adapted and generalized to other populations, such as youth at high risk for BPSD (FFT-HR; Miklowitz et al., 2020) and to address common problem areas in children with high functioning autism spectrum disorder (MF-PEP-ASD; Connolly et al., 2018). Notably, despite the manualized nature of these interventions, client satisfaction is high (Goldberg-Arnold et al., 1999; Pavuluri et al., 2004; Fristad et al., 2020), and a large emphasis is placed on maintaining a strong therapeutic alliance and providing highly individualized treatment by tailoring the material, structure, and activities of the intervention to best suit the needs of individuals, families, and groups. This flexible approach is illustrated in the following section, in which we detail how one such manual-based treatment, PEP, can be applied flexibly to achieve treatment goals.

AN ILLUSTRATION OF FLEXIBILITY WITHIN FIDELITY: PSYCHOEDUCATIONAL PSYCHOTHERAPY

Psychoeducational psychotherapy (PEP) can be delivered to multifamily groups (MF-PEP) or individual families (IF-PEP). MF-PEP and IF-PEP session content is nearly identical, with the only differences being session structure and a few unique features of IF-PEP made possible due to its individualized format. Given this similarity, only MF-PEP sessions are described in detail further on; additional IF-PEP components are presented subsequently. PEP includes psychoeducation for BPSD, but youth with depressive spectrum disorders (with or without subsyndromal manic symptoms) also can benefit. This finding is particularly important given the high rates of conversion to BPSD in children initially diagnosed with a depressive disorder (up to 50%; Cosgrove et al., 2013; Duffy et al., 2010; Luby & Navasaria, 2010). In fact, preliminary data suggest MF-PEP may reduce conversion to BPSD for youth with MDD at high risk for BPSD (Nadkarni & Fristad, 2010).

COMPONENTS REQUIRED FOR FIDELITY

Therapist requirements to deliver MF-PEP, in addition to training, include prior knowledge of and experience working with children with mood disorders and their families, as well as implementing CBT and family-based interventions. The structure and content of sessions, described in detail in the treatment manual, coupled with the use of parent/child workbooks that contain the psychoeducational information, handouts, and activities of each session, facilitate maintaining fidelity. As with any manual-based treatment, it is important to maintain fidelity by delivering the core components that have been found to be effective in clinical trials. An effectiveness study of MF-PEP indicates community clinicians are able to maintain adequate therapist adherence and provide treatment with beneficial effects following completion of a one- or two-day workshop (MacPherson et al., 2016); although dissemination/implementation research demonstrates the importance of ongoing consultation/peer supervision to maintaining fidelity (Asnaani et al., 2018).

GROUP AND SESSION STRUCTURE

Multifamily psychoeducational psychotherapy (MF-PEP) consists of eight weekly 90-minute sessions that begin and end with the family together, though parents and children meet in separate, simultaneous groups for the majority of each session. Material is presented in a manner designed to decrease stigma and blame, emphasizing that neither the child nor the family is at fault for the illness, and encouraging families to separate symptoms of the disorder from the individual. Sessions are highly formatted, with specific content and skills to be introduced and practiced within parent and child groups. Importantly, groups are designed to be interactive and elicit discussion between members—a necessary component to obtain the full effects of social support, a major benefit of the group format. Optimal group size is six to eight children, with one clinician running the parent group and two clinicians running the child group. One of the child clinicians can be a trainee who assists with behavioral management, making this an ideal opportunity to learn a new evidence-based treatment. The main activities and "lessons of the day" are provided to families in the form of handouts included in the parent/child workbooks. Finally, the program includes a weekly family "Take-Home Project" that provides families the opportunity to apply information and skills learned in-session.

Each session begins with a brief check-in with parents and children together to review the take-home project from the previous week. Families then separate into parent and child groups. Child groups begin with identifying and rating feelings ("Sharing Feelings") and sharing experiences that have occurred in the past week ("News of the Week"). Then, new content and skills are provided in a "Lesson of the Day," which is interactive, activity-based, and typically thematically linked to the content that parents receive. Next, clinicians engage the children in preparation, practice, and assignment of a take-home project of the week. Child sessions end with group games, which provide children in-vivo social skills training, followed by a brief demonstration and practice of deep breathing before joining parents to review session content. In this review, three child volunteers are tasked with explaining the lesson of the day, describing the family project, and demonstrating the breathing exercise. The child therapists are available, as needed, to support the volunteers in their presentations. They also model positive behavior management strategies for the parents (e.g., calling attention to prosocial behavior, ignoring nondangerous negative behavior, quietly but firmly addressing potentially dangerous or disruptive behavior). Parent sessions cover specific topics each week, beginning with a psychoeducational focus and shifting to more skill building as the weeks progress.

SESSION CONTENT

Session content is prescribed, but flexibility and creativity in delivering this content is encouraged, because every group is different. Activities may be modified to best suit the needs and interests of the children; however, the key element of each session should be delivered. The key elements are described here.

Session One. Families are introduced to the program's structure and expectations, including the importance of attending, actively participating, completing projects, and maintaining confidentiality of other group members. Creating a cohesive and interactive group is a key aspect of this session, because the support and encouragement of other participants with shared experiences is a major benefit of a group format for both children and parents. Parents and children separately learn about mood disorders and patterns, with a particular focus on how to identify and monitor the child's unique symptoms.

Children develop, with group leaders, rules for their group (i.e., addressing confidentiality and behavior). After learning about common symptoms of depression, mania, and other frequently occurring comorbid diagnoses (i.e., ADHD, anxiety), children complete activities geared toward identifying and rating their symptoms, including naming their emotions and recognizing their intensity. The motto, "It's Not Your Fault, but It's Your Challenge," is explained and discussed. With a better understanding of the challenges they face and consequences of their symptoms, they generate a "Personal Fix-It List," which is a list of problems or behaviors they would like to change. Children end their session with an introduction to diaphragmatic breathing (Belly Breathing).

Parents receive information on depressive disorders and BPSD, including causes, course, co-occurring symptoms and associated features, brain differences in individuals with mood disorders, suicide risk factors and warning signs, and common comorbid diagnoses. This information is tailored to the sophistication of group members and the diagnoses their children have. Parents learn various strategies for mood monitoring and are tasked with deciding how they wish to keep a record of their child's mood. The family project of the week is to complete a family "Fix-It List" by integrating input from the child's and parent's requests and turning it into a document that applies to all family members.

Session Two. This session reviews treatment (medication, therapy, school-based support) and teaches children to differentiate themselves from their symptoms. Using the "Naming the Enemy" exercise, children generate a list of their positive characteristics on one side of a paper and identify their symptoms on the other side. The paper is then folded to demonstrate how symptoms can "cover up" one's true self, and the leader explains how treatment can "put the enemy behind you." Based on the clinical profiles of participating children, relevant therapy, school-based support, and medications are reviewed, including how to manage medication side effects.

The parent session aims to help parents become better consumers of health care and more active, effective members of their child's treatment team. An overview of available treatments is provided, tailored to the needs of participating families.

In particular, information is provided about various classes of medications, including benefits, side effects, and how to manage them. Parents are encouraged to think critically about their child's treatment and to complete a "cost-benefit analysis" regarding the costs of symptoms in relation to the costs and benefits of medications and other treatments. Parents are provided samples of mood medication logs to complete as the take-home project for the week and on an ongoing basis throughout the program.

Session Three. In this session, children build a "Tool Kit" to manage strong emotions. They are taught to identify situations that may elicit "bad/sad/mad" feelings, the accompanying physiological "warning signs," and the "hurtful" behaviors these feelings elicit; then, they generate ideas for a "Tool Kit" to use when strong emotions arise. The importance of developing an array of tools is emphasized, using the acronym CARS (Creative, Active, Rest & Relaxation, Social). The family project is to build an actual "Tool Kit" at home, and the children monitor its use and effectiveness. Adolescents may prefer to simply make a list of "tools" on their phone or on index cards they can keep in a school folder or in their bedroom.

Parents focus on how to be an active part of their child's treatment team. Information covered can be tailored to the needs of the families in each group. They learn about the mental healthcare system, including providers, levels of care, and how to access appropriate services. They also learn about the educational system, including an overview of special education services, their child's educational rights, legal terms, and how to work effectively with the school. Becoming an effective consumer of care, as measured by parents' understanding and beliefs about treatment leads to improved quality of services utilized, which significantly decreases children's symptom severity (Mendenhall et al., 2009).

Session Four. In Session Four, children learn the fundamentals of CBT, using a "Thinking, Feeling, Doing" cartoon that builds on their prior learning. They also are introduced to the concept of "hurtful thoughts" and learn how emotions can be affected and modified by implementing "helpful thoughts" and actions. This notion is illustrated by a cognitive behavioral activity and take-home project, which allows children to apply this concept to their own experiences and record their thoughts, feelings, and behaviors throughout the week.

Parents shift from a primarily psychoeducational approach to working specifically on family skill building. They discuss the impact mood disorders have on the family system, as well as the common negative cycles families can enter unwittingly. Empathy for the challenging role parents play is provided and strategies to break the negative cycle and institute positive interactions are presented.

Session Five. Session Five focuses on problem-solving skills. Children learn and practice five steps to utilize when they face a challenging situation: "Stop," "Think," "Plan," "Do," and "Check." These steps build upon skills developed in the prior sessions. Although the workbook provides examples, group members are encouraged to bring up issues from their own lives to work through together during the session.

The parent group includes general coping strategies, including traps to avoid (e.g., attempting to be constantly available and positive) and the importance of self-preservation. Symptoms and family conflict are recast as problems that can be solved. Family problem-solving steps are reviewed and discussed, beginning with who should be involved in the discussion, and moving on to brainstorming, choosing, and evaluating solutions together as a family. As a take-home project, parents and children identify a family problem and use their newly practiced skills to solve it.

Session Six. This session focuses on communication skills. Children are taught the components of communication, including the difference between verbal and nonverbal communication and the ways in which messages can be misinterpreted. There is an explicit focus on nonverbal communication. Therapists can model or, if the group is willing, direct the children in role-plays and charades to better understand the effects of facial expressions, body gestures, body posture, and tone of voice on communication. This is an especially important skill to practice with families, because youth with BPSD often have facial processing deficits (Schenkel & Towne, 2020), as well as an increased tendency to misinterpret neutral faces as threatening or hostile (Rich et al., 2008). These deficits can increase the probability of a negative response to a family member that may ignite conflict.

The parent session emphasizes the importance of effective communication in improving family functioning and decreasing the frequency and severity of the child's symptoms. Parents are made aware of frequent "communication traps" that are particularly relevant to mood disorders, as well as specific strategies to improve interactions. Parents are encouraged to monitor communication with their child over the subsequent week to be mindful of their use of "hurtful" language and how to remedy these interactions with "helpful" words. The weekly family project is to use charades for parents and children to guess the emotions the other is intending to convey.

Session Seven. Children learn about verbal communication in Session Seven, with a focus on transforming "hurtful" words into "helpful" words and expressing thoughts and feelings effectively. They brainstorm requests they would like to make of their parents to improve family communication.

The parent group reviews strategies to manage unique features of mood disorders, including safety planning, and how to respond to specific manic and depressive symptoms. The needs of other family members (siblings, spouses) and management of parental stress are highlighted. The family project involves parents and children making three requests of the other to improve family communication.

Session Eight. Session Eight provides an opportunity to review what has been learned, address final questions, and celebrate completion of the program. Children play a review game and redeem their points for prizes while parents have a group discussion. Toward the end of the session, children and parents come together one final time for a graduation ceremony and receipt of certificates; child therapists provide "graduation speeches" about each child's growth during group.

ADAPTATIONS AND FLEXIBILITY IN IMPLEMENTATION

MF-PEP. Structural modifications for MF-PEP can include the number of participating families, whether groups are held simultaneously, behavior management, and rules about parent/caregiver participation. It is not always feasible, for example, for groups to include six to eight families, perhaps due to the small size of the clinic or community or, at the other extreme, a large demand for treatment. In these situations, groups may contain fewer than six or more than eight families, with proper consideration and preparation for the challenges that could arise by having a group that is quite small (e.g., decreased participation/interaction) or very large (e.g., difficulty maintaining a controlled environment). Clinicians may serve as both the parent and child therapist and alternate weeks for child and parent groups rather than hold the groups simultaneously. Potential reasons for this might be to address billing constraints, lack of staffing, space, or other practical limitations. Behavior management strategies employed may differ, based on the physical layout of the clinic (e.g., If a child is disrupting group, can the co-therapist sit in the hall with the child until their behavior warrants return to the group?) and the composition of group members (e.g., If a child with type 1 diabetes is in the group, use stickers or other little tchotchkes rather than small candies as an immediate reinforcer.). Finally, flexibility in rules and expectations regarding attendees and family participation is often necessary. Although it is preferable that the same parent (or, ideally, two parents) attend each session, this is not always feasible, and parents may need to alternate sessions. When this occurs, therapists are advised to emphasize the importance of communication between family members between sessions, particularly regarding the weekly and ongoing take-home projects. The exception to this is that at least one parent or caregiver should be present at each session. Each parent group can "vote" whether or not they would like to include other family members. Older siblings, even those who are college-aged and provide supervision for the child with the mood disorder, are usually not "voted in" to participate in sessions.

Due to the nature of an interactive, personalized multigroup format, no two groups are truly identical, and no two families receive the exact same benefits from the program. Each group differs in terms of demographic make-up as well as degree of participation, talkativeness, and cohesion. Children generally present with a wide array of comorbid diagnoses (e.g., 100% of children in a 165 family RCT; Fristad et al., 2009) and features, as well as degree of concentration, which frequently influences the focus of psychoeducational content as well as group dynamics and structure. It is beneficial, when possible, to arrange groups to be similar with regard to age of the child (e.g., offering an elementary school group, a middle school group, and a high school group).

In the same way that no two groups are identical, each family presents with a unique set of challenges, goals, motivations, and expectations. Thus, while the workbook-driven approach provides a framework and structure for evidence-based content to deliver, the unique presentation and contributions of group members, as well as the personalized nature of the treatment in terms of structure, resources, and activities, ensures that treatment is individualized to families in order to provide the highest quality care. This individualization necessitates substantial flexibility and creativity on the part of therapists, but it is a crucial aspect of treatment that benefits both the individual family and the group as a whole, because families are exposed to a variety of challenges that they may not yet have faced, as well as additional resources and solutions to these problems. It is important to be aware of any specific challenges (e.g., cognitive, developmental, learning, or physical impairments) that group members may have, and to modify the complexity of the session material to be developmentally appropriate, so that participants find it understandable and engaging.

IF-PEP. IF-PEP was created to meet the needs of families and clinicians for whom a group format is either not feasible (e.g., limited resources, staff, space, or time; few eligible families in small communities or clinics) or not desirable (e.g., family prefers the privacy of an individual format or does not wish to wait until a group session begins). IF-PEP typically includes 20 to 24 weekly 50-minute sessions, alternating between parent and child sessions. IF-PEP does not provide the benefit of additional social support and in-vivo social skills training provided in MF-PEP, but it does allow for increased flexibility/personalization of delivery. IF-PEP can accommodate sibling and school consultation sessions and covers healthy habits (i.e., nutrition, sleep, exercise) in greater detail. The logic of proceeding through sessions in a prescribed order makes good clinical sense in general, but sessions can be scheduled flexibly if needed. For example, if a family comes in with a school crisis, that can be focused on immediately, then sessions can revert back to the usual order of delivery.

The modifications described above for MF-PEP also apply to IF-PEP. Moreover, as noted, the single-family format of IF-PEP allows for additional flexibility in content delivery. As families enter treatment with varying levels of knowledge, experience, and expectations, some sessions can be combined and/or others repeated, as needed. The therapist may choose to combine content. On the other hand, some families may require additional time and assistance to learn or practice a skill, or may not have had time to apply the lesson.

Flexibility within Specific Activities and Take Home Projects. The PEP manual and workbooks provide suggested activities and handouts, but it is important to remember that the overarching goal of each session is for children and families to learn the "theme" or "take-away" of the session. Therapists are best when mindful of any limitations or challenges that specific children face when choosing which activities to implement in the effort to have activities be educational and enjoyable. This effort is important because failure to do so may cause frustration or disengagement. For example, children with mood disorders have a higher rate of learning difficulties than the general public (Arnold et al., 2005; Lagace & Kutcher, 2005). If a child is struggling with reading or writing, the child can create drawings rather than writing out examples. Group games that require fine or large motor skills can be modified so that all participants can experience success.

Finally, flexibility is allowed in the delivery and assignment of parent and family take home projects. For example, a complex and a simple mood-tracking log are provided as examples to parents, who also are encouraged to design their own system, if preferred. No one system is "better" than another; the "better" system is the one each family will actually use.

CONCLUSIONS

Much has been learned in the past two decades about pediatric BPSD, and this increased awareness has led to the development of a class of psychosocial interventions that significantly improves outcomes for these children and their families. Family psychoeducation plus skills building represents a class of well-established interventions that have been successfully implemented and adapted to improve mood symptoms and family functioning within a wide variety of settings, ages, and presenting problems. Despite fears that evidence-based protocols might be rigid, difficult to implement, and insensitive or unaccommodating to the individual needs of children and families, such treatments repeatedly have been found to be implemented with flexibility and to be efficacious at improving symptom severity and outcomes in children and families affected by the disorder. Therapists are encouraged to use their clinical expertise and creativity in delivering these family psychoeducation plus skill building interventions but not to diverge from fidelity to the core features of the treatment.

DECLARATION OF INTEREST

Mary A. Fristad receives research funding from Janssen and royalties from American Psychiatry Publishing, Child & Family Psychological Services, Guilford Press, and JK Seminars, editorial stipend from Evidence-Based Practice in Child and Adolescent Mental Health, and is a co-author of the commercially available treatment manual reviewed in this chapter. Haley M. Brickman has no conflict of interest to report.

REFERENCES

Arnold, E. M., Goldston, D. B., Walsh, A. K., Reboussin, B. A., Daniel, S. S., Hickman, E., & Wood, F. B. (2005). Severity of emotional and behavioral problems among poor and typical readers. *Journal of Abnormal Child Psychology, 33*(2), 205–217. https://doi.org/10.1007/s10802-005-1828-9

Asnaani, A., Gallagher, T., & Foa, E. B. (2018). Evidence-based protocols: Merits, drawbacks, and potential solutions. *Clinical Psychology: Science and Practice, 25*(4), 1–13. https://doi.org/10.1111/cpsp.12266

Belardinelli, C., Hatch, J. P., Olvera, R. L., Fonseca, M., Caetano, S. C., Nicoletti, M., Pliszka, S., & Soares, J. C. (2008). Family environment patterns in families with bipolar children. *Journal of Affective Disorders, 107*(1–3), 299–305. https://doi.org/10.1016/j.jad.2007.08.011

Birmaher, B., Gill, M. K., Axelson, D. A., Goldstein, B. I., Goldstein, T. R., Yu, H., Liao, F., Iyengar, S., Diler, R. S., Strober, M., Hower, H., Yen, S., Hunt, J., Merranko, J. A., Ryan, N. D., & Keller, M. B. (2014). Longitudinal trajectories and associated baseline predictors in youths with bipolar spectrum disorders. *The American Journal of Psychiatry, 171*(9), 990–999. https://doi.org/10.1176/appi.ajp.2014.13121577795–804. https://doi.org/10.1176/appi.ajp.2009.08101569

Connolly, S., Grasser, K. C., Chung, W., Tabern, K., Guiou, T., Wynn, J., & Fristad, M. (2018). Multi-family Psychoeducational Psychotherapy (MF-PEP) for children with high functioning autism spectrum disorder. *Journal of Contemporary Psychotherapy: On the Cutting Edge of Modern Developments in Psychotherapy, 48*(3), 115–121. https://doi.org/10.1007/s10879-018-9386-y

Cosgrove, V. E., Roybal, D. & Chang, K. D. (2013). Bipolar depression in pediatric populations. *Pediatric Drugs, 15*, 83–91. https://doi.org/10.1007/s40272-013-0022-8

Duffy, A., Alda, M., Hajek, T., Sherry, S. B., & Grof, P. (2010). Early stages in the development of bipolar disorder. *Journal of Affective Disorders, 121*(1–2), 127–135. https://doi.org/10.1016/j.jad.2009.05.022

Estrada, P. X., Van Meter, A. R., Camprodon, R. E., Batlle, V. S., Goldstein, B. I., & Birmaher, B. (2019). Childhood factors associated with increased risk for mood episode recurrences in bipolar disorder—A systematic review. *Bipolar Disorders, 21*(6), 483–502. https://doi.org/10.1111/bdi.12785

Faraone, S. V., Glatt, S. J., & Tsuang, M. T. (2003). The genetics of pediatric-onset bipolar disorder. *Biological Psychiatry, 53*(11), 970–977. https://doi.org/10.1016/S0006-3223(02)01893-0

Freeman, A. J., Youngstrom, E. A., Michalak, E., Siegel, R., Meyers, O. I., & Findling, R. L. (2009). Quality of life in pediatric bipolar disorder. *Pediatrics, 123*(3), e446–e452. https://doi.org/10.1542/peds.2008-0841

Fristad, M. A. (2006). Psychoeducational treatment for school-aged children with bipolar disorder. *Development and Psychopathology, 18*(4), 1289–1306. https://doi.org/10.1017/S0954579406060627

Fristad, M. A., Ackerman, J. P., & Nick, E. A. (2018). Adaptation of Multi-Family Psychoeducational Psychotherapy (MF-PEP) for adolescents with mood disorders: Preliminary findings. *Evidence-based Practice in Child and Adolescent Mental Health, 3*(4), 252–262. https://doi.org/10.1080/23794925.2018.1509031

Fristad, M. A., Gavazzi, S. M., & Soldano, K. W. (1998). Multi-family psychoeducation groups for childhood mood disorders: A program description and preliminary efficacy data. *Contemporary Family Therapy: An International Journal, 20*(3), 385–402. https://doi.org/10.1023/A:1022477215195

Fristad, M. A., Goldberg-Arnold, J. S., & Gavazzi, S. M. (2003). Multi-family psychoeducation groups in the treatment of children with mood disorders. *Journal of Marital and Family Therapy, 29*(4), 491–504. https://doi.org/10.1111/j.1752-0606.2003.tb01691.x

Fristad, M. A., Roley-Roberts, M. E., Black, S. R., & Arnold, L. E. (2021). Moody kids years later: Long-term outcomes of youth from the Omega-3 and therapy

(OATS) studies. *Journal of Affective Disorders, 281*, 24–32. https://doi.org/10.1016/j.jad.2020.11.115

Fristad, M. A., Verducci, J. S., Walters, K., & Young, M. E. (2009). Impact of multifamily psychoeducational psychotherapy in treating children aged 8 to 12 years with mood disorders. *Archives of General Psychiatry, 66*(9), 1013–1020. https://doi.org/10.1001/archgenpsychiatry.2009.112

Fristad, M. A., Young, A. S., Vesco, A. T., Nader, E. S., Healy, K. Z., Gardner, W., Wolfson, H. L., & Arnold, L. E. (2015). A randomized controlled trial of individual family psychoeducational psychotherapy and omega-3 fatty acids in youth with subsyndromal bipolar disorder. *Journal of Child and Adolescent Psychopharmacology, 25*(10), 764–774. https://doi.org/10.1089/cap.2015.0132

Goldberg-Arnold, J. S., Fristad, M. A., & Gavazzi, S. M. (1999). Family psychoeducation: Giving caregivers what they want and need. *Family Relations: An Interdisciplinary Journal of Applied Family Studies, 48*(4), 411–417. https://doi.org/10.2307/585249

Goldstein, T. R., Fersch-Podrat, R. K., Rivera, M., Axelson, D. A., Merranko, J., Yu, H., Brent, D. A., & Birmaher, B. (2015). Dialectical behavior therapy for adolescents with bipolar disorder: Results from a pilot randomized trial. *Journal of Child and Adolescent Psychopharmacology, 25*(2), 140–149. https://doi.org/10.1089/cap.2013.0145

Goldstein, T. R., Merranko, J., Krantz, M., Garcia, M., Franzen, P., Levenson, J., Axelson, D., Birmaher, B., & Frank, E. (2018). Early intervention for adolescents at-risk for bipolar disorder: A pilot randomized trial of Interpersonal and Social Rhythm Therapy (IPSRT). *Journal of Affective Disorders, 235*, 348–356. https://doi.org/10.1016/j.jad.2018.04.049

Hauser, M., Galling, B., & Correll, C. U. (2013). Suicidal ideation and suicide attempts in children and adolescents with bipolar disorder: A systematic review of prevalence and incidence rates, correlates, and targeted interventions. *Bipolar Disorders, 15*(5), 507–523. https://doi.org/10.1111/bdi.12094

Hlastala, S. A., Kotler, J. S., McClellan, J. M., & McCauley, E. A. (2010). Interpersonal and social rhythm therapy for adolescents with bipolar disorder: Treatment development and results from an open trial. *Depression and Anxiety, 27*(5), 457–464. https://doi.org/10.1002/da.20668

Johnson, S. L., Gershon, A., & McMaster, K. J. (2017). Environmental risk and protective factors in bipolar disorder. In R. J. DeRubeis & D. R. Strunk (Eds.), *The Oxford Handbook of Mood Disorders* (pp. 132–141). Oxford University Press.

Kendall, P. C., & Beidas, R. (2007). Smoothing the trail for dissemination of evidence-based practices for youth: Flexibility within fidelity. *Professional Psychology: Research and Practice, 38*, 13–20.

Kendall, P. C. & Frank, H. (2018). Implementing evidence-based treatment protocols: Flexibility within fidelity. *Clinical Psychology: Science and Practice, 25*, 1–12. doi: 10.1111/cpsp.12271.

Kieseppä, T., Partonen, T., Haukka, J., Kaprio, J., & Lönnqvis, J. (2004). High concordance of bipolar I disorder in a nationwide sample of twins. *The American Journal of Psychiatry, 161*(10), 1814–1821. https://doi.org/10.1176/appi.ajp.161.10.1814

Lagace, D. C., & Kutcher, S. P. (2005). Academic performance of adolescents with bipolar disorder. *Directions in Psychiatry, 25*(2), 111–117.

Luby, J. L., & Navsaria, N. (2010). Pediatric bipolar disorder: Evidence for prodromal states and early markers. *Journal of Child Psychology and Psychiatry, 51*(4), 459–471. https://doi.org/10.1111/j.1469-7610.2010.02210.x

MacPherson, H. A., Algorta, G. P., Mendenhall, A. N., Fields, B. W., & Fristad, M. A. (2014). Predictors and moderators in the randomized trial of multifamily psychoeducational psychotherapy for childhood mood disorders. *Journal of Clinical Child and Adolescent Psychology, 43*(3), 459–472. https://doi.org/10.1080/15374416.2013.807735'

MacPherson, H. A., Mackinaw-Koons, B., Leffler, J. M., & Fristad, M. A. (2016). Pilot effectiveness evaluation of community-based multi-family psychoeducational psychotherapy for childhood mood disorders. *Couple and Family Psychology: Research and Practice, 5*(1), 43–59. https://doi.org/10.1037/cfp0000055

Mendenhall, A. N., Fristad, M. A., & Early, T. J. (2009). Factors influencing service utilization and mood symptom severity in children with mood disorders: Effects of multifamily psychoeducation groups (MFPGs). *Journal of Consulting and Clinical Psychology, 77*(3), 463–473. https://doi.org/10.1037/a0014527

Miklowitz, D. J. (2008). Adjunctive psychotherapy for bipolar disorder: State of the evidence. *The American Journal of Psychiatry, 165*(11), 1408–1419. https://doi.org/10.1176/appi.ajp.2008.08040488

Miklowitz, D. J., Axelson, D. A., Birmaher, B., George, E. L., Taylor, D. O., Schneck, C. D., Beresford, C. A., Dickinson, L. M., Craighead, W. E., & Brent, D. A. (2008). Family-focused treatment for adolescents with bipolar disorder: Results of a 2-year randomized trial. *Archives of General Psychiatry, 65*(9), 1053–1061. https://doi.org/10.1001/archpsyc.65.9.1053

Miklowitz, D. J., Axelson, D. A., George, E. L., Taylor, D. O., Schneck, C. D., Sullivan, A. E., Dickinson, L. M., & Birmaher, B. (2009). Expressed emotion moderates the effects of family-focused treatment for bipolar adolescents. *Journal of the American Academy of Child & Adolescent Psychiatry, 48*(6), 643–651. https://doi.org/10.1097/CHI.0b013e3181a0ab9d

Miklowitz, D. J., Chang, K. D., Taylor, D. O., George, E. L., Singh, M. K., Schneck, C. D., Dickinson, L. M., Howe, M. E., & Garber, J. (2011). Early psychosocial intervention for youth at risk for bipolar I or II disorder: A one-year treatment development trial. *Bipolar Disorders, 13*(1), 67–75. https://doi.org/10.1111/j.1399-5618.2011.00890.x

Miklowitz, D. J., George, E. L., Axelson, D. A., Kim, E. Y., Birmaher, B., Schneck, C., Beresford, C., Craighead, W. E., & Brent, D. A. (2004). Family-focused treatment for adolescents with bipolar disorder. *Journal of Affective Disorders, 82*(Suppl1), S113–S128. https://doi.org/10.1016/j.jad.2004.05.020

Miklowitz, D. J., Schneck, C. D., George, E. L., Taylor, D. O., Sugar, C. A., Birmaher, B., Kowatch, R. A., DelBello, M. P., & Axelson, D. A. (2014). Pharmacotherapy and family-focused treatment for adolescents with bipolar I and II disorders: A 2-year randomized trial. *The American Journal of Psychiatry, 171*(6), 658–667. https://doi.org/10.1176/appi.ajp.2014.13081130

Miklowitz, D. J., Schneck, C. D., Singh, M. K., Taylor, D. O., George, E. L., Cosgrove, V. E., Howe, M. E., Dickinson, L. M., Garber, J., & Chang, K. D. (2013). Early intervention for symptomatic youth at risk for bipolar disorder: A randomized trial of family-focused therapy. *Journal of the American Academy of Child & Adolescent Psychiatry, 52*(2), 121–131. https://doi.org/10.1016/j.jaac.2012.10.007

Miklowitz, D. J., Schneck, C. D., Walshaw, P. D., Singh, M. K., Sullivan, A. E., Suddath, R. L., Forgey Borlik, M., Sugar, C. A., & Chang, K. D. (2020). Effects of family-focused therapy vs enhanced usual care for symptomatic youths at high risk for bipolar disorder: A randomized clinical trial. *JAMA Psychiatry, 77*(5), 455–463. https://doi.org/10.1001/jamapsychiatry.2019.4520

Moos, R., & Moos, B. (1994). *Family Environment Scale Manual: Development, Applications, Research* (3rd ed.). Consulting Psychologist Press.

Nadkarni, R. B., & Fristad, M. A. (2010). Clinical course of children with a depressive spectrum disorder and transient manic symptoms. *Bipolar Disorders, 12*(5), 494–503. https://doi.org/10.1111/j.1399-5618.2010.00847.x

Nussbaum, L., Ogodescu, A., Hogea, L., & Zetu, I. (2017). Risk factors and resilience in the offspring of psychotic parents. *Revista de Cercetare si Interventie Sociala, 56*, 114–122.

O'Donnell, L. A., Axelson, D. A., Kowatch, R. A., Schneck, C. D., Sugar, C. A., & Miklowitz, D. J. (2017). Enhancing quality of life among adolescents with bipolar disorder: A randomized trial of two psychosocial interventions. *Journal of Affective Disorders, 219*, 201–208. https://doi.org/10.1016/j.jad.2017.04.039

O'Donnell, L. A., Weintraub, M. J., Ellis, A. J., Axelson, D. A., Kowatch, R. A., Schneck, C. D., & Miklowitz, D. J. (2020). A randomized comparison of two psychosocial interventions on family functioning in adolescents with bipolar disorder. *Family Process, 59*(2), 376–389. https://doi.org/10.1111/famp.12521

Pavuluri, M. N., Graczyk, P. A., Henry, D. B., Carbray, J. A., Heidenreich, J., & Miklowitz, D. J. (2004). Child- and family-focused cognitive-behavioral therapy for pediatric bipolar disorder: Development and preliminary results. *Journal of the American Academy of Child & Adolescent Psychiatry, 43*(5), 528–537. https://doi.org/10.1097/00004583-200405000-00006

Rich, B. A., Fromm, S. J., Berghorst, L. H., Dickstein, D. P., Brotman, M. A., Pine, D. S., & Leibenluft, E. (2008). Neural connectivity in children with bipolar disorder: Impairment in the face emotion processing circuit. *Journal of Child Psychology and Psychiatry, 49*(1), 88–96. https://doi.org/10.1111/j.1469-7610.2007.01819.x

Roley-Roberts, M. E., & Fristad, M. A. (2020). Moderators of treatment for pediatric bipolar spectrum disorders. *Journal of Clinical Child and Adolescent Psychology.* https://doi.org/10.1080/15374416.2020.1772082

Schenkel, L. S., & Towne, T. L. (2020). Errors in identifying emotion in body postures and facial expressions among pediatric patients with bipolar disorder. *Journal of Clinical and Experimental Neuropsychology, 42*(7), 735–746. https://doi.org/10.1080/13803395.2020.1799946

Stapp, E. K., Mendelson, T., Merikangas, K. R., & Wilcox, H. C. (2020). Parental bipolar disorder, family environment, and offspring psychiatric disorders: A systematic review. *Journal of Affective Disorders, 268*, 69–81. https://doi.org/10.1016/j.jad.2020.03.005

Sullivan, A. E., Judd, C. M., Axelson, D. A., & Miklowitz, D. J. (2012). Family functioning and the course of adolescent bipolar disorder. *Behavior Therapy, 43*(4), 837–847. https://doi.org/10.1016/j.beth.2012.04.005

Vance, Y. H., Jones, S. H., Espie, J., Bentall, R., & Tai, S. (2008). Parental communication style and family relationships in children of bipolar parents. *British Journal of Clinical Psychology, 47*(3), 355–359. doi:http://dx.doi.org.proxy.library.nd.edu/10.1348/014466508X282824

Van Meter, A., & Cosgrove, V. E. (2019). Overhauling technology-based interventions for young people with bipolar disorder: Lessons learned from adults. *Bipolar Disorders, 21*(1), 86–87. https://doi.org/10.1111/bdi.12716

Weintraub, M. J., Axelson, D. A., Kowatch, R. A., Schneck, C. D., & Miklowitz, D. J. (2019). Comorbid disorders as moderators of response to family interventions among adolescents with bipolar disorder. *Journal of Affective Disorders, 246,* 754–762. https://doi.org/10.1016/ j.jad.2018.12.125

West, A. E., Henry, D. B., & Pavuluri, M. N. (2007). Maintenance model of integrated psychosocial treatment in pediatric bipolar disorder: A pilot feasibility study. *Journal of the American Academy of Child & Adolescent Psychiatry, 46*(2), 205–212. https://doi.org/10.1097/01.chi.0000246068.85577.d7

West, A. E., Jacobs, R. H., Westerholm, R., Lee, A., Carbray, J., Heidenreich, J., & Pavuluri, M. N. (2009). Child and family-focused cognitive-behavioral therapy for pediatric bipolar disorder: Pilot study of group treatment format. *Journal of the Canadian Academy of Child and Adolescent Psychiatry / Journal de l'Académie Canadienne de Psychiatrie de L'enfant et de L'adolescent, 18*(3), 239–246.

West, A. E., Weinstein, S. M., Peters, A. T., Katz, A. C., Henry, D. B., Cruz, R. A., & Pavuluri, M. N. (2014). Child- and family-focused cognitive-behavioral therapy for pediatric bipolar disorder: A randomized clinical trial. *Journal of the American Academy of Child & Adolescent Psychiatry, 53*(11), 1168–1178. https://doi.org/10.1016/j.jaac.2014.08.013

Youngstrom, E., & Algorta, G. P. (2014). Features and course of bipolar disorder. In I. H. Gotlib & C. L. Hammen (Eds.), *Handbook of Depression.* (3rd ed.; pp. 142–161). The Guilford Press.

10

How to Bend but Not Break an Empirically Supported Treatment for Anxiety in Youth

LARA S. RIFKIN, LINDSAY MYERBERG,
ELIZABETH A. GOSCH, LESLEY A. NORRIS,
MARGARET E. CRANE, AND PHILIP C. KENDALL ■

Anxiety is common in youth and adolescents (Cartwright-Hatton et al., 2006; Merikangas et al., 2010). Left untreated, anxiety can lead to educational under-achievement, poor social relationships, suicidality, and substance abuse (Swan & Kendall, 2016; Wolk et al., 2015; Woodward & Fergusson, 2001). Research evidence documents that cognitive behavioral therapy (CBT) is an effective treatment for youth anxiety (Weisz et al., 2017), but the majority of youth with mental health problems do not receive mental health treatment (Merikangas et al., 2011), and fewer receive evidence-based treatments (Shafran et al., 2009).

Treatments found to be effective within a controlled setting may be less effective when implemented in less controlled community settings (Kazak et al., 2010; Kumpfer et al., 2002). Reduced efficacy may suggest that the treatment does not work as expected, that it has not been implemented properly, or that manualized treatments do not fit the needs of clients in the community (Sherrill, 2016). Conversely, service providers who do not adhere to the protocol (omit key treatment components) may undermine outcomes. Therein lies the tension between following a manual while adapting it to the needs of an individual client (Kendall & Frank, 2018). Adapting treatment manuals is a necessary part of using evidence-based treatments, but not all adaptations maintain treatment fidelity (Stirman et al., 2019). Indeed, evidence-based practice requires clinicians to balance implementing empirically supported treatments and patient needs. To achieve balance, we encourage therapists to use *flexibility within fidelity*. Within this approach, therapists implement the active ingredients of an intervention (Campbell et al., 2000), while flexibly tailoring the "adaptable periphery" (Damschroder et al., 2009). Therapists distinguish between "form" (e.g., an activity, a structure) and the function (i.e., the purpose, activity, or process by which an outcome is achieved) of a strategy (Hawe et al., 2004; Kirk et al., 2019; Wandersman et al., 2008).

We discuss how therapists can adapt treatments to fit individual clients. Although our considerations apply to CBT for anxious youth in general, we use the *Coping Cat* CBT program as an example (Kendall & Hedtke, 2006a). We first review various ways (i.e., forms) that the core components of the program (i.e., functions) can be implemented. We then discuss considerations needed when implementing the program with youth with various age/developmental levels, comorbidities, and socioeconomic and cultural backgrounds.

ESSENTIAL COMPONENTS IN COGNITIVE BEHAVIORAL THERAPY FOR ANXIOUS YOUTH

The essential components of CBT for anxious youth include (a) building rapport, (b) providing psychoeducation about anxiety, (c) addressing anxious self-talk, (d) conducting exposures, (e) assigning homework, and (f) providing rewards including praise.

Building Rapport

The goal of Session 1 is for the client to return for Session 2. Start with building rapport to foster a collaborative relationship. Research indicates that alliance is associated with improved outcomes in youth across diagnoses and therapy modalities (Shirk et al., 2011). Research examining CBT for anxious youth indicates that improvement in alliance over the course of treatment is associated with reduction in anxiety-symptom severity at posttreatment (e.g., Chiu et al., 2009; Marker et al., 2013). Rapport building can take numerous forms. Younger youth frequently enjoy playing a "get to know you" game in which the therapist and child take turns drawing cards that pose questions (e.g., "Do you have any pets?" "What is your least favorite food?"). This may be turned into a memory game where the therapist and youth go back through the cards to remember one another's answers and have the option to keep score. Older youth can be given the choice of using the cards or simply chatting. Youth also may be provided with an opportunity in the initial sessions to decorate their therapy workbook with stickers or drawings. Therapists reserve five to ten minutes at the end of each therapy session to engage in a fun activity selected by the youth (e.g., play a game, watch a YouTube video). Importantly, during exposure tasks completion is paired with a reward (e.g., watch a video, eat ice cream) to celebrate brave behavior.

Psychoeducation

Psychoeducation is provided at the start of treatment making it difficult to assess the added benefit beyond other components. Research examining pharmacological interventions for anxious adults has found, however, that psychoeducation leads to greater gains in the first few weeks of treatment (Dannon et al., 2002). In addition, psychoeducation is nearly always included in CBT for anxious youth (Becker et al., 2012). Part of psychoeducation is to normalize anxiety and set expectations for treatment. Youth are told that the goal of treatment is manage anxiety not to "get rid" of it. Modest degrees of anxiety are adaptive: They are useful warnings. A useful metaphor is an oversensitive fire alarm that sounds when cookies are getting crispy in the oven (not needed) rather than only when the curtains are on fire (needed). Psychoeducation includes discussion of the various physical expressions of emotions and physiological symptoms of anxiety. The therapist and youth can name as many feelings as possible and then discuss physical expressions of various emotions using family members as examples, or play feelings charades during which they take turns acting out and guessing emotions. Some youth enjoy creating a collage of various emotions by cutting out images from magazines. Younger youth typically enjoy drawing an outline of their body on a large sheet of paper and decorating it with the physical symptoms of anxiety that they commonly experience (e.g., butterflies in stomach, racing heart). Older youth may prefer to label a stick figure or to circle symptoms they frequently experience from a common list.

Addressing Anxious Self-Talk

Research indicates that the introduction of cognitive restructuring is associated with a significant acceleration in the rate of symptom reduction and improvement in global functioning (Peris et al., 2015). Research also has found that increases in use of cognitive restructuring during treatment are associated with anxiety-symptom reduction and a decrease in negative emotions in anxious youth (Ruocco et al., 2018), and that changes in cognition mediate symptom reduction in anxious youth (Chu & Harrison, 2007; Lau et al., 2010). More specifically, some work suggests that decreases in negative self-talk mediate outcome for anxious youth (Kendall & Treadwell, 2007; Treadwell & Kendall, 1996), and other work suggests that increases in positive self-talk mediate outcome (Hogendoorn et al., 2014). Anxious self-talk can be identified and addressed in a variety of ways; drawings with empty thought bubbles is a favorite. Worry can be externalized and labeled as the "worry monster" or "worry thoughts." The therapist might help the youth identify their worry thoughts by asking the youth to describe the worst case scenario and asking questions such as, "Then what?" and "What would be the worst part about that?"

Once youth have identified their anxious self-talk they are ready to learn to challenge it. Youth might be asked to answer a set of questions designed specifically to challenge anxious self-talk: How likely is an event to occur? Has it occurred before? After these questions are answered, youth are left with more realistic statements that they can use to construct a coping thought. Older youth sometimes find "thinking traps" helpful for identifying and challenging their negative self-talk. The therapist and the youth also might role play a dialogue with the worry monster. If the youth is amenable the therapist can play the worry monster, which provides the youth with the opportunity to "argue back" with coping thoughts. Youth who struggle to identify and challenge their negative self-talk may prefer to use general coping statements, which can be applied across feared situations (e.g., "I can do it!"). Finally, self-talk can be challenged directly during exposure tasks. Such behavioral experiments can allow the youth to "collect data" to test the validity of a worry thought. Alternatively, the therapist might have the youth write out a highly specific and measurable prediction about a feared situation and then compare the outcome to the initial prediction, noting any surprises.

Exposure

Science indicates that a crucial component in CBT for anxious youth is exposure (e.g., Peris et al., 2015; 2017). A recent meta-analysis examining 75 randomized controlled trials (RCTs) of CBT for anxious youth found that the amount of in-session exposure was positively associated with larger effect sizes both from pre- to post-treatment and between CBT and waitlist control conditions (Whiteside et al., 2020). In addition, other findings indicate that change occurs after initiation of exposure tasks in CBT for anxious youth (Kendall et al., 1997). During exposure tasks, youth are asked to engage with a feared situation, which facilitates learning that the situation is not as bad as they thought and that they can handle it. Exposure tasks help youth learn that they can be flexible in their responses to somatic and cognitive cues of anxiety (i.e., "I can be anxious and do something anyway." "Often, the more I do something hard the easier it gets.").

The therapist introduces gradual exposure by using metaphors such as slowly entering a cold swimming pool. The therapist might draw a graph using an example the youth is not fearful of (e.g., elevators) to illustrate the habituation curve while being clear that one must allow themselves to experience anxiety for it to decrease. The therapist and youth collaboratively develop the exposure hierarchy beginning with a fear that the youth is motivated to work on. Providing the youth with agency (choosing the exposure task) can increase engagement, so the therapist and youth collaboratively decide where to begin on the hierarchy. The therapist also may have a conversation with the youth stating that they will push the youth to engage in challenging tasks because they know that the youth can do them, but that they also invite the youth to push back if something is too hard. Youth do not always progress up their hierarchy in a linear fashion, often jumping to more difficult items, doing easier items, and repeating items.

Homework

The assignment of psychoeducation homework tasks is useful for shaping compliance with later at-home exposure tasks. Two studies have failed to find an association between homework adherence and treatment outcome for anxious youth (Arendt et al., 2016; Hughes & Kendall, 2007), but a third study examining the relationship between symptoms of autism spectrum disorder and treatment outcome for anxiety found that family CBT was more effective than individual CBT likely due to a greater number of at-home exposures that were conducted (Puleo & Kendall, 2011). Other work indicates that active participation from youth early in treatment (which includes completion of homework) is positively associated with outcome (Chu & Kendall, 2004; Tobon et al., 2011), again suggesting that early active participation may increase compliance with at-home exposures later in treatment. Completion of at-home exposures allow gains made in session to be solidified and facilitates generalization (Swan et al., 2016). For example, youth with difficulty separating from a caregiver might practice having their caregiver leave the clinic during session and then generalize this to a real situation in which the caregiver runs an errand without the child. Engaging in out-of-session exposures reinforces the idea of engaging in activities despite being anxious—making the shift to an "exposure lifestyle," where they view anxiety-provoking situations that occur in life as opportunities to practice "facing the worry monster" or "being brave."

Rewards/Praise

The use of rewards and praise encourages treatment engagement, which is associated with symptom remission and reduced functional impairment at posttreatment (Chu & Kendall, 2009; Gordon-Hollingsworth et al., 2015). Specifically, rewards and praise encourage both in- and out-of-session exposure completion (Houlding et al., 2010; Hudson & Kendall, 2002). Silverman and colleagues (1999) compared exposure with skills training including cognitive restructuring, self-evaluation, and reward to exposure with contingency management, including training parents in positive reinforcement, shaping, and consistency. Results indicated significant differences in disorder remission at posttreatment with 88% of youth who received the skills training including self-evaluation and reward achieving remission and 55% of youth whose parents received contingency management achieving remission (Silverman et al., 1999), providing additional evidence about the importance of including rewards.

The therapist might initially provide an example of training a dog to speak to illustrate that one rewards the dog for noise at first rather than for a perfect bark. Note that rewards are given for *effort* rather than the results. The therapist and youth collaboratively develop a list of rewards the youth can earn for entering feared situations and decide before exposure tasks which rewards will be earned for task completion. Reward lists contain a combination of material and social items (e.g., choose dinner pick an activity). The therapist asks the youth to describe how they think they did after each exposure task and thus reinforces effort. The therapist also encourages the youth to evaluate and reward themselves when faced with challenging tasks on their own (e.g., tell myself that I gave it a try). Finally, the therapist provides praise for and verbally reinforces brave behavior. The parent also may collaborate with the therapist and youth to structure exposure tasks and provide agreed upon rewards outside of session.

COMMONLY INCLUDED COMPONENTS IN COGNITIVE BEHAVIORAL THERAPY FOR ANXIOUS YOUTH

The treatment components discussed thus far are essential to maintain fidelity. The following components are often part of treating anxiety in youth but may or may not be included while still providing the empirically supported program.

Relaxation Training

Two meta-analyses that coded 111 CBT conditions (Whiteside et al., 2020) and 165 CBT conditions (Higa-McMillan et al., 2016) both indicated that roughly 50% of protocols did not include relaxation. Whiteside and colleagues (2020) found that treatment conditions that contained relaxation were associated with smaller effect sizes from pre- to post-treatment compared to treatment conditions that did not include relaxation. Other research indicates that relaxation is not associated with acceleration in symptom improvement over the course of treatment (Peris et al., 2015). In addition, relaxation is not included in some empirically supported CBT protocols for anxious youth, such as the Cool Kids Program (Lyneham et al., 2003; Rapee, 2000), indicating that it is not necessary to include it for effective change. Youth may be taught progressive muscle relaxation following scripts that are recorded for at-home practice. Youth also may be taught deep breathing as another alternative to calm their physiological responses.

Caregiver Psychoeducation

Caregiver psychoeducation is sometimes included in CBT for anxious youth, with one meta-analysis, which coded 165 CBT conditions for anxious youth, indicating that caregiver psychoeducation was included in 30% of protocols (Higa-McMillan et al., 2016). A key portion of caregiver education includes discussion of accommodation, during which time caregivers are encouraged to look for ways in which they may be assisting their child in avoiding feared situations. Research indicates that significant reductions in accommodation occur from pre- to posttreatment in CBT for anxious youth (Kagan, 2019; Kagan et al., 2016) and that reductions in accommodation are associated with posttreatment anxiety severity (Kagan et al., 2016). Caregiver psychoeducation about accommodation may be provided by illustrating the cycle of avoidance (which can be done by drawing an avoidance graph) and providing the rationale for building an exposure hierarchy. In addition, caregivers are encouraged to reward brave behavior. In some cases, caregivers may be explicitly trained to be an exposure coach, first by watching the therapist conduct exposures with the youth and later by leading exposures with the therapist present. Caregivers are encouraged to look for feared situations in real life (natural exposure opportunities) and think of ways to break them down and encourage approach with reward.

Coping Modeling

Coping modeling is a way for the therapist to demonstrate coping for the youth. It is a therapist style and often is included in CBT for anxious youth. Higa-McMillan and colleagues (2016) indicated that coping modeling was included in 35% of 165 coded CBT for anxious youth, and research suggests that increased coping efficacy mediates treatment gains in CBT for anxious youth (Kendall et al., 2016; Lau et al., 2010). When serving as a coping model, therapists describe how they themselves cope with anxiety. The therapist specifies an anxiety-provoking situation (e.g., teaching a class), describes the associated somatic responses and negative automatic thoughts, and then describes coping thoughts and models brave behavior. The therapist shares differences in somatic responses, cognitions, and coping strategies in both low and high anxiety-provoking situations (e.g., raising hand to answer a question in class, being a class instructor).

LESS COMMONLY INCLUDED COMPONENTS IN COGNITIVE BEHAVIORAL THERAPY FOR ANXIOUS YOUTH

Problem Solving

Problem solving is sometimes included in CBT protocols for anxious youth and was included in between 25% and 30% of the 165 study conditions of CBT for child anxiety coded by (Higa-McMillan et al., 2016). Some research indicates that problem solving is associated with increased coping efficacy (i.e., "There is something I can do to help myself when feeling overwhelmed."), which predicts outcome (Hogendoorn et al., 2014; Kendall et al., 2016). One study found that an increase in direct problem solving mediated decreases in anxiety symptoms from pre- to post-treatment (Hogendoorn et al., 2014). Problem solving helps youth generate and identify adaptive ways of coping with anxiety. First, the therapist introduces the idea of nonjudgmental brainstorming—select a common situation (e.g., you need to leave the house for school but can only find one shoe) as an example and take turns coming up with solutions. The therapist offers silly suggestions (e.g., walk on your hands all day) to keep it fun and to remind the youth to reserve judgment. Next, the youth and therapist go through each option discussing the pros, cons, and likely outcomes. Finally, the youth and therapist pick an option to try. Once this process has been illustrated to the youth through a lower-level example, the youth and therapist can practice applying it in different higher anxiety-provoking situations.

Maintenance/Relapse Prevention

Maintenance and relapse prevention strategies were included in around 25% of the 165 CBT study conditions for anxious youth coded by Higa-McMillan and colleagues (2016). There is insufficient research examining the association between inclusion of maintenance/relapse prevention in CBT for anxious youth and treatment outcome. However, one meta-analysis examining CBT for youth with internalizing disorders more broadly found that maintenance/relapse prevention was not significantly related to effect sizes at posttreatment or follow-up (Sun et al., 2019).

The purpose of relapse prevention is to consolidate learning and anticipate future challenges. The therapist may ask the youth to reflect on what they have learned in therapy by designing a "commercial" using video, drawing, song, or another means of creative expression. The youth also may describe to the therapist what they would tell a friend who is coming to the clinic for the first time about what to expect. The therapist normalizes the fact that there will continue to be times when coping with anxiety is difficult but that continued practice will lead to continued improvement.

FLEXIBLE APPLICATIONS WHILE MAINTAINING FIDELITY

Treatment can be flexibly applied based on age/developmental level and the presence of comorbid disorders including multiple anxiety disorders, Obsessive-Compulsive Disorder (OCD), Attention-Deficit/Hyperactivity Disorder (ADHD), Major Depressive Disorder (MDD), Disruptive Behavior Disorders, and Post-Traumatic Stress Disorder (PTSD). We will also discuss adaptations based on socioeconomic status and culture.

AGE/DEVELOPMENTAL LEVEL

The evidence supports that CBT strategies are effective for anxious youth of different ages (Kendall & Peterman, 2015). Across randomized controlled trials evaluating CBT for the treatment of anxiety in youth, age has not emerged as a meaningful predictor of differential outcomes (Compton et al., 2014; Manassis et al., 2014; Bennett et al., 2013). These "cross-age" positive treatment effects may be due to the fact that the treatments have been designed specifically for children and adolescents with developmental considerations in mind (e.g., the *Coping Cat*, Kendall & Hedtke 2006a; the *C.A.T Project*, Kendall et al., 2002). Although age can be a starting point for estimating a child's capabilities, youth vary widely in their cognitive, emotional, and social development. It is incumbent on clinicians to understand developmental norms and how to match intervention strategies to youth's abilities (Frankel et al., 2012). Cognitive, emotional, and social developmental levels impact children's ability to acquire and implement the various strategies taught in CBT.

A comparison between the *Coping Cat* (ages 8 to 13 years) and the *C.A.T. Project* (ages 14 to 17 years) illustrates how CBT strategies are adapted for different ages. Both protocols employ the same key CBT components; however, the CAT Project provides more detailed psychoeducational information about the causes of anxiety, and it spends less time on affective education and more time on cognitive skills (e.g., thinking traps). In addition, the CAT project places greater emphasis on encouraging adolescent autonomy (e.g., discussing differences between parent and child perspectives). In the following section, we provide examples of how to adapt a few key CBT anxiety treatment components to meet the needs of youth at varying developmental levels.

Cognitive Restructuring

A key CBT component involves the identification and modification of dysfunctional thought patterns (self-talk). Cognitive restructuring requires some level of metacognition (the ability to think about one's own thinking) as well as self-reflection (the ability to apply reasoning and metacognitive skills to one's own beliefs and actions; Frankel et al., 2012). As they age, children develop the ability to monitor their own thoughts and gain the capacity to report their thoughts to others. The ability to report on one's thoughts in the present develops before the ability to reflect on one's thoughts in the past or future (Frankel et al., 2012). Children's ability to see multiple aspects of a situation and examine contradictory evidence develops over time. Although problem-solving and metacognitive skills emerge in middle childhood, logical thinking remains somewhat concrete and tied to observable events (Kingery et al., 2006). As youth mature into adolescence, they develop more sophisticated reasoning and problem-solving abilities. They are better able to engage in conditional and hypothetical reasoning as well as consider multiple perspectives (Frankel et al., 2012). Adolescents, unlike children, may develop the capacity to distinguish theory from facts and logically test hypotheses by thinking about conflicting evidence simultaneously (Holmbeck et al., 2006).

Adaptations facilitate cognitive restructuring with children who exhibit developmentally appropriate cognitive limitations (e.g., more time devoted to teaching about thoughts with younger children). The *Coping Cat* suggests that caregivers and therapists provide scaffolding to help children reflect on their thinking—such as encouraging children to use concrete cues (e.g., somatic sensations or emotional reactions) to prompt thinking about thinking. It can be helpful to use other concrete, visual tools such as cartoons and thought bubbles applied to specific situations. For example, presenting children with a cartoon of a child in school taking a test helps them connect to the thoughts and feelings they may experience in that situation. Given that children with less mature cognitive abilities find it easier to reflect on their thoughts in the here-and-now, the use of role plays or games that induce some anxiety may help them "catch" their thoughts in the moment. Like Frankel and colleagues (2012), we recommend the use of more concrete role-play strategies based on actual situations from the child's life rather than hypothetical, abstract (e.g., "what if") future-oriented scenarios. It is also wise to avoid "if-then" language with children who display limited conditional and hypothetical reasoning abilities (e.g., "If I think I will fail, I will feel anxious."). We have found that using short, incomplete sentences to simplify the cognitive load when teaching about thoughts and feelings can be helpful (e.g., "When it is storming outside, I feel _____. I think _____."). The use of puppets and toys can facilitate the process of identifying children's beliefs. One young girl who had difficulty considering alternative perspectives was able to counter her own anxious self-talk when her therapist used a puppet to play the child's perspective while the child's puppet took on the role of "talking back" to anxiety with coping self-talk. Although understanding cognitive distortions may be beyond some children's abilities, we have found acting out one or two "mind-traps" (e.g., wearing dark-colored glasses, fortune telling) with props that are familiar to the child can facilitate understanding. Some children may not be able to identify their thoughts and may benefit from a few specific self-instructions (e.g., "Remember, I can do this."). We have created "coping key chains" (laminated coping statements and actions on a key ring) to provide concrete reminders of self-instructions for children to facilitate the use of coping strategies when experiencing anxiety.

For adolescents or youth with more advanced cognitive abilities, less time is needed to teach thought identification and evaluation. These youth are better equipped to engage in the metacognitive and reasoning processes. However, developmental characteristics associated with adolescence such as burgeoning identity formation, needs for autonomy, and the ability to hold more strongly entrenched beliefs can be a challenge (Frankel et al., 2012). These factors may impact adolescents' willingness to learn and participate in CBT (e.g., cognitive restructuring, therapeutic exposures). We have worked with many adolescents who can identify thinking patterns and beliefs that maintain their anxiety but are loathe to question them. They experience the evaluation of their beliefs, even in the spirit of collaboration, as a threat to their tenuous sense of identity and of autonomy. When adolescents reject evaluating thoughts (e.g., Socratic questioning, examining the evidence), we have found the use of motivational interviewing helpful (e.g., reflective listening, engaging in cost-benefit analyses, developing discrepancies between values and behavior; Naar-King & Suarez, 2011). Evaluating the helpfulness of a particular belief is more acceptable than questioning the veracity of the belief.

Relaxation

Relaxation training can follow progressive muscle relaxation scripts such as those by Koeppen (1974) for young children and Ollendick for older children (Ollendick & Cerny, 1981). We often provide a digital voice recording geared to the youth's age and interests with directions for relaxation exercises to practice at home. Younger children may prefer imagery (e.g., pretend you are squeezing lemons, now let your hand relax) or breathing exercises (e.g., blowing bubbles, take a breath so your belly rises) rather than progressive muscle relaxation. For young, active, or cognitively impaired children, shortened versions of these exercises and the rationale for relaxation are suggested. To support an adolescent's autonomy, we try several types of relaxation exercises (e.g., imagery, body scans, Progressive Muscle Relaxation [PMR], meditation) as well as provide a rationale that incorporates their interests. For example, one adolescent soccer player became interested in meditation when the therapist brought in examples of famous professional soccer players who used meditation techniques in their training. We typically provide more detailed information to adolescents regarding the brain processes involved in fear and anxiety as well as the body's stress response to facilitate their engagement with relaxation exercises.

Exposure

The concept of different levels of anxiety may be difficult to grasp for some children. Providing concrete, visual representations of different situations with anxiety ratings on cards arranged on a ladder helps the child begin to perceive differences in their anxiety levels. Depending on the child, the hierarchy may be limited to easy, medium, and difficult or may contain eight levels of difficulty. Parental input can be helpful.

For younger children or those with limited cognitive abilities, modifications can be made to exposure tasks to increase the probability that the child will remain engaged. For example, a concrete plan to use during the exposure phase can be developed, which may include one coping thought (e.g., "I can do it.") and a simplified problem-solving step (e.g., take deep breaths) followed by reward. Simplified pre- and post-exposure processing may occur. The child is asked how anxious they predict they will be on a simplified Subjective Units of Distress Scale (SUDS) (e.g., feelings thermometer) prior to and once during an exposure, comparing the visual representation of the two ratings after the exposure. To provide a concrete reminder of their success at being brave, photographs can be taken and printed of the child facing each of their fears. Parents may be more involved in the implementation and reinforcement of exposure activities with younger children.

With regard to adolescents, adaptations to exposure procedures involve greater efforts to promote engagement, motivation, and autonomy. Adolescents have greater input in the development of their anxiety hierarchy and treatment goals. They are given greater choice in their selection and implementation of exposures. We talk with adolescents about their values, how anxiety/avoidance is interfering with their ability to engage in activities they enjoy, and how engaging in exposures helps them act in accord with their beliefs. When processing exposures, adolescents are better able to generate predictions about how distressing the experience will be and the likelihood of various harmful outcomes, which they can compare to their actual experience following the exposure. When appropriate, we make more efforts to elicit adolescents' thoughts and what they learned from exposure activities (e.g., expectancy violations). We support adolescents in adapting an "exposure lifestyle" in which they plan how they will continue to engage in exposures posttreatment and how they will find reinforcement for doing so. Despite growing needs for autonomy, age-appropriate parental support may be required to help adolescents engage in exposure activities outside of sessions. For example, an adolescent with a fear of speaking to strangers had difficulty with an initial exposure (e.g., placing a food order) but found it helpful for her parents to prompt her to order her food and to reinforce her. Later in treatment, she independently completed exposures, but the initial support provided by her parents contributed to her success.

COMORBIDITY

Multiple Anxiety Disorders

Comorbidity across youth anxiety disorders is the norm, with 78% of one sample meeting criteria for two or more of the "big three" disorders (separation anxiety disorder [SAD], social anxiety disorder [SoP], or generalized anxiety disorder [GAD]; Kendall et al., 2010). Presence of comorbid anxiety disorders does not consistently predict or moderate differential treatment outcomes (Compton et al., 2014; Knight, McLellan, Jones, & Hudson, 2014; Nilsen, Eisemann, & Kvernmo, 2013; Norris & Kendall, in press), although there is some suggestion youth with primary SoP, while responding favorably to treatment, may be less responsive than others (see Knight et al., 2014; Nilsen et al., 2013). Other analyses have suggested that youth with SoP may respond optimally to treatments including medication, although findings are inconsistent across studies and may be driven by symptom severity more globally (Norris et al., 2020).

Cognitive Behavioral Therapy for youth anxiety was developed to target the range of anxiety disorders, so minimal modifications are needed when treating co-occurring anxiety disorders. We typically teach coping skills using examples that tap core fears of the principal disorder so that skills generalize across situations. For example, cognitive restructuring can be applied to both what the "worry monster" says in social situations and when more generalized anxious self-talk arises. For exposures, we collaboratively build hierarchies to target worries associated with each presenting disorder and implement graduated exposure along each hierarchy. For example, for youth who present with both social worries and generalized intolerance of uncertainty (IU), exposures to social evaluative situations (e.g., sending a text message to a peer, talking with a stranger, giving a presentation, ordering a snack) can also target IU by having the youth choose the exposure of the day out of a hat, rather than planning in advance. We typically implement this later on in treatment as "buy in" to the exposure model increases, with some reminders from the therapist that "exposure is something I do *with* you, not *to* you."

Obsessive-Compulsive Disorder

Obsessive-Compulsive Disorder (OCD) is often comorbid with anxiety disorders, with research indicating that roughly 40% of youth with OCD meet diagnostic criteria for another anxiety disorder (Ivarsson et al., 2008; Swedo et al., 1989). CBT is an empirically supported treatment for childhood OCD, but the cognitive restructuring and exposures are applied differently (Piacentini et al., 2002; Piacentini & Langley, 2004). Storch and colleagues (2008) found that treatment response in CBT for OCD was not impacted by anxiety comorbidity, suggesting that CBT for OCD is appropriate for youth with principal OCD and comorbid anxiety disorders. It remains unclear, however, whether comorbid OCD impacts treatment response in CBT for anxious youth. For youth with a principal anxiety diagnosis and comorbid OCD a traditional CBT protocol can be applied with several important adaptations taken from CBT for OCD protocols (e.g., Piacentini et al., 2007).

In cognitive restructuring we focus on helping the youth identify anxious thoughts and label them as worry thoughts or OCD thoughts. We provide basic education on obsessions and compulsions (see Franklin OCD chapter) and illustrate differences between obsessions that necessitate a rigid response and other worries using specific examples relevant to the youth. We focus on identifying and labeling obsessions and anxious thoughts (Piacentini et al., 2002) rather than generating adaptive responses to OCD thoughts (i.e., arguing with the OCD).

We note caution when teaching relaxation, given that it can become ritualized. We may teach progressive muscle relaxation but emphasize that it is not to be used in response to OCD thoughts. Finally, exposures that target OCD focus on response prevention and may include behavioral experiments to target specific obsessive thought. We may elect to begin assigning exposure and response prevention tasks to target OCD earlier in treatment (e.g., Sessions 3 to 8), particularly if anxiety and OCD are co-principal.

Attention-Deficit/Hyperactivity Disorder

Epidemiological studies indicate that approximately 25% of youth diagnosed with anxiety disorders exhibit comorbid Attention-Deficit/Hyperactivity

Disorder (ADHD; Lawrence et al., 2015; Larson, Russ, Kahn, & Halfon, 2011). Although a strong evidence base supports the effectiveness of CBT for anxiety, there have been mixed findings regarding the effectiveness of CBT for children with both anxiety and ADHD. Findings from the Child/ Adolescent Multisite Study (CAMS) suggest that children with anxiety and ADHD did not respond as favorably to CBT alone at posttreatment, although these differences were not evident at six-month follow-up (Halldorsdottir et al., 2015). Several small studies, however, have demonstrated the efficacy of CBT programs specifically designed for the treatment of comorbid anxiety and ADHD in children (Sciberras et al., 2018; Jarrett & Ollendick, 2012) and adolescents (Houghton et al., 2017). Parental involvement may be important for children experiencing attentional and behavioral impairments common to ADHD (Maric et al., 2018).

It appears that youth with anxiety and ADHD can benefit from CBT for anxiety with some adaptations. The adaptations include an activity schedule and positive reinforcement to support on-task behavior, one-minute breaks between activities, shorter directions and descriptions of major concepts, greater repetition of instructions and key concepts, and visual aids to facilitate skills practice and exposure activities (Sciberras et al., 2018). When delivering the *Coping Cat* to children with ADHD, we use similar strategies to address the attentional, motivational, and behavioral impairments characteristic of ADHD. We meet with these children in a room with few distractions, sitting next to the child at a table that has only a few items on it. We use a whiteboard on which the child writes the tasks we will accomplish in session and checks them off as they are accomplished. Depending on the child's needs, we provide opportunities to earn points and direct reinforcement for on-task behavior (e.g., take five minutes to play after completing two tasks). Although we always try to incorporate a child's interests into our discussion of CBT concepts, we make an even greater effort to do so with these children to support their engagement. We attempt to facilitate learning through concrete visual aids and hands-on practice as much as possible (e.g., illustrating their somatic symptoms on a life-sized body drawing). Some children find fidget toys helpful while attending sessions; other children may find them too distracting. When using the *Coping Cat Workbook*, we may cover all the material on a page except for the particular item we are discussing. We provide information to the child in small, manageable chunks and have the child frequently repeat back what they have heard or understood.

Children with ADHD require greater support from their parents to cue and reinforce the skills they learn in CBT as well as to engage in therapeutic exposures. We typically invite parents in for a portion of a session, allowing the child to tell the parents what they learned. For example, we have the child teach the parent a short relaxation exercise to help the child remember the skill and to encourage a sense of mastery. We provide short, visually clear instructions for completing homework activities that are reviewed with both the child and the parent. In some cases, we might use visual prompts and text messages to cue out-of-session exposure exercises. We may help parents implement a home reward program, often with a visual reward chart. We have found these youth to benefit from CBT when we partner with parents to support them in this endeavor.

Disruptive Behavior Disorders

The co-occurrence of anxiety and symptoms of disruptive behavior disorders (i.e., oppositional defiant disorder [ODD] and conduct disorder [CD]) in youth occurs across developmental periods (e.g., Cunningham & Ollendick, 2010; Drabick et al., 2010; Marmorstein, 2007; Martin et al., 2014; Suveg et al., 2009). Co-occurring DBD may affect treatment, although research is mixed and studies typically include attention-deficit/hyperactivity disorder (ADHD) in the category of externalizing disorders along with ODD and CD (e.g., Kreuze et al., 2018). Findings indicate that the presence of externalizing disorders does not moderate anxiety outcomes (e.g., Compton et al., 2014; Flannery-Schroeder et al., 2004; Ginsburg et al., 2011; Ollendick et al., 2015; Southam-Gerow et al., 2001; Thirlwall et al., 2017; Wergeland et al., 2016), but other studies have found that co-occurring DBDs were associated with poorer anxiety outcomes (e.g., Hudson et al., 2013; Ginsburg et al., 2014; Hudson et al., 2015). Research suggests it is difficult to treat anxiety in the context of coercive parent-child interactions, which are often present in the context of DBDs (Rahman et al., 2013).

We make adaptations when treating youth with co-occurring disruptive behavior disorders and anxiety using *Coping Cat*. First, we may conduct a functional behavioral analysis (FBA) to determine how the anxiety and DBD symptoms interact and what factors maintain each set of symptoms (Rahman et al., 2013). We regularly incorporate parent management training (PMT), one of the most commonly used empirically supported interventions for DBDs (Eyberg et al., 2008), which provides caregivers with strategies to increase compliance and decrease disruptive behaviors (Dedousis-Wallace et al., 2020). During psychoeducation we provide caregivers with information about the causes of disruptive behavior to help them differentiate between oppositionality that functions to avoid anxiety from oppositionality that functions for other reasons (e.g., attention-seeking). This knowledge can increase caregivers' awareness of the ways in which they accommodate their child's anxiety by "giving in" to disruptive behaviors (e.g., allowing their child to opt out of an exposure due to refusal to participate), thereby helping caregivers limit accommodation of anxiety while also reducing the likelihood of reinforcing the disruptive behavior. We also emphasize differential attention (e.g., positive attending, ignoring minor undesired behaviors), effective commands, limit setting, and developmentally appropriate contingency management programs, which can be done in the first parent session of the *Coping Cat* program. We frequently ask caregivers to complete Antecedent–Behavior–Consequence charts to provide the therapist with more data to inform treatment adaptations. Finally, we focus on using behavioral strategies ourselves within sessions, such as setting an agenda at the start of each session and setting clear limits within sessions. During sessions with the child, we incorporate the same skills we encourage caregivers to use, including differential attention, labelled praise, effective commands, limit setting, and reward systems.

Depression

Anxiety disorders frequently co-occur with depression in youth (Cummings et al, 2014; Garber & Weersing, 2010); however, findings examining treatment outcome in anxious youth with comorbid depression are mixed. One review found that five out of seven studies indicated that the presence of a comorbid major depressive episode predicted worse treatment outcome, with effect sizes ranging from small to large (Walczak et al., 2018). A recent study directed at clarifying the role of depression in outcomes for youth anxiety found that youth with anxiety disorders and comorbid depression had significantly higher anxiety disorder severity and poorer overall functioning at pretreatment compared to those without comorbid depression (Frank et al., 2020), but there were no significant differences between groups in the amount of improvement on overall symptoms, functioning, and anxiety severity at posttreatment. Interestingly, youth with comorbid depression had more severe overall symptoms, functioning, and anxiety severity at posttreatment compared to those without comorbid depression, indicating that although symptoms improved proportionally, these youth may benefit from additional treatment. Overall, it appears that CBT is effective for youth with comorbid anxiety and depression.

When delivering *Coping Cat* to youth with depression, we address the cognitive and behavioral impairments characteristic of anxiety and depression concurrently. First, lack of enjoyment and motivation may interfere with completion of assigned tasks. We may elect to assign a "fun" activity for the youth to engage in over the week, encourage the youth (with support of parents) to participate in the activity regardless of how they feel beforehand and to observe how they feel after. We also strive to include enjoyable activities in session (e.g., go for a walk while discussing particular principles) to illustrate to the youth that activities they did not initially think would be pleasurable may be.

Given that depressed youth focus on past negative events and create negative internal attributions to these events, addressing cognition is important. We address and challenge depressed self-talk. Self-evaluation and reward can be important for depressed youth who often have unrealistic expectations; we shift these unrealistic expectations by prompting the youth to set measurable objective goals for exposure tasks and to self-evaluate and reward themselves.

Trauma

Approximately two thirds of youth reported one or more traumatic events by age 16 (Copeland et al., 2007). Longitudinal studies suggest that post-traumatic stress disorder (PTSD) following such events can be associated with subsequent anxiety disorders (Cortes et al., 2005). Youth trauma histories are important in the treatment of youth anxiety yet few studies have examined whether history of traumatic experiences is associated with differential treatment response among anxious youth, although the experience of negative life events more broadly have been associated with negative long-term outcomes (Casline et al., 2021; Ginsburg et al., 2014; Ginsburg et al., 2018; Kendall et al., 2004) and childhood trauma has been associated with poorer outcomes for youth with depression (e.g., Asarnow et al., 2009; Barbe et al., 2004; Lewis et al., 2010). It is worth noting that some youth anxiety treatment studies exclude primary PTSD (Nilsen et al., 2013), which may preclude examination of traumatic experiences as a predictor or moderator of outcome.

The common elements across well-established treatments for youth who have been exposed to traumatic events (i.e., psychoeducation, training in emotion regulation strategies, imaginal and in-vivo exposure, cognitive processing and problem solving; Dorsey et al., 2017) overlap with core components of youth anxiety treatments, and we implement them flexibly to address both anxiety symptoms and symptoms of post-traumatic stress. First, we include information about trauma prevalence during psychoeducation (Dorsey et al., 2017) to both youth and caregivers (keep in mind that youth may not have disclosed their trauma to caregivers [Cohen et al., 2010a; Dorsey et al., 2017; Gerson & Rappaport, 2013]). We may integrate cognitive processing during cognitive restructuring. For example, while putting the "anxiety monster" on trial in other anxiety domains, self-blame or overgeneralizations can also be critically examined and negative misappraisals are addressed (Smith et al., 2019), emphasizing youth resiliency throughout. We may consider discussion of true versus false anxiety alarms in these sections through a "trauma lens" (i.e., a true alarm may occur in the presence of an offending individual vs. a false alarm safety concern that is generalized to all adults).

We implement in-vivo and imaginal exposures flexibly to address post-traumatic stress. For example, we may encourage youth to gradually write a booklet with different chapters discussing the traumatic event (Pine & Cohen, 2002) and to begin to approach innocuous trauma reminders (Cohen et al., 2010a; Cohen et al., 2010b). We implement this simultaneously with other exposures targeting different anxiety domains. For example, youth who present with co-occurring GAD and trauma may experience safety concerns. The hierarchy can be built to target both nontrauma-related fears (e.g., taking the subway) and those that stem from traumatic experiences (e.g., being in an environment that leads to trauma reminders). Of note, some research suggests that explicit exposure (i.e., trauma narratives) may not be necessary for efficacious treatment (David et al., 2012; Deblinger et al., 2011; Salloum & Overstreet, 2012) and that lower-level exposures to the traumatic event via other treatment components may be sufficient (Dorsey et al., 2017).

SOCIOECONOMIC STATUS

As of 2019, 10.5% of the population in the United States are living in poverty (U.S. Census Bureau, 2019) and socioeconomic inequality continues to increase

(Saez & Zucman, 2020). It is important to adapt CBT to address youth anxiety across socioeconomic backgrounds (Hittner et al., 2019). That said, socioeconomic status (SES) is not a consistent predictor of outcomes following CBT for youth anxiety. Whereas some studies suggest lower SES predicts poorer long-term CBT outcomes (Ginsburg et al., 2014; Kodal et al., 2018; Nevo et al., 2014; Taylor et al., 2018; Weisz et al., 2013; Wergeland et al., 2016), other studies have not found an association between SES and CBT outcomes (e.g., Compton et al., 2014; Kennedy et al., 2018; Southam-Gerow et al., 2001). A review of short-term follow-up studies found that SES did not predict CBT outcomes, suggesting perhaps the role of SES in CBT outcomes may depend on timing of posttreatment assessment (Knight et al., 2014). This difference between short- and long-term outcomes may be related to the pervasive influence of low SES on youth anxiety over time (Kessler et al., 2012; Najman et al., 2010). In addition, limited financial resources may impact a family's ability to engage in treatment. For example, low-income families may not be able to implement reward systems comparable to their higher-income counterparts. The likelihood that a low SES family may not follow through with homework is increased, which is problematic given that some research suggests homework adherence predicts CBT outcomes (e.g., Arendt et al., 2016). Our treatment adaptations are·rooted in a sensitivity to family resources: for families with less financial resources we help caregivers incorporate more social rewards or privileges (e.g., watch a favorite TV show; pick a game or activity for family to play; stay up past bedtime on weekends). Given individuals from low-SES backgrounds are more frequently exposed to barriers, negative events, and uncertainties (Roy et al., 2004), it is essential to understand how this applies to one's client.

CULTURE

Research on cultural adaptations of interventions often defines culture as either a set of "practices" or a set of "values" held by the client (Frese, 2015). Other research differentiates between culturally informed modifications to *content* (e.g., language, use of concepts) versus *process* (e.g., involvement of family members; Lau, 2006). Cultural groups exhibit different "levels of identification" within a common culture and individuals are impacted by intersecting identities (Marsiglia & Booth, 2015). We invite clients to share anything about their own or their family's background they think would be important for us to know, such as race or ethnic background, gender, sexual orientation, faith or religion, communities to which one belongs, languages spoken, and where one or one's family is from.

Research suggests cultural factors impact presentation and expression of symptoms, treatment-seeking behaviors, and treatment delivery of mental health problems among children and adolescents (Koydemir & Essau, 2018). Intervention adaptation is therefore necessary to fit the needs of populations differing in cultural or ethnic/racial backgrounds.

Cultural Variations in Anxiety Treatment Outcomes

Some research findings suggest that demographic factors predict youth adherence to anxiety treatment, although findings are mixed. For instance, ethnic minority youth and youth from single-parent households are more likely to prematurely terminate CBT treatment (Kendall & Sugarman, 1997), whereas others have found no significant associations between demographics and youth adherence to treatment (Chu & Kendall, 2004). Given that treatment adherence is related to treatment outcomes (Lee et al., 2019), these findings have implications for when cultural adaptations are needed. There are also mixed findings regarding whether cultural factors moderate treatment outcomes for youth participating in CBT for anxiety disorders. Among a diverse sample (40.9% Caucasian, 59.1% Hispanic/ Latinx), anxiety outcomes did not vary by Latinx ethnicity or Spanish language use in the intervention (Pina et al., 2012). Note that Pina and colleagues (2012) examined a "culturally sensitive" intervention. Likewise, African American/Black and white youth have been found to be similar with respect to baseline anxiety symptoms and CBT outcomes (Gordon-Hollingsworth et al., 2015).

Other findings suggest race and ethnicity are linked to CBT outcomes for anxiety among children and adolescents. For example, a randomized controlled trial comparing parent-involved CBT and peer-involved group CBT found parental acculturation level moderated CBT outcomes among Latinx youth with anxiety disorders (Vaclavik et al., 2017). Specifically, at low levels of parental acculturation, youth anxiety ratings were lower following the peer-involved group intervention than the parent-involved intervention. At high levels of parental acculturation, however, anxiety ratings at posttreatment were lower among youth who had received the parent-involved intervention than youth who had received the peer-involved group intervention (Vaclavik et al., 2017).

Effectiveness of Culturally Adapted Cognitive Behavioral Therapy for Youth Anxiety

Although there is limited research comparing the effectiveness of culturally adapted CBT versus nonadapted ("regular") CBT (Ishikawa et al., 2019; Koydemir & Essau, 2018), there are a growing, albeit limited, number of studies examining the effectiveness of adapted evidence-based CBT programs for treating anxiety among youth across the globe. In fact, adaptations of the *Coping Cat* program (Kendall & Hedtke, 2006a; 2006b) have been tested in numerous RCTs across various countries (Lenz, 2015).

Japan

A Japanese translation of the *Coping Cat* program was tested among clinic-referred youth ($N = 45$; ages 6 to 11 years) randomly assigned to treatment or waitlist (Lau et al., 2010). Findings indicated significant improvements in youth self-report and caregiver report of anxiety symptoms, and 65% of youth diagnosed with an anxiety disorder at pretreatment no longer met diagnostic criteria at posttreatment (Lau et al., 2010). The adaptations to the program included replacing the "FEAR" acronym used to help youth remember skills with a more culturally relevant acronym and incorporating culturally specific analogies (e.g., kung fu) throughout (Lau et al., 2010). The authors also incorporated culturally specific illustrations as well as vignettes in which Japanese children tend to experience anxiety (Lau et al., 2010). Likewise, the language used to describe emotions was informed by research on the relation between self-statements and anxiety symptoms in Japanese youth (Ishikawa & Sakano, 2005). Given that it is uncommon in Japanese culture for children to be seen by a health professional without a caregiver present, caregivers remained in the same room as their child during psychoeducational portions of the protocol (Lau et al., 2010).

The Netherlands

A Dutch version of *Coping Cat* (*Dappere Kat*; Nauta & Scholing, 1998) has been found to be effective in reducing anxiety symptoms among Dutch youth (Nauta et al., 2003). Children with anxiety disorders ($N = 79$; ages 7 to 18 years) randomly assigned to treatment showed significant reductions in anxiety symptoms following the intervention compared to children on waitlist (Nauta et al., 2003). Several adaptations were made while maintaining fidelity to the core components of the program (Nauta et al., 2003). Adaptations included reducing the original 16 sessions to 12 sessions, beginning exposures in Session 4, teaching skills in parallel to exposures rather than beforehand, and adding additional workbook pages for adolescents with more "profound" explanations of cognitive strategies (Nauta et al., 2003).

Canada

Mendlowitz and colleagues (1999) examined *The Coping Bear* program (Scapillato & Mendlowitz, unpublished, 1993). The 16-session individual Coping Cat was restructured into a 12-session group program. Three conditions were compared: (1) parent and child groups, (2) child-only groups, and (3) parent-only groups. Children with anxiety disorders ($N = 62$; ages 7 to 12 years) and their caregivers were randomly assigned and all groups exhibited a decrease in anxiety symptoms following treatment (Mendlowitz et al., 1999). Children in the parent-child groups, however, demonstrated more frequent use of active coping skills posttreatment, and parents of these children reported greater improvements in their children's emotional well-being compared to the other two conditions (Mendlowitz et al., 1999).

Norway

Examining the effectiveness of the Coping Cat program in routine clinical settings, Villabø and colleagues (2018) evaluated a Norwegian version of the manual (Kendall & Martinsen, 2008; Kendall, Martinsen, & Neumer, 2006) among youth throughout Norway. Children ($N = 165$; ages 7 to 13 years) were randomly assigned to the individual treatment, group treatment, or a waitlist. Findings revealed that for children with a primary diagnosis of generalized anxiety or separation anxiety, individual and group CBT were equally effective, whereas the group-based format was more effective than the individual format for children with social anxiety disorder at immediate follow-up. By two-year follow-up, however, both treatments were comparable in terms of youth anxiety symptoms (Villabø et al., 2018).

Pakistan

Khan and colleagues (2020) translated the Coping Cat program into Urdu for Pakistani children and adapted the protocol based on cultural factors. The protocol was tested among 24 Pakistani children (ages 8 to 13 years) in an orphanage setting and participants were randomly assigned to either treatment or waitlist. Given the context, caregiver-only sessions (Session 4 and Session 9) were unable to be conducted. Nevertheless, findings indicated significant positive effect on reducing anxiety sensitivity and anxiety symptoms in children (Khan et al., 2020).

Following Lee and colleagues' (2008) "planned adaptation approach," which resolves the tension between implementing programs with fidelity and the need to tailor programs to fit the target population, a literature review was conducted to understand the program's theoretical basis and to maintain the fidelity of the core components of the program. The workbook name was translated to *Bahdur Billi* in Urdu and "simple everyday language" was used to translate the various components of the program. The "FEAR" acronym was revised into an Urdu language poem (while still representing the core principles of CBT). Other "surface level" modifications included changing some of the pictures and names of characters in the workbook so that the content was more relatable to Pakistani children (e.g., Abraham Lincoln was replaced with Quaid-i-Azam). The authors reported that special consideration was given to translating the emotional expressions, cultural jargon, and culturally specific information by bearing in mind the developmental perspective of Pakistani children (Khan et al., 2020).

Iran

Dadsetan and colleagues (2011) tested an Iranian version of Coping Cat among 80 third to fifth grade youth randomly assigned to a treatment or no-treatment group. Findings demonstrated significant posttreatment reductions in anxiety symptoms with over 30% of youth ($N = 80$; 3rd to 5th grade) no longer meeting criteria for a diagnosis following the intervention (Dadsetan et al., 2011). Shokri Mirhosseini and colleagues (2018) also tested an adapted version of Coping Cat in Iranian youth (ages 9 to 11 years). Children were randomly assigned to the Coping Cat or a no-treatment condition and results demonstrated significant reductions in anxiety disorder symptoms at posttreatment and after one-month follow-up (Shokri Mirhosseini et al., 2018).

Brazil

A Brazilian adaptation of Coping Cat demonstrated substantial treatment effects for anxiety symptoms among youth ($N = 28$; ages 10 to 17 years) in an open trial (de Souza et al., 2013). The authors conducted a pilot study to assess "suitability" in a Brazilian population and the Brazilian protocol included two additional caregiver sessions. Families reported that the extra sessions were very important in understanding and learning how to respond to their child's anxiety (de Souza et al., 2013).

Australia

Barrett, Dadds, and Rapee (1996) tested *The Coping Koala* (Barrett, Dadds, & Holland, 1994; adapted *Coping Cat*) among Australian youth with one or more anxiety disorders ($N = 79$; ages 7 to 14 years). Participants were randomly assigned to one of three conditions: The Coping Koala, the Coping Koala plus family management, or a waitlist control group. The name and context within illustrative examples were changed, while the order, content, and processes of skills modules remained intact across adaptations (Lenz, 2015). Results indicated that both treatment conditions demonstrated greater benefits than the control group, although the treatment condition with family management demonstrated some added benefits (Barrett et al., 1996).

Overall, the findings from various cultures provide support for the flexibility within fidelity framework; evidence-based interventions for anxiety among youth can be adapted, remain true to the core components, and have beneficial outcomes. That said, cultural adaptations are not only important when implementing a program in a different country. We implement the *Coping Cat* program flexibly based on cultural factors including race/ethnicity, religion, and child-rearing practices.

Race/Ethnicity

Given that barriers to treatment are greater among marginalized racial/ethnic minority groups, it is worthwhile to promote session attendance. The role of intergenerational trauma and systemic racism in anxiety symptoms is important to assess among youth from racial/ethnic minority backgrounds, such as those from African descent (Gregory, 2019). We are careful to consider the ways in which cognitive restructuring is used with marginalized groups, whose worry thoughts in many cases are not irrational and are, in fact, based on lived experiences. For instance, advising youth from marginalized groups to question the likelihood of a feared outcome may not only be particularly unhelpful, but also quite invalidating to youth (Graham, Sorenson, & Hayes-Skelton, 2013) and damaging to the alliance. Instead, we focus on validating the youth's experience while helping the youth decipher between irrational negative automatic thoughts and more realistic ones.

Religious or Spiritual Beliefs

At times, a child's religious or spiritual beliefs are incorporated into treatment. For instance, religious beliefs may be used in developing effective coping statements. The degree to which an exposure is aligned with a family's cultural values and practices is also considered. In other words, we parse apart anxiety that is consistent with cultural norms versus anxiety that exceeds cultural norms. For example, an appropriate social anxiety exposure for an adolescent from a nonreligious background, such as introducing oneself and shaking the hand of someone of the opposite sex would be inappropriate for a child from an orthodox religious background whose practices would preclude touching of the opposite sex.

Child-Rearing Practices

Cultural differences in parenting can impact anxiety symptoms in youth (Varela & Hensley-Maloney, 2009) and influence aspects of treatment. For example, a family may not feel comfortable allowing their child to tolerate distress and are therefore more likely to accommodate their child's anxiety, which has negative implications for likelihood of following through with at-home exposures. In these cases, parental psychoeducation may need to be expanded upon to include conversations with caregivers regarding their overarching long-term goals for their child and how treatment is consistent with these larger goals. Information about child-rearing practices can be assessed at the onset of treatment (Besteiro & Quintanilla, 2017; Lindhout et al., 2009).

CONCLUSION

Cognitive Behavioral Therapy for youth anxiety, as illustrated by The *Coping Cat* program, is implemented flexibly based on considerations including age/developmental level, co-occurring disorders, SES, and cultural factors to enhance outcomes. For fidelity, the program adheres to key components: building rapport, providing psychoeducation about anxiety, addressing anxious self-talk, conducting exposures, assigning homework, and providing rewards/praise. The essential components, however, are applied with flexibility.

Research is needed to evaluate strategies to increase continued fidelity to the core components of treatment. Sadly, approximately three years after receiving training, less than 10% of therapists used the full protocol, with exposures and homework being the least commonly used (Chu et al., 2015). This finding is noteworthy because homework and exposures are essential components of effective CBT (e.g., Higa-McMillan et al., 2016; Kazantzis et al., 2016). Peer consultation and supervision may be valuable for maintaining fidelity while flexibly applying the program to a specific client (Becker-Haimes et al., 2020). Funding agencies may consider enhanced reimbursement rates for those who use evidence-based practices with fidelity as a way to encourage their proper use (Powell et al., 2016).

REFERENCES

Arendt, K., Thastum, M., & Hougaard, E. (2016). Homework adherence and cognitive behaviour treatment outcome for children and adolescents with anxiety disorders. *Behavioural and Cognitive Psychotherapy, 44,* 225–235.

Asarnow, J. R., Emslie, G., Clarke, G., Wagner, K. D., Spirito, A., Vitiello, B., Iyengar, S., Shamseddeen, W., Ritz, L., Birmaher, B., Ryan, N., Kennard, B., Mayes, T., DeBar, L., McCracken, J., Strober, M., Suddath, R., Leonard, H., Porta, G., . . . & Brent, D. (2009). Treatment of selective serotonin reuptake inhibitor—resistant depression in adolescents: Predictors and moderators of treatment response. *Journal of the American Academy of Child & Adolescent Psychiatry, 48,* 330–339.

Barbe, R. P., Bridge, J. A., Birmaher, B., Kolko, D. J., & Brent, D. A. (2004). Lifetime history sexual abuse, clinical presentation, and outcome in a clinical trial for adolescent depression. *The Journal of Clinical Psychiatry, 65,* 77–83.

Barrett, P. M., Dadds, M. R., & Holland, D. E. (1994). *The Coping Koala: Prevention manual* [Unpublished manuscript]. The University of Queensland, Queensland, Australia.

Barrett, P. M., Dadds, M. R., & Rapee, R. M. (1996). Family treatment of childhood anxiety: A controlled trial. *Journal of Consulting and Clinical Psychology, 64,* 333–342.

Becker, E. M., Becker, K. D., & Ginsburg, G. S. (2012). Modular cognitive behavioral therapy for youth with anxiety disorders: A closer look at the use of specific modules and their relation to treatment process and response. *School Mental Health, 4,* 243–253.

Becker-Haimes, E. M., Byeon, Y. V., Frank, H. E., Williams, N. J., Kratz, H. E., & Beidas, R. S. (2020). Identifying the organizational innovation-specific capacity needed for exposure therapy. *Depression and Anxiety, 37*, 1007–1016.

Bennett, K., Manassis, K., Walter, S. D., Cheung, A., Wilansky-Traynor, P., Diaz-Granados, N., Duda, S., Rice, M., Baer, S., Barrett, P., Bodden, D., Cobham, V. E., Dadds, M. R., Flannery-Schroeder, E., Ginsburg, G., Heyne, D., Hudson, J. L., Kendall, P. C., Liber, J., . . . Wood, J. J. (2013). Cognitive behavioral therapy age effects in child and adolescent anxiety: An individual patient data meta-analysis. *Depression and Anxiety, 30*, 829–841.

Besteiro, E. M., & Quintanilla, A. J. (2017). The relationship between parenting styles or parenting practices, and anxiety in childhood and adolescence: A systematic review. *Revista Española de Pedagogía, 75*, 337–351.

Campbell, M., Fitzpatrick, R., Haines, A., Kinmonth, A. L., Sandercock, P., Spiegelhalter, D., & Tyrer, P. (2000). Framework for design and evaluation of complex interventions to improve health. *BMJ, 321*, 694–696.

Cartwright-Hatton, S., McNicol, K., & Doubleday, E. (2006). Anxiety in a neglected population: Prevalence of anxiety disorders in pre-adolescent children. *Clinical Psychology Review, 26*, 817–833.

Casline, E., Ginsburg, G., Piacentini, J., Compton, S., & Kendall, P. C. (2021). Negative life events as predictors of anxiety outcomes: An examination of event type. *Journal of Abnormal Child Psychology* (now *Research in Child and Adolescent Psychopathology*), *49*, 91–102. https://doi.org/10.1007/s10802-020-00711-x

Chiu, A. W., McLeod, B. D., Har, K., & Wood, J. J. (2009). Child–therapist alliance and clinical outcomes in cognitive behavioral therapy for child anxiety disorders. *Journal of Child Psychology and Psychiatry, 50*, 751–758.

Chu, B. C., & Harrison, T. L. (2007). Disorder-specific effects of CBT for anxious and depressed youth: A meta-analysis of candidate mediators of change. *Clinical Child and Family Psychology Review, 10*, 352–372.

Chu, B. C., & Kendall, P. C. (2004). Positive association of child involvement and treatment outcome within a manual-based cognitive-behavioral treatment for children with anxiety. *Journal of Consulting and Clinical Psychology, 72*, 821.

Chu, B. C., & Kendall, P. C. (2009). Therapist responsiveness to child engagement: Flexibility within manual-based CBT for anxious youth. *Journal of Clinical Psychology, 65*, 736–754.

Chu, B. C., Crocco, S. T., Arnold, C. C., Brown, R., Southam-Gerow, M. A., & Weisz, J. R. (2015). Sustained implementation of cognitive-behavioral therapy for youth anxiety and depression: Long-term effects of structured training and consultation on therapist practice in the field. *Professional Psychology: Research and Practice, 46*, 70–79.

Cohen, J. A., The Work Group on Quality Issues and the AACAP Work Group on Quality Issues (2010a). Practice parameter for the assessment and treatment of children and adolescents with posttraumatic stress disorder. *Journal of the American Academy of Child & Adolescent Psychiatry, 49*, 414–430.

Cohen, J. A., Mannarino, A. P., & Deblinger, E. (2010b). Trauma-focused cognitive-behavioral therapy for traumatized children. *Evidence-Based Psychotherapies for Children and Adolescents, 2*, 295–311.

Compton, S. N., Peris, T. S., Almirall, D., Birmaher, B., Sherrill, J., Kendall, P. C., March, J. S., Gosch, E. A., Ginsburg, G. S., Rynn, M. A., Piacentini, J. C., McCracken, J. T.,

Keeton, C. P., Suveg, C. M., Aschenbrand, S. G., Sakolsky, D., Iyengar, S., Walkup, J. T., & Albano, A. M. (2014). Predictors and moderators of treatment response in childhood anxiety disorders: Results from the CAMS trial. *Journal of Consulting and Clinical Psychology, 82,* 212–224.

Copeland, W. E., Keeler, G., Angold, A., & Costello, E. J. (2007). Traumatic events and posttraumatic stress in childhood. *Archives of General Psychiatry, 64,* 577–584.

Cortes, A. M., Saltzman, K. M., Weems, C. F., Regnault, H. P., Reiss, A. L., & Carrion, V. G. (2005). Development of anxiety disorders in a traumatized pediatric population: A preliminary longitudinal evaluation. *Child Abuse & Neglect, 29,* 905–914.

Cummings, C., Caporino, N., & Kendall, P. C. (2014). Comorbidity of anxiety and depression in children and adolescents: 20 years after. *Psychological Bulletin, 140,* 816–845.

Cunningham, N. R., & Ollendick, T. H. (2010). Comorbidity of anxiety and conduct problems in children: Implications for clinical research and practice. *Clinical Child and Family Psychology Review, 13,* 333–347.

Dadsetan, P., Tehranizadeh, M., Tabatabaee, K. R., Fallah, P. A., & Ashtiani, A. F. (2011). Effectiveness of the Coping Cat therapy program in decreasing internalized symptoms of Iranian children. *Developmental Psychology: Journal of Iranian Psychologists, 7,* 313–322.

Damschroder, L. J., Aron, D. C., Keith, R. E., Kirsh, S. R., Alexander, J. A., & Lowery, J. C. (2009). Fostering implementation of health services research findings into practice: A consolidated framework for advancing implementation science. *Implementation Science, 4,* 50.

Dannon, P. N., Iancu, I., & Grunhaus, L. (2002). Psychoeducation in panic disorder patients: Effect of a self-information booklet in a randomized, masked-rater study. *Depression and Anxiety, 16,* 71–76.

David, R., Nixon, V., Sterk, J., & Pearce, A. (2012). A randomized trial of cognitive behavior therapy and cognitive therapy for children with Posttraumatic Stress Disorder following single-incident trauma. *Journal of Abnormal Child Psychology, 40,* 327.

de Souza, M. A. M., Salum, G. A., Jarros, R. B., Isolan, L., Davis, R., Knijnik, D., et al. (2013). Cognitive-behavioral group therapy for youths with anxiety disorders in the community: Effectiveness in low and middle income countries. *Behavioural and Cognitive Psychotherapy, 41,* 255–264.

Deblinger, E., Mannarino, A. P., Cohen, J. A., Runyon, M. K., & Steer, R. A. (2011). Trauma-focused cognitive behavioral therapy for children: Impact of the trauma narrative and treatment length. *Depression and Anxiety, 28,* 67–75.

Dedousis-Wallace, A., Drysdale, S. A., McAloon, J., & Ollendick, T. H. (2020). Parental and familial predictors and moderators of parent management treatment programs for conduct problems in youth. *Clinical Child and Family Psychology Review,* 1–28.

Dorsey, S., McLaughlin, K. A., Kerns, S. E., Harrison, J. P., Lambert, H. K., Briggs, E. C., Revillion Cox, J., & Amaya-Jackson, L. (2017). Evidence base update for psychosocial treatments for children and adolescents exposed to traumatic events. *Journal of Clinical Child & Adolescent Psychology, 46,* 303–330.

Drabick, D. A., Ollendick, T. H., & Bubier, J. L. (2010). Co-occurrence of ODD and anxiety: Shared risk processes and evidence for a dual-pathway model. *Clinical Psychology: Science and Practice, 17,* 307–318.

Eyberg, S. M., Nelson, M. M., & Boggs, S. R. (2008). Evidence-based psychosocial treatments for children and adolescents with disruptive behavior. *Journal of Clinical Child & Adolescent Psychology, 37*, 215–237.

Flannery-Schroeder, E., Suveg, C., Safford, S., Kendall, P. C., & Webb, A. (2004). Comorbid externalising disorders and child anxiety treatment outcomes. *Behaviour Change, 21*, 14–25.

Frank, H. E., Titone, M. K., Kagan, E. R., Alloy, L. B., & Kendall, P. C. (2020). The role of comorbid depression in youth anxiety treatment outcomes. *Child Psychiatry & Human Development, 88*, 1–8.

Frankel, S. A., Gallerani, C. M., & Garber, J. (2012). Developmental considerations across childhood. In E. Szigethy, J. R. Weisz, & R. L. Findling (Eds.), *Cognitive-behavior therapy for children and adolescents* (pp. 29–73). American Psychiatric Publishing.

Frese, M. (2015). Cultural practices, norms, and values. *Journal of Cross-Cultural Psychology, 46*, 1327–1330.

Garber, J., & Weersing, V. R. (2010). Comorbidity of anxiety and depression in youth: Implications for treatment and prevention. *Clinical Psychology, 17*, 293–306.

Gerson, R., & Rappaport, N. (2013). Traumatic stress and posttraumatic stress disorder in youth: Recent research findings on clinical impact, assessment, and treatment. *Journal of Adolescent Health, 52*, 137–143.

Ginsburg, G. S., Becker, E. M., Keeton, C. P., Sakolsky, D., Piacentini, J. C., Albano, A. M., Compton, S. N., Iyengar, S., Caporino, N., Peris, T., Birmaher, B., Rynn, M., March, J., & Kendall, P. C. (2014). Naturalistic follow-up of youths treated for pediatric anxiety disorders. *JAMA Psychiatry, 71*, 310–318.

Ginsburg, G. S., Becker-Haimes, E. M., Keeton, C., Kendall, P. C., Iyengar, S., Sakolsky, D., Albano, A. M., Peris, T., Compton, S. N., & Piacentini, J. (2018). Results from the child/adolescent anxiety multimodal extended long-term study (CAMELS): Primary anxiety outcomes. *Journal of the American Academy of Child & Adolescent Psychiatry, 57*, 471–480.

Ginsburg, G. S., Sakolsky, D., Piacentini, J., Walkup, J. T., Coffey, K. A., Keeton, C. P., Iyengar, S., Kendall, P. C., Compton, S. N., Albano, A. M., Sherrill, J., Ryann, M. A., McCracken, J. T., Bergman, L., Birmaher, B., & March, J. (2011). Remission after acute treatment in children and adolescents with anxiety disorders: Findings from the CAMS. *Journal of Consulting and Clinical Psychology, 79*, 806.

Gordon-Hollingsworth, A. T., Becker, E. M., Ginsburg, G. S., Keeton, C., Compton, S. N., Birmaher, B. B., Sakolsky, D. J., Piacentini, J., Albano, A. M., & Kendall, P. C. (2015). Anxiety disorders in Caucasian and African American children: A comparison of clinical characteristics, treatment process variables, and treatment outcomes. *Child Psychiatry & Human Development, 46*, 643–655.

Graham, J. R., Sorenson, S., & Hayes-Skelton, S. A. (2013). Enhancing the cultural sensitivity of cognitive behavioral interventions for anxiety in diverse populations. *The Behavior Therapist, 36*, 101–108.

Gregory Jr, V. L. (2019). Cognitive-behavioral therapy for anxious symptoms in persons of African descent: A meta-analysis. *Journal of Social Service Research, 45*, 87–101.

Halldorsdottir, T., Ollendick, T. H., Ginsburg, G., Sherrill, J., Kendall, P. C., Walkup, J., Sakolsky, D. J., & Piacentini, J. (2015). Treatment outcomes in anxious youth with and without comorbid ADHD in the CAMS. *Journal of Clinical Child and Adolescent Psychology, 44*, 985–991.

Hawe, P., Shiell, A., & Riley, T. (2004). Complex interventions: How "out of control" can a randomised controlled trial be? *British Medical Journal, 328*, 1561–1563.

Higa-McMillan, C. K., Francis, S. E., Rith-Najarian, L., & Chorpita, B. F. (2016). Evidence base update: 50 years of research on treatment for child and adolescent anxiety. *Journal of Clinical Child & Adolescent Psychology, 45*, 91–113.

Hittner, E. F., Rim, K. L., & Haase, C. M. (2019). Socioeconomic status as a moderator of the link between reappraisal and anxiety: Laboratory-based and longitudinal evidence. *Emotion, 19*, 1478–1489.

Hogendoorn, S. M., Prins, P. J., Boer, F., Vervoort, L., Wolters, L. H., Moorlag, H., Nauta, M. H., Garst, H., Hartman, C. A., & de Haan, E. (2014). Mediators of cognitive behavioral therapy for anxiety-disordered children and adolescents: Cognition, perceived control, and coping. *Journal of Clinical Child & Adolescent Psychology, 43*, 486–500.

Holmbeck, G. N., O'Mahar, K., Abad, M., Colder, C., & Updegrove, A. (2006). Cognitive-behavioral therapy with adolescents: Guides from developmental psychology. In P. C. Kendall (Ed.), *Child and adolescent therapy: Cognitive-behavioral procedures* (3rd ed.; pp. 429–470). Guilford Press.

Houghton, S., Alsalmi, N., Tan, C., Taylor, M., & Durkin, K. (2017). Treating comorbid anxiety in adolescents with ADHD using a cognitive behavior therapy program approach. *Journal of Attention Disorders, 21*, 1094–1104.

Houlding, C., Schmidt, F., & Walker, D. (2010). Youth therapist strategies to enhance client homework completion. *Child and Adolescent Mental Health, 15*, 103–109.

Hudson, J. L., & Kendall, P. C. (2002). Showing you can do it: Homework in therapy for children and adolescents with anxiety disorders. *Journal of Clinical Psychology, 58*, 525–534.

Hudson, J. L., Keers, R., Roberts, S., Coleman, J. R. I., Breen, G., Arendt, K., Bögels, S., Cooper, P., Creswell, C., Hartman, C., Heiervang, E. R., Hötzel, K., In-Albon, T., Lavallee, K., Lyneham, H. J., Marin, C. E., McKinnon, A., Meiser-Stedman, R., Morris, T., . . . Eley, T. C. (2015). Clinical predictors of response to cognitive-behavioral therapy in pediatric anxiety disorders: The Genes for Treatment (GxT) Study. *Journal of the American Academy of Child and Adolescent Psychiatry, 54*, 454–463.

Hudson, J. L., Lester, K. J., Lewis, C. M., Tropeano, M., Creswell, C., Collier, D. A., Cooper, P., Lyneham, H. J., Morris, T., Rapee, R. M., Roberts, S., Donald, J. A., & Eley, T. C. (2013). Predicting outcomes following cognitive behaviour therapy in child anxiety disorders: The influence of genetic, demographic and clinical information. *Journal of Child Psychology and Psychiatry, 54*, 1086–1094.

Hughes, A. A., & Kendall, P. C. (2007). Prediction of cognitive behavior treatment outcome for children with anxiety disorders: Therapeutic relationship and homework compliance. *Behavioural and Cognitive Psychotherapy, 35*, 487.

Ishikawa, S. I., Kikuta, K., Sakai, M., Mitamura, T., Motomura, N., & Hudson, J. L. (2019). A randomized controlled trial of a bidirectional cultural adaptation of cognitive behavior therapy for children and adolescents with anxiety disorders. *Behaviour Research and Therapy, 120*, 103432.

Ishikawa, S., & Sakano, Y. (2005). Investigation on the relationship between self-statement and anxiety symptoms in children. *Japanese Journal of Behavior Therapy, 31*, 45–57.

Ivarsson, T., Melin, K., & Wallin, L. (2008). Categorical and dimensional aspects of co-morbidity in Obsessive-Compulsive Disorder (OCD). *European Child & Adolescent Psychiatry, 17*, 20–31.

Jarrett, M. A., & Ollendick, T. H. (2012). Treatment of comorbid Attention-Deficit/Hyperactivity Disorder and anxiety in children: A multiple baseline design analysis. *Journal of Consulting and Clinical Psychology, 80*, 239–244.

Kagan, E. (2019). *Targeting parental accommodation in the treatment of youth with anxiety: A comparison of two cognitive behavioral treatments* [Doctoral dissertation. Temple University]. https://search.proquest.com/docview/2297180233/abstract/CA108215D86048CCPQ/1

Kagan, E. R., Peterman, J. S., Carper, M. M., & Kendall, P. C. (2016). Accommodation and treatment of anxious youth. *Depression and Anxiety, 33*, 840–847.

Kazak, A. E., Hoagwood, K., Weisz, J. R., Hood, K., Kratochwill, T. R., Vargas, L. A., & Banez, G. A. (2010). A meta-systems approach to evidence-based practice for children and adolescents. *American Psychologist, 65*, 85–97.

Kazantzis, N., Whittington, C., Zelencich, L., Kyrios, M., Norton, P. J., & Hofmann, S. G. (2016). Quantity and quality of homework compliance: A meta-analysis of relations with outcome in cognitive behavior therapy. *Behavior Therapy, 47*, 755–772.

Kendall, P. C., Choudhury, M., Hudson, J., & Webb, A. (2002). *The C.A.T. project manual for the Cognitive-Behavioral Treatment of anxious adolescents*. Workbook Publishing.

Kendall, P. C., Compton, S. N., Walkup, J. T., Birmaher, B., Albano, A. M., Sherrill, J., Ginsburg, G., Rynn, M., McCracken, J., Gosch, E., Keeton, C., Bergman, L., Sakolsky, D., Suveg, C., March, J., & Piacentini, J. (2010). Clinical characteristics of anxiety disordered youth. *Journal of Anxiety Disorders, 24*, 360–365.

Kendall, P. C., Cummings, C. M., Villabø, M. A., Narayanan, M. K., Treadwell, K., Birmaher, B., Compton, S., Piacentini, J., Sherrill, J., Walkup, J., Gosch, E., Keeton, C., Ginsburg, G., Suveg, C., & Albano, A. M. (2016). Mediators of change in the Child/Adolescent Anxiety Multimodal Treatment Study. *Journal of Consulting and Clinical Psychology, 84*, 1–14.

Kendall, P. C., Flannery-Schroeder, E., Panichelli-Mindel, S. M., Southam-Gerow, M., Henin, A., & Warman, M. (1997). Therapy for youths with anxiety disorders: A second randomized clinical trial. *Journal of Consulting and Clinical Psychology, 65*, 366.

Kendall, P. C., & Frank, H. E. (2018). Implementing evidence-based treatment protocols: Flexibility within fidelity. *Clinical Psychology: Science and Practice, 25*, e12271.

Kendall, P. C., & Hedtke, K. A. (2006a). *Cognitive-behavioral therapy for anxious children: Therapist manual* (3rd ed.). Workbook Publishing.

Kendall, P. C., & Hedtke, K. A. (2006b). *The Coping Cat workbook* (2nd ed.). Workbook Publishing.

Kendall, P. C., & Martinsen, K. D. (2008). *Mestringskatten (Coping cat): kognitiv atferdsterapi for barn med angst: gruppemanual: manualen er et tillegg som skal brukes sammen med den individuelle manualen for Mestringskatten*. Universitetsforlaget.

Kendall, P. C., Martinsen, K. D., & Neumer, S. P. (2006). Mestringskatten (Coping Cat). *Kognitiv atferdsterapi for barn med angst. Terapeutmanual. Oslo: Universitetsforlaget.*

Kendall, P. C., & Peterman, J. (2015). CBT for anxious adolescents: Mature yet still developing. *American Journal of Psychiatry, 172*, 519–530.

Kendall, P. C., Safford, S., Flannery-Schroeder, E., & Webb, A. (2004). Child anxiety treatment: Outcomes in adolescence and impact on substance use and depression at 7.4-year follow-up. *Journal of Consulting and Clinical Psychology, 72*, 276–287.

Kendall, P. C., & Sugarman, A. (1997). Attrition in the treatment of childhood anxiety disorders. *Journal of Consulting and Clinical Psychology, 65*, 883–888.

Kendall, P. C., & Treadwell, K. R. (2007). The role of self-statements as a mediator in treatment for youth with anxiety disorders. *Journal of Consulting and Clinical Psychology, 75*, 380.

Kennedy, S. M., Tonarely, N. A., Sherman, J. A., & Ehrenreich-May, J. (2018). Predictors of treatment outcome for the unified protocol for transdiagnostic treatment of emotional disorders in children (UP-C). *Journal of Anxiety Disorders, 57*, 66–75.

Kessler, R. C., Petukhova, M., Sampson, N. A., Zaslavsky, A. M., & Wittchen, H. U. (2012). Twelve-month and lifetime prevalence and lifetime morbid risk of anxiety and mood disorders in the United States. *International Journal of Methods in Psychiatric Research, 21*, 169–184.

Khan, A., Malik, T. A., Ahmed, S., & Riaz, A. (2020). Translation, adaptation and implementation of Coping Cat program with Pakistani children. *Child & Youth Care Forum, 49*, 23–41.

Kingery, J. N., Roblek, T. L., Suveg, C., Grover, R. L., Sherrill, J. T., & Bergman, R. L. (2006). They're not just "little adults": Developmental considerations for implementing cognitive-behavioral therapy with anxious youth. *Journal of Cognitive Psychotherapy, 20*, 263–273.

Kirk, M. A., Haines, E. R., Rokoske, F. S., Powell, B. J., Weinberger, M., Hanson, L. C., & Birken, S. A. (2019). A case study of a theory-based method for identifying and reporting core functions and forms of evidence-based interventions. *Translational Behavioral Medicine*. doi:10.1093/tbm/ibz178.

Knight, A., McLellan, L., Jones, M., & Hudson, J. (2014). Pre-treatment predictors of outcome in childhood anxiety disorders: A systematic review. *Psychopathology Review, 1*, 77–129.

Kodal, A., Fjermestad, K., Bjelland, I., Gjestad, R., Öst, L. G., Bjaastad, J. F., Haugland, B. S. M., Havik, O. E., Heiervang, E., & Wergeland, G. J. (2018). Long-term effectiveness of cognitive behavioral therapy for youth with anxiety disorders. *Journal of Anxiety Disorders, 53*, 58–67.

Koeppen, A. S. (1974). Relaxation training for children. *Elementary School Guidance & Counseling, 9*, 14–21.

Koydemir, S., & Essau, C. A. (2018). Anxiety and anxiety disorders in young people: A cross cultural perspective. In *Understanding uniqueness and diversity in child and adolescent mental health* (pp. 115–134). Academic Press.

Kreuze, L. J., Pijnenborg, G. H. M., de Jonge, Y. B., & Nauta, M. H. (2018). Cognitive-behavior therapy for children and adolescents with anxiety disorders: A meta-analysis of secondary outcomes. *Journal of Anxiety Disorders, 60*, 43–57.

Kumpfer, K. L., Alvarado, R., Smith, P., & Bellamy, N. (2002). Cultural sensitivity and adaptation in family-based prevention interventions. *Prevention Science, 3*, 241–246.

Larson, K., Russ, S. A., Kahn, R. S., & Halfon, N. (2011). Patterns of comorbidity, functioning, and service use for US children with ADHD, 2007. *Pediatrics, 127*, 462–470.

Lau, A. S. (2006). Making the case for selective and directed cultural adaptations of evidence-based treatments: Examples from parent training. *Clinical Psychology: Science and Practice, 13*, 295–310.

Lau, W., Chan, C. K., Li, J. C., & Au, T. K. (2010). Effectiveness of group cognitive-behavioral treatment for childhood anxiety in community clinics. *Behaviour Research and Therapy, 48*, 1067–1077.

Lawrence, D., Johnson, S., Hafekost, J., Boterhoven De Haan, K., Sawyer, M., Ainley, J., & Zubrick, S. R. (2015). *The mental health of children and adolescents. Report on the second Australian Child and Adolescent Survey of Mental Health and Wellbeing.* Department of Health, Canberra.

Lee, P., Zehgeer, A., Ginsburg, G. S., McCracken, J., Keeton, C., Kendall, P. C., Birmaher, B., Sakolsky, D., Walkup, J., Peris, T., Albano, A. M., & Compton, C. (2019). Child and adolescent adherence with cognitive behavioral therapy for anxiety: Predictors and associations with outcomes. *Journal of Clinical Child & Adolescent Psychology, 48*, S215–S226.

Lee, S. J., Altschul, I., & Mowbray, C. T. (2008). Using planned adaptation to implement evidence-based programs with new populations. *American Journal of Community Psychology, 41*, 290–303.

Lenz, A. S. (2015). Meta-analysis of the Coping Cat program for decreasing severity of anxiety symptoms among children and adolescents. *Journal of Child and Adolescent Counseling, 1*, 51–65.

Lewis, C. C., Simons, A. D., Nguyen, L. J., Murakami, J. L., Reid, M. W., Silva, S. G., & March, J. S. (2010). Impact of childhood trauma on treatment outcome in the Treatment for Adolescents with Depression Study (TADS). *Journal of the American Academy of Child & Adolescent Psychiatry, 49*, 132–140.

Lindhout, I. E., Markus, M. T., Hoogendijk, T. H., & Boer, F. (2009). Temperament and parental child-rearing style: Unique contributions to clinical anxiety disorders in childhood. *European Child & Adolescent Psychiatry, 18*, 439–446.

Lyneham, H. J., Abbott, M. J., Wignall, A., & Rapee, R. M. (2003). *The Cool Kids Program.* Macquarie University Anxiety Research Unit: Macquarie University, Sydney.

Manassis, K., Lee, T. C., Bennett, K., Zhao, X. Y., Mendlowitz, S., Duda, S., Saini, M., Wilansky, P., Baer, S., Barrett, P., Bodden, D., Cobham, V., Dadds, M., Flannery-Schroeder, E., Ginsburg, G., Heyne, D., Hudson, J., Kendall, P. C., Liber, J., Warner, C. M., Nauta, M., Rapee, R., Silverman, W., Siqueland, L., Spence, S., Utens, E., & Wood, J. J. (2014). Types of parental involvement in CBT with anxious youth: A preliminary meta-analysis. *Journal of Consulting and Clinical Psychology, 82*, 1163–1172.

Maric, M., van Steensel, Francisca J. A., & Bögels, S. M. (2018). Parental involvement in CBT for anxiety-disordered youth revisited: Family CBT outperforms child CBT in the long term for children with comorbid ADHD symptoms. *Journal of Attention Disorders, 22*, 506–514.

Marker, C. D., Comer, J. S., Abramova, V., & Kendall, P. C. (2013). The reciprocal relationship between alliance and symptom improvement across the treatment of childhood anxiety. *Journal of Clinical Child & Adolescent Psychology, 42*, 22–33.

Marmorstein, N. R. (2007). Relationships between anxiety and externalizing disorders in youth: The influences of age and gender. *Journal of Anxiety Disorders, 21*, 420–432.

Marsiglia, F. F., & Booth, J. M. (2015). Cultural adaptation of interventions in real practice settings. *Research on Social Work Practice, 25*, 423–432.

Martín, V., Granero, R., & Ezpeleta, L. (2014). Comorbidity of oppositional defiant disorder and anxiety disorders in preschoolers. *Psicothema, 26*, 27–32.

Mendlowitz, S. L., Manassis, K., Bradley, S., Scapillato, D., Miezitis, S., & Shaw, B. E. (1999). Cognitive-behavioral group treatments in childhood anxiety disorders: The role of parental involvement. *Journal of the American Academy of Child & Adolescent Psychiatry, 38*, 1223–1229.

Merikangas, K. R., He, J., Burstein, M. E., Swendsen, J., Avenevoli, S., Case, B., Georgiades, K., Heaton, L., Swanson, S., & Olfson, M. (2011). Service utilization for lifetime mental disorders in U.S. adolescents: Results of the National Comorbidity Survey Adolescent Supplement (NCS-A). *Journal of the American Academy of Child & Adolescent Psychiatry, 50*, 32–45.

Merikangas, K. R., He, J., Burstein, M., Swanson, S. A., Avenevoli, S., Cui, L., Benjet, C., Georgiades, K., & Swendsen, J. (2010). Lifetime prevalence of mental disorders in U.S. adolescents: Results from the national comorbidity survey replication—adolescent supplement (NCS-A). *Journal of the American Academy of Child & Adolescent Psychiatry, 49*, 980–989.

Naar-King, S., & Suarez, M. (2011). *Motivational interviewing with adolescents and young adults*. Guilford Press.

Najman, J. M., Hayatbakhsh, M. R., Clavarino, A., Bor, W., O'Callaghan, M. J., & Williams, G. M. (2010). Family poverty over the early life course and recurrent adolescent and young adult anxiety and depression: A longitudinal study. *American Journal of Public Health, 100*, 1719–1723.

Nauta, M. H., Scholing, A., Emmelkamp, P. M., & Minderaa, R. B. (2003). Cognitive-behavioral therapy for children with anxiety disorders in a clinical setting: No additional effect of a cognitive parent training. *Journal of the American Academy of Child & Adolescent Psychiatry, 42*, 1270–1278.

Nauta, M., & Scholing, A. (1998). *Dappere Kat* [Intern manuscript]. *Groningen: Rijksuniversiteit, afdeling Klinische Psychologie*.

Nevo, G. W. A., Avery, D., Fiksenbaum, L., Kiss, A., Mendlowitz, S., Monga, S., & Manassis, K. (2014). Eight years later: Outcomes of CBT-treated versus untreated anxious children. *Brain and Behavior, 4*, 765–774.

Nilsen, T. S., Eisemann, M., & Kvernmo, S. (2013). Predictors and moderators of outcome in child and adolescent anxiety and depression: A systematic review of psychological treatment studies. *European Child & Adolescent Psychiatry, 22*, 69–87.

Norris, L. A., & Kendall, P. C. (in press). Moderators of outcome for youth anxiety treatments: Current findings and future directions. *Journal of Clinical Child and Adolescent Psychology*.

Norris, L., Olino, T., Gosch, E., Compton, S., Piacentini, J., Albano, A.M., Walkup, J., Birmaher, B., & Kendall, P. C. (2020). Person-centered profiles among treatment-seeking youth with anxiety disorders. *Journal of Clinical Child and Adolescent Psychology, 49*, 626–638. doi:10.1080/15374416.2019.1602839

Ollendick, T. H., & Cerny, J. A. (1981). *Clinical Behavior Therapy with children*. Springer US.

Ollendick, T. H., Halldorsdottir, T., Fraire, M. G., Austin, K. E., Noguchi, R. J. P., Lewis, K. M., Jarrett, M. A., Cunningham, N. R., Canavera, K., Allen, K. B., & Whitmore, M. J. (2015). Specific phobias in youth: A randomized controlled trial comparing one-session treatment to a parent-augmented one-session treatment. *Behavior Therapy, 46*, 141–155.

Peris, T. S., Caporino, N. E., O'Rourke, S., Kendall, P. C., Walkup, J. T., Albano, A. M., Bergman, R. L., McCracken, J. T., Birmaher, B., Ginsburg, G. S., Sakolsky, D., Piacentini, J., & Compton, S. N. (2017). Therapist-reported features of exposure tasks that predict differential treatment outcomes for youth with anxiety. *Journal of the American Academy of Child & Adolescent Psychiatry, 56*, 1043–1052.

Peris, T. S., Compton, S. N., Kendall, P. C., Birmaher, B., Sherrill, J., March, J., Gosch, E., Ginsburg, G., Rynn, M., McCracken, J. T., Keeton, C. P., Sakolsky, D., Suveg, C., Aschenbrand, S., Almirall, D., Iyengar, S., Walkup, J. T., Albano, A. M., & Piacentini, J. (2015). Trajectories of change in youth anxiety during cognitive-behavior therapy. *Journal of Consulting and Clinical Psychology, 83*, 239–252.

Piacentini, J., & Langley, A. K. (2004). Cognitive-behavioral therapy for children who have Obsessive-Compulsive Disorder. *Journal of Clinical Psychology, 60*, 1181–1194.

Piacentini, J., Bergman, R. L., Jacobs, C., McCracken, J. T., & Kretchman, J. (2002). Open trial of cognitive behavior therapy for childhood Obsessive–Compulsive Disorder. *Journal of Anxiety Disorders, 16*, 207–219.

Piacentini, J., Langley, A., & Roblek, T. (2007). *Cognitive behavioral treatment of childhood OCD: It's only a false alarm therapist guide.* Oxford University Press.

Pina, A. A., Zerr, A. A., Villalta, I. K., & Gonzales, N. A. (2012). Indicated prevention and early intervention for childhood anxiety: A randomized trial with Caucasian and Hispanic/Latino youth. *Journal of Consulting and Clinical Psychology, 80*, 940–946.

Pine, D. S., & Cohen, J. A. (2002). Trauma in children and adolescents: Risk and treatment of psychiatric sequelae. *Biological Psychiatry, 51*, 519–531.

Powell, B. J., Beidas, R. S., Rubin, R. M., Stewart, R. E., Wolk, C. B., Matlin, S. L., Weaver, S., Hurford, M. O., Evans, A. C., Hadley, T. R., & Mandell, D. S. (2016). Applying the policy ecology framework to Philadelphia's behavioral health transformation efforts. *Administration and Policy in Mental Health, 43*, 909–926.

Puleo, C. M., & Kendall, P. C. (2011). Cognitive-behavioral therapy for typically developing youth with anxiety: Autism spectrum symptoms as a predictor of treatment outcome. *Journal of Autism and Developmental Disorders, 41*, 275–286.

Rahman, O., Ale, C. M., Sulkowski, M. L., & Storch, E. A. (2013). Treatment of comorbid anxiety and disruptive behavior in youth. In *Handbook of Treating Variants and Complications in Anxiety Disorders* (pp. 97–108). Springer.

Rapee, R. M. (2000). Group treatment of children with anxiety disorders: Outcome and predictors of treatment response. *Australian Journal of Psychology, 52*, 125–129.

Roy, K. M., Tubbs, C. Y., & Burton, L. M. (2004). Don't have no time: Daily rhythms and the organization of time for low-income families. *Family Relations, 53*, 168–178.

Ruocco, S., Freeman, N. C., & McLean, L. A. (2018). Learning to cope: A CBT evaluation exploring self-reported changes in coping with anxiety among school children aged 5–7 years. *The Educational and Developmental Psychologist, 35*, 67–87.

Saez, E., & Zucman, G. (2020). The rise of income and wealth inequality in America: Evidence from distributional macroeconomic accounts. *Journal of Economic Perspectives, 34*, 3–26.

Salloum, A., & Overstreet, S. (2012). Grief and trauma intervention for children after disaster: Exploring coping skills versus trauma narration. *Behaviour Research and Therapy, 50*, 169–179.

Scapillato, D., & Mendlowitz, S. L. (1993). *The Coping Bear workbook* [Unpublished manuscript]. Boston University.

Sciberras, E., Mulraney, M., Anderson, V., Rapee, R. M., Nicholson, J. M., Efron, D., Lee, K., Markopoulos, Z., & Hiscock, H. (2018). Managing anxiety in children with ADHD using cognitive-behavioral therapy: A pilot randomized controlled trial. *Journal of Attention Disorders, 22*, 515–520.

Shafran, R., Clark, D. M., Fairburn, C. G., Arntz, A., Barlow, D. H., Ehlers, A., Freeston, M., Garety, P. A., Hollon, S. D., Ost, L. G., Salkovskis, P. M., Williams, J. M. G., & Wilson, G. T. (2009). Mind the gap: Improving the dissemination of CBT. *Behaviour Research and Therapy, 47,* 902–909.

Sherrill, J. T. (2016). Adaptive treatment strategies in youth mental health: A commentary on advantages, challenges, and potential directions. *Journal of Clinical Child & Adolescent Psychology, 45*, 1–6.

Shirk, S. R., Karver, M. S., & Brown, R. (2011). The alliance in child and adolescent psychotherapy. *Psychotherapy, 48*, 17.

Shokri Mirhosseini, H., Alizade, H., & Fasrrokhi, N. (2018). The impact of Coping Cat program on symptoms reduction in children with anxiety disorders. *Quarterly Journal of Child Mental Health, 5*, 1–13.

Silverman, W. K., Kurtines, W. M., Ginsburg, G. S., Weems, C. F., Rabian, B., & Serafini, L. T. (1999). Contingency management, self-control, and education support in the treatment of childhood phobic disorders: A randomized clinical trial. *Journal of Consulting and Clinical Psychology, 67*, 675.

Smith, P., Dalgleish, T., & Meiser-Stedman, R. (2019). Practitioner Review: Posttraumatic stress disorder and its treatment in children and adolescents. *Journal of Child Psychology and Psychiatry, 60*, 500–515.

Southam-Gerow, M. A., Kendall, P. C., & Weersing, V. R. (2001). Examining outcome variability: Correlates of treatment response in a child and adolescent anxiety clinic. *Journal of Clinical Child Psychology, 30*, 422–436.

Stirman, S. W., Baumann, A. A., & Miller, C. J. (2019). The FRAME: An expanded framework for reporting adaptations and modifications to evidence-based interventions. *Implementation Science, 14*, 1–10.

Storch, E. A., Merlo, L. J., Larson, M. J., Geffken, G. R., Lehmkuhl, H. D., Jacob, M. L., Murphy, T. K., & Goodman, W. K. (2008). Impact of comorbidity on cognitive-behavioral therapy response in pediatric obsessive-compulsive disorder. *Journal of the American Academy of Child & Adolescent Psychiatry, 47*, 583–592.

Sun, M., Rith-Najarian, L. R., Williamson, T. J., & Chorpita, B. F. (2019). Treatment features associated with youth cognitive behavioral therapy follow-up effects for internalizing disorders: A meta-analysis. *Journal of Clinical Child & Adolescent Psychology, 48*, S269–S283.

Suveg, C., Hudson, J. L., Brewer, G., Flannery-Schroeder, E., Gosch, E., & Kendall, P. C. (2009). Cognitive-behavioral therapy for anxiety-disordered youth: Secondary outcomes from a randomized clinical trial evaluating child and family modalities. *Journal of Anxiety Disorders, 23*, 341–349.

Swan, A. J., & Kendall, P. C. (2016). Fear and missing out: Youth anxiety and functional outcomes. *Clinical Psychology: Science and Practice, 23*, 417–435.

Swan, A. J., Carper, M. M., & Kendall, P. C. (2016). In pursuit of generalization: An updated review. *Behavior Therapy, 47*, 733–746.

Swedo, S. E., Rapoport, J. L., Leonard, H., Lenane, M., & Cheslow, D. (1989). Obsessive-compulsive disorder in children and adolescents: Clinical phenomenology of 70 consecutive cases. *Archives of General Psychiatry, 46*, 335–341.

Taylor, J. H., Lebowitz, E. R., Jakubovski, E., Coughlin, C. G., Silverman, W. K., & Bloch, M. H. (2018). Monotherapy insufficient in severe anxiety? Predictors and moderators in the child/adolescent anxiety multimodal study. *Journal of Clinical Child & Adolescent Psychology, 47*, 266–281.

Thirlwall, K., Cooper, P., & Creswell, C. (2017). Guided parent-delivered cognitive behavioral therapy for childhood anxiety: Predictors of treatment response. *Journal of Anxiety Disorders, 45*, 43–48.

Tobon, J. I., Eichstedt, J. A., Wolfe, V. V., Phoenix, E., Brisebois, S., Zayed, R. S., & Harris, K. E. (2011). Group cognitive-behavioral therapy for anxiety in a clinic setting: Does child involvement predict outcome? *Behavior Therapy, 42*, 306–322.

Treadwell, K. R., & Kendall, P. C. (1996). Self-talk in youth with anxiety disorders: States of mind, content specificity, and treatment outcome. *Journal of Consulting and Clinical Psychology, 64*, 941.

U.S. Census Bureau. (2019). Income, poverty and health insurance coverage in the United States: 2019. https://www.census.gov/newsroom/press-releases/2020/income-poverty.html.

Vaclavik, D., Buitron, V., Rey, Y., Marin, C. E., Silverman, W. K., & Pettit, J. W. (2017). Parental acculturation level moderates outcome in peer-involved and parent-involved CBT for anxiety disorders in Latino youth. *Journal of Latina/o Psychology, 5*, 261–274.

Varela, R. E., & Hensley-Maloney, L. (2009). The influence of culture on anxiety in Latino youth: A review. *Clinical Child and Family Psychology Review, 12*, 217–233.

Villabø, M. A., Narayanan, M., Compton, S. N., Kendall, P. C., & Neumer, S.-P. (2018). Cognitive-behavioral therapy for youth anxiety: An effectiveness evaluation in community practice. *Journal of Consulting and Clinical Psychology, 86*, 751–764.

Walczak, M., Ollendick, T., Ryan, S., & Esbjørn, B. H. (2018). Does comorbidity predict poorer treatment outcome in pediatric anxiety disorders? An updated 10-year review. *Clinical Psychology Review, 60*, 45–61.

Wandersman, A., Duffy, J., Flaspohler, P., Noonan, R., Lubell, K., Stillman, L., Blachman, M., Dunville, R., & Saul, J. (2008). Bridging the gap between prevention research and practice: The interactive systems framework for dissemination and implementation. *American Journal of Community Psychology, 41*, 171–181.

Weisz, J. R., Ugueto, A. M., Cheron, D. M., & Herren, J. (2013). Evidence-based youth psychotherapy in the mental health ecosystem. *Journal of Clinical Child & Adolescent Psychology, 42*, 274–286.

Weisz, J. R., Kuppens, S., Ng, M. Y., Eckshtain, D., Ugueto, A. M., Vaughn-Coaxum, R., Jensen-Doss, A., Hawley, K. M., Marchette, L. K., Chu, B. C., Weersing, V. R., & Fordwood, S. R. (2017). What five decades of research tells us about the effects of youth psychological therapy: A multilevel meta-analysis and implications for science and practice. *American Psychologist, 72*, 79–117.

Wergeland, G. J. H., Fjermestad, K. W., Marin, C. E., Bjelland, I., Haugland, B. S. M., Silverman, W. K., Öst, L., Bjaastad, J. F., Oeding, K., Havik, O. E., & Heiervang, E. R. (2016). Predictors of treatment outcome in an effectiveness trial of cognitive behavioral therapy for children with anxiety disorders. *Behaviour Research and Therapy, 76,* 1–12.

Whiteside, S. P., Sim, L. A., Morrow, A. S., Farah, W. H., Hilliker, D. R., Murad, M. H., & Wang, Z. (2020). A meta-analysis to guide the enhancement of CBT for childhood anxiety: Exposure over anxiety management. *Clinical Child and Family Psychology Review, 23,* 102–121.

Wolk, C. B., Kendall, P. C., & Beidas, R. S. (2015). Cognitive-behavioral therapy for child anxiety confers long-term protection from suicidality. *Journal of the American Academy of Child & Adolescent Psychiatry, 54,* 175–179.

Woodward, L. J., & Fergusson, D. M. (2001). Life course outcomes of young people with anxiety disorders in adolescence. *Journal of the American Academy of Child & Adolescent Psychiatry, 40,* 1086–1093.

11

The Coping Power Program for Children with Aggressive Behavior Problems

JOHN E. LOCHMAN, NICOLE P. POWELL, AND SHANNON JONES ■

Aggressive behavior has been defined as an act directed toward another person or thing with the intent to hurt or frighten, where there is a consensus about the aggressive intent of the action (Shaw et al., 2000). Some forms of aggression are considered normal as a child develops and matures. A young child throwing a tantrum when he doesn't get what he wants or the horseplay of two young boys is developmentally appropriate and accepted. Neither of these examples are considered aggressive behavior due the lack of intent to hurt or frighten. However, as defined above, childhood aggressive behavior can serve as a predictor for juvenile delinquency, substance use and abuse, and disruptive behavior disorders such as Oppositional Defiant Disorder and Conduct Disorder. Examples of aggression in youth are bullying, threatening, tantrums, verbal attacks, hitting in anger, and taking part in physical fights. Children who are considered aggressive demonstrate verbal and/or physical behaviors that are atypical in their frequency, intensity, and/or duration relative to their developmental level and result in significant interference socially, behaviorally, and emotionally for the child and others in their environment. Aggressive behavior in youth has been a major focus of both research and practice efforts within clinical psychology, likely because childhood aggression has serious negative implications for children's adaptive functioning across domains (e.g., academics, peer relationships, family relationships) and has been consistently linked with negative developmental outcomes beyond childhood.

The severity of negative outcomes associated with aggressive behaviors, in addition to the chronic nature of these risks, suggest that preventative intervention during childhood is pivotal. In fact, aggressive behaviors are among the most common reasons for referrals for mental health services among children (Kazdin, 1995). To date, various evidence-based interventions have proven effective for reducing these behaviors. These interventions have been informed by theoretical models that suggest aggressive behaviors in childhood are likely the result of a combination of familial and personal factors (Lochman & Wells, 1996). A combination of social-cognitive, emotional, and neuropsychological processes contribute to the development and maintenance of aggressive behaviors in youth.

CONTEXTUAL SOCIAL-COGNITIVE MODEL

One specific theoretical model is the contextual social-cognitive model of prevention, which focuses on the interaction between child-level (e.g., poor social-cognitive skills, lack of social competence) and parent-level factors (e.g., lack of caregiver involvement with effective implementation of child discipline). The contextual social-cognitive model suggests that aggressive children demonstrate cognitive distortions in their appraisal of social information. Specifically, children with elevated aggression are more likely to attribute others' actions as threatening or hostile, suggesting that aggressive children have deficits in their interpretation of encoded social information. These deficits result in poor social problem-solving skills. For example, when aggressive youth are asked to identify potential solutions to interpersonal conflicts, they demonstrate deficits in both the overall number and quality of solutions generated, produce fewer appropriate verbal solutions (e.g., compromise), and identify more direct-action solutions, which often involve physical aggression (Lochman & Wells, 2002a). These deficiencies in social-cognitive processing are also likely accompanied by increased anger arousal and a lack of identification and use of appropriate coping methods to reduce the high level of physiological arousal (e.g., self-statements, relaxation, attention focusing; Lochman & Wells, 2002a).

Parenting behaviors also play an important role in the development and maintenance of aggressive behaviors in youth. Specifically, childhood aggression may arise from poor parenting practices including harsh or inconsistent discipline, poor problem solving, vague commands, and poor monitoring of child behavior (Lochman & Wells, 2002a; Pardini et al., 2014). Parent-level factors can exert a direct effect on aggressive behavior and an indirect effect via their association with factors such as childhood aggression, poor social competence, and academic failure. The relationship between poor parenting practices and childhood aggression is also bidirectional, which suggests the ways children engage with their parents—including the ways the child uses aggressive behaviors in the home—shape the approaches that parents subsequently incorporate to address the aggressive behavior (Pardini, 2008).

The theoretical basis for the contextual social-cognitive model relies on three assumptions: (1) aggressive behavior in childhood is a risk factor for subsequent negative outcomes across development; (2) both the child- and parent-specific factors described in the contextual social-cognitive model are related to the child's aggressive behaviors; and (3) changes in the contextual social-cognitive processes will lead to reductions in aggressive behavior and impact later outcomes across the child's development. The model and its underlying theoretical assumptions served as the guide for developing the child and parent components of the Coping Power Program (Lochman & Wells, 2002a, 2002b).

COPING POWER

Coping Power (Lochman, Wells, & Lenhart, 2008) is an empirically supported cognitive-behavioral intervention for children who demonstrate elevated aggressive behaviors. The program is both a comprehensive and multicomponent intervention based on the contextual social-cognitive model of prevention to reduce elevated aggressive behaviors in youth. Coping Power includes a 34-session Child Component, which is delivered over the course of 15 months, typically during the late elementary and early middle school years. The program is a school-based intervention that can be delivered in a group format (i.e., four to six children) or individually. Coping Power groups typically meet once a week for approximately an hour during the school day.

The Coping Power Child Component addresses social-cognitive deficits commonly experienced by children with aggressive behavior problems. Specific content includes: long-term and short-term goal setting and monitoring of progress toward goals; organization and study skills to reduce academic difficulties and conflicts with parents and teachers; emotion identification and regulation; development of prosocial coping strategies; understanding perspective-taking; social problem-solving; strategies to resist peer pressure; and how to identify and join positive peer groups. Overall, the major intervention goals for the program are to reduce aggressive attitudes and behaviors and prevent substance abuse among aggressive youth.

The Coping Power Parent Component (Wells, Lochman, & Lenhart, 2008) consists of 16 group sessions that take place separately from the child sessions. These sessions occur during the same 15-month period. Sessions typically occur on a twice-monthly basis and are 60 to 90 minutes in duration. Content for the Parent Component is based on social learning theory-based parent training programs, which were previously developed by researchers who focused on child aggression (Lochman & Wells, 2002a). Session content largely focuses on parent skills training. Specifically, parents learn the following skills over the course of the 16 sessions: (1) stress management training; (2) identifying prosocial and disruptive behavioral targets for their children using specific operational terms; (3) rewarding and attending to appropriate child behaviors; (4) giving effective instructions and commands; (5) establishing age-appropriate rules and expectations; (6) applying effective consequences to negative behaviors by the child; and, (7) establishing family communication and problem-solving structures in the home. In the Parent Component sessions, parents are also informed of the skills targeted in the Child Component and are encouraged to reinforce their children using these new skills at home and school.

FIDELITY PROCEDURES AND ASSESSMENT

To ensure that these intervention components were provided as planned, procedures were formulated for developing and evaluating intervention fidelity. Detailed intervention manuals were used for both the Coping Power Child Component and Parent Component. Staff and school counselors received a 10-hour training program prior to the start of, and during, intervention, and received weekly scheduled supervision of their intervention work. Leaders used the OLCPS (Objectives List for Coping Power Sessions) to indicate whether each objective of each session was met completely, partially, or not at all. Fidelity to session objectives were coded after each session by the delivering clinician. Trained research staff also coded each audio-recorded session and provided an independent rating as to the extent to which each objective was met. The trained staff used the 14-item MCPIQ (Measure of Coping Power Implementation Quality) to rate quality of implementation of each child session. The coders used an 11-item MCPIQ to rate parent sessions. Fidelity checklists were reviewed by the supervisors during weekly supervision sessions. Over 90% of session objectives were delivered (Lochman & Wells, 2003).

INITIAL EFFICACY STUDIES

Several trials examined the efficacy of Coping Power as a prevention program for aggressive youth. In the first (Lochman & Wells, 2002a; Lochman & Wells, 2004), 183 aggressive boys who were in the top 22% in teachers' ratings of children's aggressive and disruptive behavior were randomized to Coping Power Child Component only, combined Coping Power Child and Parent Components, or a no-treatment control. At one-year posttreatment, boys who were assigned to the Coping Power conditions demonstrated reductions in their self-reported delinquent behaviors, parent-reported marijuana use by the child, and improvements in teacher-reported school functioning relative to the control condition (Lochman & Wells, 2004). Further, Coping Power's effects on parent-reported substance use by the child and delinquent behavior were more pronounced for boys assigned to the Combined Coping Power condition. Intervention effects for the initial efficacy trial were at least partly mediated by changes in boys' social-cognitive processes and schemas as well as by changes in parenting behaviors (Lochman & Wells, 2002a).

In a second efficacy study, inclusion of a brief universal classroom-level prevention intervention component, along with Coping Power has been shown to result in reduced self-reported substance use, lower teacher-rated aggression, higher perceived social competence, and greater teacher-rated improvement in the child's behaviors compared to a control group (Lochman & Wells, 2002b). Replicating the first study, children who had received Coping Power had lower rates of substance use, delinquency, and aggressive behavior at a one-year follow-up (Lochman & Wells, 2003), and the brief universal intervention was not found to augment these follow-up effects. In a subsequent three-year follow-up, the universal intervention again no longer had effects, but Coping Power continued to lead to reductions in aggressive behavior and academic behavioral problems, along with improvements in children's abilities to anticipate consequences for their actions and in parents' supportiveness in the home (Lochman et al., 2013). When neighborhood-level moderators were examined, the Coping Power positive effect on children's aggressive behavior was more robust in problematic neighborhoods, where parents perceived lower levels of neighborhood social cohesion and organization.

FLEXIBILITY WITHIN FIDELITY

Over 10 years ago, Kendall introduced the concept of "flexibility within fidelity" as a useful way to guide effective implementation and dissemination of structured, manual-based interventions that had been found to be efficacious in rigorous controlled research (Kendall & Beidas, 2007). Kendall and Frank (2018) described how this concept fits within the Consolidated Framework for Implementation Research (CFIR; Damschroder et al., 2009). The CFIR addresses five domains that are considered to be important for meaningful implementation of psychological interventions; these include (1) the intervention itself, (2) the outer setting or factors external to the organization hosting the intervention, (3) the inner setting and characteristics of the organization, (4) the individual clinician providing the intervention, and (5) the process of the planning and execution of the implementation of the intervention. The latter process-oriented domain also includes the training and supervision processes that can affect intervention implementation (Schoenwald, Mehta, Frazier, & Shernoff, 2013).

According to the CFIR, the components of the first domain, a structured intervention, can be separated into those that are core components, which are key elements that can't be changed, and those that are adaptable periphery components, namely, parts of the intervention that can be adapted. It is precisely this distinction that is critically important for the notion of flexibility within fidelity. Fidelity involves therapist adherence to the intervention protocol components (Kendall & Frank, 2018). For example, in our Coping Power Program implementation guides for each session, we have activities nested within objectives, many of which are linked to target mechanisms designed to reduce externalizing behavior problems; the adherence to objective completion is the main indicator of adherence to the fidelity of the intervention. Applying the concept of flexibility within fidelity, the clinician implements core intervention ingredients (attaining fidelity), but adapts implementation in meaningful ways to address child engagement and variations in the child's ability to understand the purpose of activities (Kendall & Frank, 2018). Thus, adaptations of interventions are expected, but there may be important distinctions between fidelity-consistent and fidelity-inconsistent modifications (Stirman, Gamarra, Bartlett, Calloway, & Gutner, 2017).

In the remainder of this chapter, we address how elements of the CFIR model have been evident in our dissemination research with the Coping Power Program in real-world settings. We will focus especially on the issue of adaptations of evidence-based intervention (Lochman, Boxmeyer, Kassing, Powell, & Stromeyer, 2019; Lochman, Powell, Boxmeyer, Andrade, Stromeyer, & Jimenez-Camargo, 2012). We first explore how adaptations become evident and commonly occur in the practice of real-world clinicians, and how that is affected by the degree of intensity in training and the characteristics of the clinicians and of their school settings. Second, we discuss how planned adaptations can be made and tested by program developers, following concrete adaptation steps (e.g., Goldstein et al., 2012) to address variations in clients and cultures and to optimize the structure and format of the intervention.

ADAPTATIONS AND DISSEMINATION WITH REAL-WORLD COUNSELORS

Effects of Variation in Intensity of Training

Research indicates that Coping Power can be disseminated effectively to clinicians in real-world settings. Research has examined how variations in CFIR domains, including clinician training, as well as counselor and school characteristics may affect successful use of the program. Coping Power was implemented by school mental health personnel (primarily school guidance counselors) in a field trial that examined intensity of training (Lochman, Boxmeyer et al., 2009). School counselors conducted Coping Power with groups of children, as well as with the children's parents. Counselors received either basic training (CP-BT) or intensive training (CP-IT). A comparison group of counselors was included as a third condition and did not implement Coping Power.

Fifty-seven public schools in north-central Alabama were included in the study, and each school counselor was randomly assigned to the CP-BT, CP-IT, or comparison condition. Sixteen schools had a counselor who also served another school, thus schools were yoked so there were eight pairs of yoked schools, which were then randomly assigned. Stratified random assignment was used to guarantee an equal number of schools per condition (19). Children were screened for aggression by their third-grade teachers, and the top 30% of aggressive children were considered for the study. A total of 531 children and their parents participated and were roughly equally distributed across the schools and conditions. The 34-session Child Component was delivered over 18 months, corresponding to the spring semester of fourth grade and all of fifth grade. During this period, counselors also met with parents for the 16-session Coping Power Parent Component. Counselors used intervention manuals for both components and all sessions were audiotaped.

There were 17 counselors in both the CP-BT and comparison conditions, and 15 counselors in the CP-IT condition; they were equivalent in terms of ethnicity and years of experience. Counselors received training from four doctoral-level clinical psychologists. In both the CP-BT and CP-IT conditions, counselors attended three workshop trainings prior to starting the intervention. Trainers also provided two-hour training sessions every month that included concrete training for upcoming sessions, debriefing of previous sessions, and assistance in problem-solving of barriers and difficulties in implementation. Only the CP-IT counselors received individualized supervisory feedback on the quality of their intervention implementation. Trainers provided monthly written letters, and phone calls as needed, based on audiotape review of sessions. Feedback included review of completion of the intervention objectives for each session and discussion of the enthusiasm and involvement of participants, as well as feedback on the counselors' ability to stimulate discussion and elaborate and clarify material while staying on topic, engage students in positive ways, and use appropriate monitoring and consequences during sessions. Intervention fidelity was assessed by counselors' reports of whether each of the principal objectives during sessions was addressed "completely," "partially," or "not at all." Intervention sessions were also audiotaped, and trained research staff coded each session using the same measure of objective completion.

Results indicated that children in the CP-IT condition had better parent-, teacher-, and child-rated behavioral outcomes than both the CP-BT and comparison conditions. Additionally, children in the CP-IT condition demonstrated significant improvements in their expectations about the negative consequences of aggressive behavior, and teachers reported concurrent improvements in positive social behavior and study skills. A follow-up study of children's academic outcomes found that CP-IT children had significantly smaller declines in language arts grades at a two-year follow-up than did their peers in the comparison condition (Lochman, Boxmeyer, Powell, Qu, Wells, & Windle, 2012). Children in the CP-BT and comparison conditions did not have significantly different outcomes. Taken together, the results indicate that Coping Power can be effectively disseminated for use with school counselors, provided training is intensive and ongoing.

The equivalence in outcomes of students in CP-BT schools and students in control comparison schools was particularly striking, given that the training provided to counselors in the CP-BT condition was more intensive than is often provided in real-world practice settings (which typically entails one or two days of workshop training and does not include the recording of sessions or ongoing consultation while implementation is underway). The primary difference between the CP-BT and CP-IT conditions in the field trial was the provision of monthly "performance feedback" based upon supervisory review of recorded sessions. CP-IT counselors who received regular performance feedback were better at implementing Coping Power with high quality and with high child and parent engagement, as measured by independent coders' ratings. Receiving individualized performance feedback may have contributed to the counselors' enhanced engagement with child and parent participants and motivated them to better implement the program, both of which may have contributed to improved child outcomes. Not surprisingly, the findings indicate that providing ongoing, individualized supervisory feedback is a crucial training component when disseminating manualized interventions such as Coping Power.

Effects of Organizational Climate, Leadership and Counselor Characteristics on Quality of Implementation

From a CFIR framework, leadership and organizational climate are important aspects of the "support system" for developing and sustaining high fidelity implementation of cognitive-behavioral interventions (CBIs) in systems and organizations (Aarons, Ehrhart, Farahnak, & Sklar, 2014). A range of characteristics can influence the implementation and outcomes of CBIs, such as leadership style and commitment to program implementation, counselors' personalities, the social environment of the organization, and the relationships among individuals in the work setting (e.g., Aarons et al., 2014).

In the trial of Coping Power just described, the degree and quality of implementation of Coping Power was influenced by characteristics of the school staff members who were trained to provide the intervention and by the climate of the schools in which the program was delivered (Lochman, Powell et al., 2009, 2015). Counselor "agreeableness" was positively associated with several measures of program implementation, including completion of session objectives, the number of sessions scheduled, and engagement with parents. Counselor "conscientiousness" was positively associated with engagement with children. School-level characteristics also predicted implementation outcomes. Counselors who were "cynical about organizational change" had poorer quality of engagement with children and parents, in particular when they worked in schools with environments that allowed staff members limited autonomy and that had greater managerial control. Dissemination into real-world settings must take into account the social contexts (Aarons et al., 2014), especially their interaction with individual provider characteristics such as agreeableness, conscientiousness, and level of cynicism about organizational change. Dissemination of evidence-based interventions benefits from careful screening and training of clinicians.

Despite widespread concern about the frequent failure of trained prevention staff to continue to use evidence-based programs following periods of intensive training, little research has addressed the characteristics and experiences of counselors that might predict their sustained use of a program. A follow-up study of the same sample of school counselors who were trained to use Coping Power determined their levels of continued use of the program's child and parent components in the two years following the counselors' intensive training in the program (Lochman, Powell, Boxmeyer, Qu, Sallee, Wells, & Windle, 2015). By two years after the intervention, most of the counselors were continuing to use Coping Power, although not the full program. Intensively trained counselors used

83% of the objectives for the Coping Power Child Component, but only 39% of the objectives for the Coping Power Parent Component. Counselor characteristics and experiences also were examined as predictors of their sustained use of the program components. The results indicated that counselors' perceptions of interpersonal support from teachers within their schools, their perceptions of the effectiveness of the program, and their expectations for using the program were all predictive of program use over the following two years. In addition, certain counselor personality characteristics (i.e., conscientiousness) and the level of actual teacher-rated behavior change experienced by the children they worked with during training were predictors of counselors' sustained use of the program.

Adaptations Counselors Made in their Delivery of the Program

To more deeply examine the kinds of changes that counselors made spontaneously in their delivery of Coping Power during the training phase of this field trial, Boxmeyer, Lochman, Powell, Windle, and Wells (2008) examined the frequency and types of adaptations made by the field trial counselors. Research staff re-coded a random sample of 60 audiotaped sessions (45 child sessions, 15 parent sessions) using a semistructured adaptation coding system. The coding system was designed to assess the following types of potential adaptations: (1) addition of new material related to the planned session content; (2) addition of new material unrelated to the planned session content; (3) alterations to planned session activities and objectives; (4) deviations from the behavioral management system outlined in the Coping Power manual; (5) changes to the order in which the session objectives were completed; and (6) other adaptations. Thirty of the audiotapes (20 child sessions, 10 parent sessions) were double-coded to assess the reliability of the adaptation coding system.

Counselors added new material in 39 of 60 (65%) sessions. New material that was considered to be relevant to the session content was added to 24 sessions, while unrelated material was added to 15 sessions. Examples of related additions included: provision of additional examples to further elucidate the material, discussion about respective child or parent group meetings, and relation of the material to specific incidents that had occurred at school or in the intervention group. Examples of unrelated additions included: discussion of personal, school-related, or family matters, without any linkage made to the Coping Power Program content.

Counselors made changes to the session objectives in 33 of 60 (55%) sessions. The most frequent changes were restrictions, in which activities were simplified or shortened (e.g., counselor briefly mentions barriers to goals but does not elicit examples of recently encountered barriers from the group or conduct role plays to illustrate how to overcome a barrier), and alterations, in which the "rules" for an activity were not followed (e.g., counselor assigned the students personal behavioral goals rather than allowing the students to select goals themselves; counselor praises specific behavior changes the students have made but does not ask them to identify positive changes in themselves or other group members). Restrictions occurred in 47% of sessions and alterations in 40% of sessions. Expansions, in which the counselor conducted an optional activity or repeated an activity to meet an objective more comprehensively, occurred in 45% of child sessions, but in no parent sessions. No substitutions, in which the counselor replaced a session activity with his or her own activity or substantially adapted the terminology, occurred.

These findings illustrate the types of adaptations that real-world practitioners made to a manual-based intervention—and the appropriate adaptations did not detract from the favorable outcomes! Several examples of adaptations strengthened the implementation quality (e.g., repeating an activity until the skill was mastered; modifying the suggested language to make it more culturally or developmentally appropriate; using a real group problem to illustrate a lesson). There were also examples, however, of adaptations that detracted from the implementation quality (ranging from complete omission of sessions or session objectives, to an alteration or restriction of an activity so that its intended impact was dampened or lost). Feedback about the range of appropriate to inappropriate adaptations was included in the performance feedback element in the intensive training for Coping Power providers and should be an important element of future training.

PLANNED ADAPTATIONS AND OPTIMIZATION

Adaptations are common, and perhaps inevitable, when evidence-based interventions are implemented in real-world settings, and are often made in response to unique client needs and/or limited resources. Though they may be well-intended, adaptations made in this manner may compromise the effectiveness of the original program. Nonetheless, there may be advantages, in terms of credibility and efficiency, to applying an established intervention to a new population or within a different context. Ideally, adaptations made to existing intervention programs will be carefully thought out and implemented and evaluated in a systematic way. Goldstein, Kemp, Leff, and Lochman (2012) address this topic, providing a nine-step process for adapting manualized treatment programs to address clinical and contextual factors not included in the original protocol, while retaining the programs' key clinical content and active mechanisms.

Goldstein and colleagues (2012) emphasize the importance of stakeholder input in the adaptation process, basing their guidelines in Participatory Action Research. The nine steps they recommend for adaptation include: (1) choose a manual/program for adaptation; (2) conduct a focus group with the new target population; (3) make initial manual revisions; (4) pilot initial revisions of the manualized intervention; (5) conduct facilitator focus groups; (6) acquire expert review of the revised manual; (7) incorporate staff and expert feedback; (8) conduct an initial open trial of the revised manual-based intervention; and (9) conduct a randomized controlled trial of the revised manual-based intervention.

Using this process, the Coping Power Program has been adapted to target relational aggression in urban African-American girls (Friend2Friend Program; Leff et al., 2015) and with girls receiving treatment while in juvenile detention centers (Juvenile Justice Anger Management [JJAM]; Goldstein et al., 2018). Through the nine-step process, both of the adapted programs planfully incorporated culture-, gender-, and context-specific factors into the new protocols, while retaining essential program content. Subsequent evaluations of both programs demonstrated positive effects on girls' aggressive behavior (Goldstein et al., 2018; Leff et al., 2015), providing support for the newly developed programs and for the adaptation process.

Adaptations to Address Program Length

In addition to the Friend2Friend and JJAM adaptations of Coping Power, which aim to address the unique needs of girls with externalizing behavior problems, the program also has been modified to address other practical and clinical concerns. For example, an abbreviated version has been developed in response to concerns about the program's length, which spans two academic years in the full program. While preserving all of the program's focal clinical content, Lochman and colleagues (2014) reduced the number of sessions from 34 to 24 for children, and from 16 to 12 for parents, with the new curriculum designed for implementation within a single school year. Results from a randomized controlled trial (RCT) involving 240 fifth-grade students indicated improvements in teacher-rated externalizing problems at posttreatment, which were maintained at a three-year follow-up (Lochman et al., 2014).

   Similar concerns about length of treatment and, for school-based administration, time required away from the classroom, led to the development of another abbreviated adaptation, Internet-Enhanced Coping Power (CP-IE; Lochman et al., 2017). CP-IE is a hybrid program in which half of the intervention sessions are administered in-person to small groups of students, while the other half of the sessions are completed individually online. This arrangement allows all of the original program content to be delivered with only half as much out-of-class time required. Additionally, the hybrid design preserves opportunities for group interaction with peers and for attention and support from the group leader. CP-IE also has a parent component that follows the same model of alternating in-person groups with independent completion of online modules in the intervening weeks. In an evaluation involving 91 fifth graders, children in a care-as-usual comparison condition had significantly greater increases in conduct problems than did the CP-IE children, demonstrating the program's preventive effects. Although implementation of CP-IE required less time and resources, the program delivered results similar to those found in trials of the full Coping Power Program. By successfully addressing implementation concerns about length of treatment, these two adapted programs increase the likelihood of wider dissemination and greater public health impact.

Adaptations to Address Program Targets

Several intervention outcome studies of Coping Power have shown stronger program effects on proactive aggression (e.g., planned, unemotional, reward-driven) than on reactive aggression (e.g., emotion-driven, impulsive). In an effort to enhance and broaden the program's effectiveness, Miller and colleagues (2020) adapted Coping Power by incorporating mindfulness techniques shown to impact reactive mechanisms (e.g., attentional, cognitive, emotional, and behavioral dysregulation) in other populations. Onto the existing Coping Power curriculum, Mindful Coping Power (MCP) added mindfulness activities such as breathing exercises, yoga, and loving-kindness meditation, while also reframing standard Coping Power activities to have a mindfulness focus. For example, standard Coping Power teaches students to identify angry cognitions and substitute "coping statements," while MCP encourages students to notice and accept their angry thoughts and let them pass. A similar adaptation process was completed for the MCP parent component. The relative merits of this adaptation await the results of research evaluations.

Optimization of Format Delivery

Across multiple trials of Coping Power, the program has demonstrated positive effects, and iatrogenic effects have not been identified. For some children, however, program benefits are small, and one line of Coping Power research has sought to identify factors predictive of children's differential response. With this information, future intervention modifications can be planned to optimize outcome effects.

Lochman and colleagues (2015) studied 360 fourth- and fifth-grade students to evaluate a version of Coping Power, adapted for individual administration versus the standard group-based program. Overall results were positive for both programs, but effects were stronger for the individual version, particularly for children with certain characteristics. Children who started the project with low ratings of inhibitory control were less responsive to the group-based program than the individual program, based on teacher ratings of externalizing behavior at a one-year follow-up (Lochman et al., 2015). Psychophysiological measurements and genotype traits similarly moderated the effects of individual versus group delivery (Glenn et al., 2019; Glenn et al., 2018; Lochman et al., 2019). Children's respiratory sinus arrhythmia (RSA), a measure of parasympathetic nervous system activity (i.e., arousal reduction), and skin conductance level (SCL), a measure of sympathetic nervous system activity (i.e., "fight of flight" response), were measured at baseline. The individual version of Coping Power proved to be a better fit for students whose preintervention RSA scores were low, based on teacher ratings of aggression one year after intervention. Similarly, students who started the program with high levels of SCL showed more improvement in the individual intervention, based on teacher ratings of externalizing behavior at a four-year follow-up. Finally, the individual version of Coping Power produced stronger effects on teacher ratings at the four-year follow-up for a group of children with a genotype for an Oxytocin receptor gene associated with social bonding, suggesting that such children may have benefitted less from group Coping Power because they were distracted by peers or influenced by negative peer behaviors. Results from moderator analyses demonstrate how programs can be adapted, in this case from group delivery to individual administration, to optimize effects for samples with specific characteristics and/or clinical needs.

International Adaptations for Specific Populations and Intervention Settings

Other adaptations embodying the principles of "flexibility within fidelity" involve cultural modifications for delivery in international settings. The program has been implemented around the globe, in countries including the Netherlands, Italy, Sweden, and Pakistan.

The Netherlands. Van de wiel, Matthys, Cohen-Kettenis, and van Engeland (2003) translated the program into Dutch and modified it for implementation in outpatient clinics with children receiving treatment for Conduct Disorder (CD) or Oppositional Defiant Disorder (ODD). To address this population's behavioral issues, sessions were reconfigured to rely less on discussion and to include more hands-on activities. The parent and child components also were condensed into fewer sessions, to more closely approximate standard outpatient treatment length. Results indicated that this version was comparably effective as the clinic's standard treatment, but Coping Power was delivered at lower cost and by less experienced therapists. Additional analyses found that Coping Power produced greater effects on parent-reported aggression than family therapy, though results were equivalent with behavior therapy (van de Wiel et al., 2007). At a four-year follow-up, students who had participated in Coping Power had lower rates of smoking and marijuana use, as compared to the treatment as usual group, and the Coping Power group's use of these substances was not different from that of typically developing controls (Zonnevylle-Bender et al., 2007).

Others in the Netherlands adapted Coping Power for use with children with mild-to-borderline intellectual disability (MBID). The program was revised to accommodate the children's learning abilities by including more repetition, simplified language, more visual cues, more activities with a physical component, and a reduced amount of content in each session. For parents, new psychoeducational information concerning children with MBID was added to the core content. Evaluation of the program indicated reductions in teacher ratings of externalizing behavior, improvements in positive parenting, and improvements in the parent-child relationship (Schuiringa et al., 2017).

Italy. A team developed several adaptations of Coping Power, including versions for classroom implementation (preschool, elementary, and middle school) and for clinic-based administration.

Classroom adaptations. Class-wide versions of the program were developed in response to teacher concerns about high rates of disruptive behavior in their classrooms and challenges with general classroom behavior management (Muratori et al., 2015). Adapting the program for classroom use has advantages including broader reach, the opportunity for children who are socially skilled to positively influence those experiencing challenges, and, because teachers are the main implementers, increased likelihood of sustainability. In addition, because students' regular classroom teachers implement the program, teachers can coach and reinforce program skills throughout the school day, providing greater opportunity for integration and generalization.

To modify the program for classroom use, adaptations were made to make small group activities inclusive for the whole class. For example, in the regular program student goals are tracked on "goal sheets" kept by students in personal notebooks and each student works toward earning individual rewards. For the classroom version, students work toward a group reward and a poster is used to track all students' goals, heightening accountability to the group. Students also are divided into teams for activities, allowing more participation across the class (Muratori et al., 2015). Providing an exemplar of flexibility within fidelity, class-wide administration is further supported by illustrated storybooks developed for each of the Italian classroom versions (preschool, elementary, middle; Muratori et al., 2020; Muratori, Bertacchi, et al., 2019; Muratori, Giuli, et al., 2017). Each story conveys Coping Power's key concepts with fidelity to the model, doing so within a developmental context appropriate for the target students' level (e.g., a bumble bee is the main character for preschoolers, while a rock band is the background for early adolescents).

Cultural adaptations were made to enhance program relevance for Italian students. For example, in the original program, students are evaluated on progress toward goals on a "yes-no" basis, while the Italian version also includes a "so-so" option in recognition that it is possible to "somewhat" respect a norm in Italian culture (Muratori, Bertacchi, et al., 2017). The adapted program also advised a stronger degree of teasing in an activity designed for practice managing strong feelings, noting that gentle teasing is culturally normative and unlikely to provoke a significant emotional reaction useful for applying anger management skills.

Outcome evaluations of the Italian classroom versions of Coping Power provide support for the programs. When compared to children in elementary classrooms receiving the standard social-emotional learning curriculum in Italy, Coping Power students have been shown to decrease teacher-rated problem behaviors and to increase prosocial behaviors (Muratori et al., 2015; Muratori et al., 2016). Although the classroom programs do not include a parenting component, positive results have been found to generalize to the home setting, as indicated by improvements in parent-rated conduct problems (Muratori, Bertacchi et al., 2019). Positive outcomes for middle school students include decreased internalizing symptoms and improvements in prosocial behavior, compared to students receiving standard instruction (Muratori et al., 2020). Preschoolers in Coping Power classrooms have shown improvements in parent and teacher ratings of externalizing behaviors across two samples (Muratori, Giuli et al., 2017; Muratori, Lochman et al., 2019).

Clinic-based adaptations. Coping Power has been adapted and evaluated for delivery in Italian outpatient settings. For both the parent and child components, the program content and length are consistent with the original curricula; however, the program was adapted to address children's attentional needs by reducing the emphasis on discussion and incorporating hands-on activities and play into the sessions. When compared to two different active treatments (multicomponent intervention, child psychotherapy) at a one-year follow-up, Coping Power was more effective in reducing aggressive behaviors and callous-unemotional traits (Muratori, Milone et al., 2017).

Sweden. A Swedish version of Coping Power also has been shown to have promise for outpatient populations (Helander et al., 2018). Children diagnosed with CD or ODD and their parents were randomly assigned to participate in Coping Power and Parent Management Training (PMT) or PMT only. Instead of the standard one-hour sessions, children met for 15 two-and-a-half hour sessions, during which breaks were scheduled for children to interact and practice social skills. Other adaptations addressed the children's attentional difficulties (e.g., more frequent breaks, completing activities orally rather than in writing). At posttreatment, children from both conditions demonstrated reduced behavior problems, with greater increases in prosocial behavior for the children who received Coping Power. For children with high levels of baseline ODD symptoms, the combined Coping Power and PMT treatment produced significantly stronger effects on behavior problems and prosocial behavior than PMT alone.

Pakistan. In Pakistan, Mushtaq and colleagues (2017) made cultural adaptations to Coping Power for school-based administration to small groups of boys. The manual was translated into Urdu, and modifications were made to reflect religious beliefs and cultural practices related to anger management and communication skills. A parenting intervention was planned, but due to poor response, only the child component was implemented. An RCT involved randomization of 112 highly aggressive fourth grade boys to Coping Power or waitlist control conditions, with Coping Power students participating in 25 sessions at their schools. In postintervention analyses, Coping Power boys showed significant reductions in teacher- and parent-reported aggression, and also demonstrated improved teacher-reported prosocial skills (Mushtaq et al., 2017).

CONCLUSION

"Flexibility within fidelity" (Kendall & Frank, 2018) plays an important role in how the cognitive-behavioral intervention, Coping Power, can be implemented successfully in real-world school and clinic settings. Dissemination requires use of implementation science methods, including careful attention to the intensity of training provided to service providers, and to the characteristics of the providers and their work settings. Clinicians in real-world settings can make acceptable and appropriate adaptations of the structured Coping Power activities, but also can make unacceptable adaptations. To prevent unacceptable adaptations, intense training with performance feedback helps service providers to see the difference. Coping Power is not a stagnant program, but one that evolves with planned adaptations to address various types of clients and delivery methods. We anticipate that a future direction for research on cognitive-behavioral programs such as Coping Power will be further exploration of moderators of intervention effects, leading to planful steps to optimize and tailor interventions for various types of children (Lochman, Boxmeyer et al., 2019).

REFERENCES

Aarons, G. A., Ehrhart, M. G., Farahnak, L. R., & Sklar, M. (2014). Aligning leadership across systems and organizations to develop a strategic climate for evidence-based practice implementation. *Annual Review of Public Health, 35*, 255–274.

Boxmeyer, C. L., Lochman, J. E., Powell, N. R., Windle, M., & Wells, K. (2008). School counselors' implementation of Coping Power in a dissemination field trial: Delineating the range of flexibility within fidelity. *Report on Emotional and Behavioral Disorders in Youth, 8*, 79–95.

Damschroder, L. J., Aron, D. C., Keith, R. E., Kirsh, S. R., Alexander, J. A., & Lowery, J. C. (2009). Fostering implementation of health services research findings into practice: A consolidated framework for advancing implementation science. *Implementation Science, 4(1)* doi: 10.1186/1748-5908-4-50

Glenn, A. L., Lochman, J. E., Dishion, T., Powell, N. P., Boxmeyer, C., Kassing, F., Qu, L., & Romero, D. (2019). Toward tailored interventions: Sympathetic and parasympathetic functioning predicts responses to an intervention for conduct problems delivered in two formats. *Prevention Science, 20*(1), 30–40.

Glenn, A. L., Lochman, J. E., Dishion, T., Powell, N. P., Boxmeyer, C., & Qu, L. (2018). Oxytocin receptor gene variant interacts with intervention delivery format in predicting intervention outcomes for youth with conduct problems. *Prevention Science, 19*(1), 38–48.

Goldstein, N. E. S., Giallella, C. L., Haney-Caron, E., Peterson, L., Serico, J., Kemp, K., Romaine, C. R., Zelechoski, A. D., Holliday, S. B., Kalbeitzer, R., Kelley, S. M., Hinz, H., Sallee, M., Pennacchia, D., Prelic, A., Burkard, C., Grisso, T., Heilbrun, K., Núñez, A., . . . Lochman, J. (2018). Juvenile Justice Anger Management (JJAM) Treatment for Girls: Results of a randomized controlled trial. *Psychological Services, 15*(4), 386–397. https://doi.org/10.1037/ser0000184

Goldstein, N. E. S., Kemp, K. A., Leff, S. S., & Lochman, J. E. (2012). Guidelines for adapting manualized treatments for new target populations: A step-wise approach using anger management as a model. *Clinical Psychology: Science and Practice, 19*, 385–401.

Helander, M., Lochman, J., Högström, J., Ljótsson, B., Hellner, C., & Enebrink, P. (2018). The effect of adding Coping Power Program-Sweden to Parent Management Training-effects and moderators in a randomized controlled trial. *Behaviour Research and Therapy, 103*, 43–52. https://doi.org/10.1016/j.brat.2018.02.001

Kazdin, A. E. (1995). *Conduct disorders on childhood and adolescence* (2nd ed.). Sage.

Kendall, P. C., & Beidas, R. S. (2007). Smoothing the trail for dissemination of evidence-based practices for youth: Flexibility within fidelity. *Professional Psychology: Research and Practice, 58*, 13–20.

Kendall, P. C., & Frank, H. E. (2018). Implementing evidence-based treatment protocols: Flexibility within fidelity. *Clinical Psychology: Science and Practice, 25 (4),* doi: 10.1111/cpsp.12271

Leff, S. S., Paskewich, B. S., Waasdorp, T. E., Waanders, C., Bevans, K. B., & Jawad, A. F. (2015). Friend to friend: A randomized trial for urban African American relationally aggressive girls. *Psychology of Violence, 5*(4), 433–443. https://doi.org/10.1037/a0039724

Lochman, J. E., Baden, R. E., Boxmeyer, C. L., Powell, N. P., Qu, L., Salekin, K. L., & Windle, M. (2014). Does a booster intervention augment the preventive effects of an abbreviated version of the Coping Power Program for aggressive children? *Journal of Abnormal Child Psychology, 42*(3), 367–381.

Lochman, J. E., Boxmeyer, C. L., Jones, S., Qu, L., Ewoldsen, D., & Nelson III, W. M. (2017). Testing the feasibility of a briefer school-based preventive intervention with aggressive children: A hybrid intervention with face-to-face and internet components. *Journal of School Psychology, 62*, 33–50.

Lochman, J. E., Boxmeyer, C. L., Kassing, F. L., Powell, N. P., & Stromeyer, S. L. (2019). Cognitive-behavioral intervention for youth at-risk for conduct problems: Future directions. *Journal of Clinical Child and Adolescent Psychology, 48*, 799–810.

Lochman, J. E., Boxmeyer, C., Powell, N., Qu, L., Wells, K., & Windle, M. (2009). Dissemination of the Coping Power Program: Importance of intensity of counselor training. *Journal of Consulting and Clinical Psychology, 77*, 397–409.

Lochman, J. E., Boxmeyer, C. L., Powell, N. P., Qu, L., Wells, K., & Windle, M. (2012). Coping Power dissemination study: Intervention and special education effects on academic outcomes. *Behavioral Disorders, 37*, 192–205.

Lochman, J. E., Dishion, T. J., Powell, N. P., Boxmeyer, C. L., Qu, L., & Sallee, M. (2015). Evidence-based preventive intervention for preadolescent aggressive children: One-year outcomes following randomization to group versus individual delivery. *Journal of Consulting and Clinical Psychology, 83*(4), 728.

Lochman, J. E., Glenn, A. L., Powell, N. P., Boxmeyer, C. L., Bui, C., Kassing, F., Qu, L., Romero, D., & Dishion, T. (2019). Group versus individual format of intervention for aggressive children: Moderators and predictors of outcomes through 4 years after intervention. *Development and Psychopathology, 31*(5), 1757–1775.

Lochman, J. E., Powell, N., Boxmeyer, C., Andrade, B., Stromeyer, S., & Jimenez-Camargo, L. A. (2012). Adaptations to the Coping Power Program's structure, delivery settings, and clinician training. *Psychotherapy, 49*, 135–142.

Lochman, J. E., Powell, N. P., Boxmeyer, C. L., Qu, L., Sallee, M., Wells, K. C., & Windle, M. (2015). Counselor-level predictors of sustained use of an indicated preventive intervention for aggressive children. *Prevention Science, 16*, 1075–1085.

Lochman, J. E., Powell, N., Boxmeyer, C., Qu, L., Wells, K., & Windle, M. (2009). Implementation of a school-based prevention program: Effects of counselor and school characteristics. *Professional Psychology: Research and Practice, 40*, 476–497.

Lochman, J. E., & Wells, K. C. (1996). A social–cognitive intervention with aggressive children: Prevention effects and contextual implementation issues. In R. D. Peters & R. J. McMahon (Eds.), *Prevention and early intervention: Childhood disorders, substance use and delinquency* (pp. 111–143). Sage.

Lochman, J. E., & Wells, K. C. (2002a). Contextual social-cognitive mediators and child outcome: A test of the theoretical model in the Coping Power Program. *Development and Psychopathology, 14*, 971–993.

Lochman, J. E., & Wells, K. C. (2002b). The Coping Power Program at the middle school transition: Universal and indicated prevention effects. *Psychology of Addictive Behaviors, 16*, S40–S54.

Lochman, J. E., & Wells, K. C. (2003). Effectiveness study of Coping Power and classroom intervention with aggressive children: Outcomes at a one-year follow-up. *Behavior Therapy, 34*, 493–515.

Lochman, J. E., & Wells, K. C. (2004). The Coping Power program for preadolescent aggressive boys and their parents: Outcome effects at the one-year follow-up. *Journal of Consulting and Clinical Psychology, 72*, 571–578.

Lochman, J. E., Wells, K. C., & Lenhart, L. A. (2008*). Coping Power child group program: Facilitator guide.* Oxford University Press.

Lochman, J. E., Wells, K. C., & Lenhart, L. A. (2008*). Coping Power parent group program: Facilitator guide.* Oxford University Press.

Lochman, J. E., Wells, K. C., Qu, L., & Chen, L. (2013). Three year follow-up of Coping Power intervention effects: Evidence of neighborhood moderation? *Prevention Science, 14*, 364–376.

Miller, S., Boxmeyer, C., Romero, D., Powell, N., Jones, S., & Lochman, J. (2020). Theoretical model of Mindful Coping Power: Optimizing a cognitive behavioral program for high-risk children and their parents by integrating mindfulness. *Clinical Child and Family Psychology Review, 23*, 393–406.

Muratori, P., Bertacchi, I., Catone, G., Mannucci, F., Nocentini, A., Pisano, S., & Lochman, J. E. (2020). Coping Power Universal for middle school students: The first efficacy study. *Journal of Adolescence, 79*, 49–58. https://doi.org/10.1016/j.adolescence.2019.12.014

Muratori, P., Bertacchi, I., Giuli, C., Lombardi, L., Bonetti, S., Nocentini, A., Manfredi, A., Polidori, L., Ruglioni, L., Milone, A., & Lochman, J. E. (2015). First adaptation of Coping Power Program as a classroom-based prevention intervention on aggressive behaviors among elementary school children. *Prevention Science, 16*(3), 432–439. https://doi.org/10.1007/s11121-014-0501-3

Muratori, P., Bertacchi, I., Giuli, C., Nocentini, A., & Lochman, J. E. (2017). Implementing Coping Power adapted as a universal prevention program in Italian primary schools: A randomized control trial. *Prevention Science, 18*(7), 754–761. https://doi.org/10.1007/s11121-016-0715-7

Muratori, P., Bertacchi, I., Giuli, C., Nocentini, A., Ruglioni, L., & Lochman, J. E. (2016). Coping Power adapted as universal prevention program: Midterm effects on children's behavioral difficulties and academic grades. *The Journal of Primary Prevention, 37*(4), 389–401. https://doi.org/10.1007/s10935-016-0435-6

Muratori, P., Bertacchi, I., Masi, G., Milone, A., Nocentini, A., Powell, N. P., Lochman, J. E., Jones, S., Kassing, F., & Romero, D. (2019). Effects of a universal prevention program on externalizing behaviors: Exploring the generalizability of findings across school and home settings. *Journal of School Psychology, 77*, 13–23. https://doi.org/10.1016/j.jsp.2019.09.002

Muratori, P., Giuli, C., Bertacchi, I., Orsolini, L., Ruglioni, L., & Lochman, J. E. (2017). Coping Power for preschool-aged children: A pilot randomized control trial study. *Early Intervention in Psychiatry, 11*(6), 532–538. https://doi.org/10.1111/eip.12346

Muratori, P., Lochman, J. E., Bertacchi, I., Giuli, C., Guarguagli, E., Pisano, S., Gallani, A., & Mammarella, I. C. (2019). Universal Coping Power for pre-schoolers: Effects on children's behavioral difficulties and pre-academic skills. *School Psychology International, 40*(2), 128–144.

Muratori, P., Milone, A., Manfredi, A., Polidori, L., Ruglioni, L., Lambruschi, F., Masi, G., & Lochman, J. E. (2017). Evaluation of improvement in externalizing behaviors and callous-unemotional traits in children with disruptive behavior disorder: A 1-year follow up clinic-based study. *Administration and Policy in Mental Health and Mental Health Services Research, 44*(4), 452–462. https://doi.org/10.1007/s10488-015-0660-y

Mushtaq, A., Lochman, J. E., Tariq, P. N., & Sabih, F. (2017). Preliminary effectiveness study of Coping Power Program for aggressive children in Pakistan. *Prevention Science, 18*(7), 762–771. https://doi.org/10.1007/s11121-016-0721-9

Pardini, D. A. (2008). Novel insights into longstanding theories of bidirectional parent–child influences: Introduction to the special section. *Journal of Abnormal Child Psychology, 36*, 627–631.

Pardini, D. A., Waller, R., & Hawes, S. W. (2014). Familial influences on the development of serious conduct problems and delinquency. In J. Morizot & L. Kazemian (Eds.), *The development of criminal and antisocial behavior: Theoretical foundations and practical applications* (pp. 201–220). Springer.

Schoenwald, S. K., Mehta, T. G., Frazier, S. L., & Shernoff, E. S. (2013). Clinical supervision in effectiveness and implementation research. *Clinical Psychology: Science and Practice, 20*, 44–59.

Schuiringa, H., van Nieuwenhuijzen, M., Orobio de Castro, B., Lochman, J. E., & Matthys, W. (2017). Effectiveness of an intervention for children with externalizing behavior and mild to borderline intellectual disabilities: A randomized trial. *Cognitive Therapy and Research, 41*(2), 237–251. https://doi.org/10.1007/s10608-016-9815-8

Shaw, D. S., Gilliom, M., & Giovannelli, J. (2000). Aggressive behavior disorders. In C. H. Zeanah, Jr. (Ed.), *Handbook of infant mental health* (pp. 397–411). The Guilford Press.

Stirman, S. W., Gamarra, J. M., Bartlett, B. A., Calloway, A., & Gutner, C. A. (2017). Empirical examinations of modifications and adaptations to evidence-based psychotherapies: Methodologies, impact, and future directions. *Clinical Psychology: Science and Practice, 24*, 396–420.

van de Wiel, N. M. H., Matthys, W., Cohen-Kettenis, P. T., Maassen, G. H., Lochman, J. E., & van Engeland, H. (2007). The effectiveness of an experimental treatment when compared to care as usual depends on the type of care as usual. *Behavior Modification, 31*(3), 298–312. https://doi.org/10.1177/0145445506292855

van De Wiel, N. M., Matthys, W., Cohen-Kettenis, P., & Van Engeland, H. (2003). Application of the Utrecht Coping Power Program and care as usual to children with disruptive behavior disorders in outpatient clinics: A comparative study of cost and course of treatment. *Behavior Therapy, 34*(4), 421–436.

Wells, K. C., Lochman, J. E., & Lenhart, L. A. (2008). *Coping Power parent group program: Facilitator guide.* New York, NY: Oxford.

Zonnevylle-Bender, M. J. S., Matthys, W., Van De Wiel, N. M. H., & Lochman, J. E. (2007). Preventive effects of treatment of Disruptive Behavior Disorder in middle childhood on substance use and delinquent behavior. *Journal of the American Academy of Child & Adolescent Psychiatry, 46*(1), 33–39. https://doi.org/10.1097/01.chi.0000246051.53297.57

12

Delivering Treatment for Adolescent Panic Disorder with Flexibility and Fidelity

DONNA B. PINCUS, LAURA NELSON DARLING, AND OVSANNA LEYFER ■

INTRODUCTION

Panic disorder is one of the most impairing of the anxiety disorders to affect youth, with adolescence being its peak period of onset (American Psychiatric Association, 2013). Given that panic disorder is characterized by the recurrence of unexpected surges of somatic and/or cognitive symptoms that develop quite abruptly, and without any readily identifiable cause, it is not surprising that individuals experiencing panic disorder often worry about the onset of these feelings and tend to avoid any situations they think might trigger them. For adolescents with panic disorder, the symptoms of panic, as well as the associated fears about the possible catastrophic causes or outcomes of these symptoms, can disrupt many aspects of their lives, including their academic, family, social, and vocational functioning. Panic in adolescents has been referred to as one of the most debilitating and impairing psychological disorders to affect youth (Ollendick & Pincus, 2008; Pincus et al., 2017).

Many adolescents who experience a sudden rush of feelings that appear "out of the blue" (e.g., shortness of breath, nausea, dizziness, trembling, heart palpitations, feelings of "unreality" and sweating) tend to avoid situations that they believe could potentially elicit these feelings. Developmentally appropriate activities such as going to movies, malls, school, concerts, restaurants, school functions, parties are often avoided due to the fear that these activities might cause panic symptoms to reoccur. As adolescents' avoidance of positive and reinforcing activities increases, feelings of depression may ensue. Family members may understandably be frightened by the adolescents' symptoms, and may be unsure how to help. In an effort to prevent panic from occurring, parents may inadvertently facilitate adolescents' avoidance, which can further exacerbate the frequency of panic. Given that adolescence is a developmental stage when youth should be seeking greater independence and peer interaction, the onset of panic disorder can detrimentally impact an adolescent's developmental trajectory. In fact, numerous studies show that if panic disorder is left untreated, it tends to persist throughout adolescence and it is commonly associated with agoraphobia and other mental health disorders such as mood disorders in adolescence and adulthood (Merikangas et al., 2010).

Fortunately, the development of psychological treatments to address panic disorder in adolescence has progressed significantly over the past three decades (Ollendick, 1995; Pincus et al., 2008, 2010, 2014). These manual-based treatments have demonstrated efficacy in helping decrease the severity and frequency of panic attacks and, most importantly, have helped youth decrease their avoidance practices and return to healthy developmental activities. Decades of research on panic informed the manual-based treatment; the goal of these protocols is to equip adolescents with education about the nature of panic and anxiety, and to provide them with a set of core tools for learning to recognize the triggers of panic, to manage maladaptive thoughts about panic, and to re-enter situations previously avoided (Pincus et al., 2008). Among their many benefits empirically supported, manual-based treatments provide guidelines for therapists on how to frame and deliver treatment, and they provide a standardized way to deliver the treatment (Kendall et al., 1998, 2008). Just as with other manual-based treatments, however, treatment for panic disorder should not be delivered in a rigid fashion; rather, it should be delivered flexibly, with the core treatment components taught but tailored to each individual and family.

Several "core ingredients" or "core skills" are necessary for implementation of panic treatment for adolescents, the cognitive behavioral protocol for treating panic. Clinical practice also includes tailoring the delivery of the treatment to the individual and using the manual as a guide that can be implemented flexibly (Kendall et al., 1998). Using the model and theoretical framework upon which the manual is based, the therapist can tailor the treatment based on the client's individual characteristics, the treatment setting, and other relevant variables, while fostering a strong alliance and trust. Being flexible allows the therapist to adapt and tailor skills for therapy to the teen's particular likes and interests, which could foster rapport and facilitate engagement (e.g., devising a "mountain of accomplishments" rather than a "fear ladder" when a youth is interested in mountain climbing, or using surfing analogies about "riding the wave" of panic with a teen who is interested in surfing). This tailoring of aspects of the treatment can foster the adolescent's increased engagement, an improved therapeutic alliance between the therapist and patient, and can "breathe life into a manual," a concept introduced by Kendall and colleagues (Kendall et al., 1998). As another example, while some youth with high levels of motivation might progress quickly to the top of their exposure hierarchy with just four to six exposure sessions, others might require more exposure sessions due to their persistent levels of avoidance. Youth with comorbid conditions might benefit from the therapist using the panic treatment protocol in a flexible manner. For example, an adolescent with comorbid depression and panic who has sleep disturbance might need to have additional sessions that are focused solely on behavioral activation or sleep hygiene, and may need to be educated about the relationship between sleep and anxiety. Thus, careful consideration of the teen's comorbid conditions, individual characteristics, and background can help guide a practitioner in knowing how to deliver a particular treatment flexibly, but while maintaining fidelity (Kendall et al., 1998; Kendall & Frank, 2018).

When treating adolescents with panic disorder, it is recommended that practitioners consider both the "critical" treatment components that must be delivered to be sure that youth receive the core ingredients of Cognitive Behavioral Therapy (CBT) for panic, as well as the variety of ways that being flexible facilitates positive patient outcomes and client-focused implementation. In the first section of the chapter we describe each of the treatment components required to maintain fidelity, as well as those components that are considered "optional" or "supplemental." We then turn to a review of data on important factors to be considered as well as how information about those factors can inform the flexible, patient-focused implementation.

ESSENTIAL COMPONENTS TO MAINTAIN FIDELITY

Psychoeducation

Teaching the adolescent about the nature of panic and anxiety, the external and internal triggers of panic attacks, and the relationship between one's thoughts, feelings, and behavior is a core component. Psychoeducation is aimed at helping the adolescent dispel any myths or misconceptions about the impact of panic attacks (e.g., that panic symptoms will last forever, or that they will cause one to have a heart attack or to vomit). Regardless of the format of treatment delivery (e.g., intensive or weekly, group or individual), evidence-based treatment for panic typically begins with one or more sessions devoted to education about the cycle of panic (Angelosante et al., 2009; Pincus et al., 2008, 2010).

It is crucial for the adolescent to know that fear and anxiety are normal, necessary, yet harmless emotions that are not only part of the human (and animal) experience, but they are also emotions that can help optimize one's performance (e.g., anxiety before a race can help one run faster; panic when crossing the street as a car is coming can protect us from harm). During an early session, the adolescent learns that there can be identifiable triggers for panic attacks, which do not come on "out of the blue." It is important for the adolescent to learn to identify and become more aware of potential triggers for their panic attacks (including thoughts, physical feelings, or behaviors) so that they can learn that these feelings are actually under their control and need not be feared. Adolescents also are taught that there are various ways one might react to these panic triggers that could help to reduce panic and anxiety. During psychoeducation, the adolescent learns that the goal of treatment is not to completely eliminate all feelings of fear and anxiety, but to reduce the unnecessary or unhelpful "alarm reactions." The adolescent learns to outline the "three components of anxiety: What I Think, What I Feel, and What I Do," and breaks down one of their panic attacks into these three parts. This process allows the adolescent to identify the antecedents and consequences of panic and teaches them to become an "objective observer" of their panic and anxiety rather than a passive "victim."

Taking on the role of objective observer, or scientist who is investigating the patterns of panic attacks allows the adolescent to begin taking control of the "cycle" of panic. Every adolescent is taught to recognize that the panic cycle can fluctuate; while "dizziness" may be the prominent triggering sensation for some panic attacks, a maladaptive thought may be most prominent trigger for other panic attacks. Although some youth may be unable to readily identify the patterns in their panic, or may need some assistance with developing this ability, others may more easily begin to identify situations, feelings, or behaviors that tend to trigger feelings of panic. Thus, as we will illustrate for all core components of panic treatment, it is essential that the delivery of the psychoeducation be tailored to the developmental level of the youth as well as in consideration with other variables (e.g., setting, cognitive ability, motivation).

Another important element of the psychoeducation component of panic treatment is communicating an understanding of the physiology of panic and anxiety. The therapist explains the adaptive and protective purposes of the activation of the "fight or flight" response and the impact this fight or flight reaction has on many systems in the body. For example, as a result of the fight or flight response, the cardiovascular system is affected, because blood is directed toward large muscle groups needed for running, and away from the skin and smaller muscles. The respiratory system also is affected, because we often breathe faster and deeper to circulate more oxygen throughout the body in reaction to fear; this can cause the common feelings of dizziness, lightheadedness, and tingling/numbness in the fingers. Persons in the midst of a panic attack might sweat, might experience a decrease in their salivation (resulting in dry mouth), and might have tense muscles; all of these reactions are part of the fight or flight system, and this is adaptive and normal. The patient is taught the differences between the sympathetic and parasympathetic nervous system, and all the reasons why the physiological sensations that accompany panic are actually all quite normal and adaptive. Patients are taught about why it takes some time for the physical sensations to dissipate, as well as the "survival value" of the fight or flight system. The information taught during the psychoeducation component of panic treatment will be used throughout treatment (e.g., cognitive component, exposure component) (Pincus et al., 2008).

Cognitive Work: Recognizing and Changing Anxious Thoughts

Cognitive strategies are a core component of most child and adolescent CBT for anxiety (e.g., Kendall & Hedtke, 2006a; Kendall & Hedtke, 2006b; Rapee et al., 2006a) and are also critical components of treatments designed specifically to treat panic in adolescents (Pincus et al., 2008). Adolescents are taught to recognize the ways their thoughts can trigger physiological feelings of anxiety, and they are also taught to recognize the fact that many panic-related maladaptive thoughts are not necessarily true or accurate (e.g., "I will faint if I feel panic," "This panic is damaging my heart," "What if these panic sensations last forever and never stop"). Once adolescents are introduced to the rationale for taking a closer look at one's thoughts, they are also taught how anticipating the possibility of a future panic attack makes one feel hypervigilant, overly focused on one's physical sensations, and constantly on the "lookout" for signs of danger.

As one step toward identifying anxious cognitions (self-talk), youth are taught two of the most common cognitive distortions—(1) probability overestimation and (2) catastrophizing—and how they relate to panic disorder. It is essential that youth realize that overestimating the likelihood that something negative will happen inadvertently causes unnecessary anxiety and panic. Using homework sheets and illustrative metaphors, the therapist helps the teen to determine whether they are engaging in any probability overestimations related to panic. For example, if the adolescent interprets a beating heart as an indication of an impending cardiac issue, their emotion will be charged toward panic, whereas if the adolescent interpreted that same beating heart as a sign of excitement or something positive that was about to happen, then their emotion might be less fearful and more relaxed. Similarly, catastrophic thinking, or thinking the worst thing imaginable is going to happen, is a cognitive error that is a very common trigger for panic attacks. For example, thoughts such as "If it comes on, my panic will be intolerable" or "If a panic attack happens at the school dance, it will be a total catastrophe and the worst thing in the world," only further fuels panic. Adolescents are taught to put the panic feelings into a context—and to evaluate whether it would truly be as "catastrophic" as imagined if the event were to happen. Patients are taught how cognitive errors can inadvertently intensify anxiety and panic-like physical sensations.

A key component of the cognitive work is to help adolescents examine the facts and situations and see a more realistic probability of a feared outcome actually occurring. Using facts, past experiences, the real probabilities of events, and data from the experiences from others, adolescents are asked to evaluate their panic-related thinking to explore whether there is sufficient evidence to support the idea as being a "true fact." For example, an adolescent might ask themselves, "Is it a fact that if I go to the dance I definitely will have a panic attack and people will notice? Is there any evidence that it might not happen? Even if it happened, could I cope with it, or would it really be the end of the world? Even if people did notice, would people be talking about this forever, or is it more likely that people would move on and talk about other things eventually?" By learning to counter catastrophic thoughts, adolescents begin to ask themselves, "What is the worst that can happen, and even if that did happen, could I cope?" Through this exercise of examining panic-related cognitions, adolescents learn that in most cases, panic and its effects (e.g., embarrassment), even at their worst are time limited and very manageable. They learn common "myths and misconceptions" about anxiety (e.g., that the panic symptoms mean that they are losing control, having a heart attack, going crazy, or at risk of fainting or vomiting), and they learn information to counter these myths. Challenging anxious cognition helps adolescents replace maladaptive anxious thoughts about panic with more adaptive coping thoughts.

Exposure

Within empirically supported treatments for panic, exposure is a core component, and there are several types of exposure.

Interoceptive Exposure. Avoiding the internal bodily symptoms associated with anxiety and panic is known as *interoceptive avoidance* (Bouton et al., 2001; Rapee et al., 1995). Patients with panic disorder often avoid activities or situations that could elicit the bodily sensations associated with symptoms of panic. Given that a core feature of panic disorder is that patients have heightened sensitivity to and fear of physical sensations of anxiety, it is critical that adolescents acquire the concept of *interoceptive conditioning*—the form of conditioning that occurs when associations develop between specific physical sensations and a response of fear or panic. Furthermore, youth are taught about how interoceptive conditioning can cause panic to occur, even in response to subtle physical sensations. By giving illustrative examples of all of the activities that could result in a conditioned fear reaction, such as running or exercising at the gym, going on an amusement park ride, or perspiring, adolescents become aware that fear reactions in fact do not always "come out of the blue" but might be triggered by a physical sensation. Likewise, it is essential for youth with panic not to avoid these benign and sometimes subtle physical sensations. As a result, a core component of panic treatment involves *interoceptive exposure*, or learning to gradually bring on feared physical sensations in a controlled way (Schmidt & Trakowski, 2004). By practicing bringing on these physical sensations through a series of symptom-induction exercises, the adolescent gradually learns that these situations dissipate relatively quickly on their own and are not harmful. By not avoiding the feared sensations, and by purposefully causing them to increase, adolescents gain exposure to their fear and to the sensations until they begin to habituate to the sensations. It is essential for adolescents to fully engage in these symptom-induction exercises, without engaging in safety behaviors, or behaviors that are intended to avoid disaster. Some of the exercises on the list of interoceptive exposure exercises in the panic treatment protocol for adolescents include: running in place for one minute, holding one's breath for 30 seconds, shaking one's head from side to side for

30 seconds, tensing one's muscles for one minute, spinning in a chair quickly for one minute, or breathing through a thin cocktail straw for two minutes with the nostrils held closed. After engaging in each of these exercises, the adolescent then chooses the exercises that produce the sensations that are most similar to those that occur naturally during a panic attack, and these are the exercises that are practiced for homework. Therapists can combine exercises or create new ones to personalize and tailor treatment so that the exercise produces physical sensations that are most similar to their panic. To keep track of the interoceptive exposure practice, the therapist assigns a record sheet for teens to record the exercise they engaged in, the intensity of the resulting physical sensation, and the intensity of the anxiety, as well as a rating of its similarity to naturally occurring panic (Pincus et al., 2008).

Situational Exposure. Perhaps the most important and core component of panic treatment is having the adolescent engage in situational exposure challenges. Exposure is a central component to most all CBT anxiety treatments for youth (Beidas et al., 2010; Chorpita et al., 2002; Seligman & Ollendick, 2011). To prepare teens for conducting exposures for panic, the therapist engages the patient in a discussion about the concept of *avoidance* and how it relates to panic attacks. Youth are taught the differences between overt avoidance (e.g., walking out of anxiety-provoking situations or refusing to engage in activities due to panic sensations) and subtle avoidance or safety behaviors (e.g., engaging in distraction, excessively drinking water, or carrying a good luck charm to try to ward off panic). Youth are taught the ways that both types of avoidance only further perpetuate panic, and the ways that avoidance can generalize, or spread to other situations. Although avoidance typically eliminates or reduces fear in the short term, it only prolongs the cycle of panic in the long term. This concept of avoidance is critical to learn prior to engaging in exposures, because safety behaviors can make exposures less effective and can interfere with the formation of new learning that the imagined and feared outcome is unlikely to happen.

After learning the importance of nonavoidance, the *rationale for exposure* is described, along with the benefits of facing one's fears. The patient is taught about *habituation*—the ways that anxiety tends to increase upon immediately entering a new situation, and how it gradually decreases over time—by drawing out the habituation curve and describing how repeated exposure practices help the brain create new learning to replace the old "automatic fear response." Importantly, the patient is taught how important it is to maximize the efficacy of exposure practice by repeating variations of exposures within different contexts, consistent with Craske and colleagues' inhibitory learning approach (Craske et al., 2014). Collaboratively, the therapist and teen develop a *fear hierarchy*, which is a list of avoided situations arranged in order from least anxiety provoking to most anxiety provoking. For patients with panic, the situations listed on the hierarchy should be situations that will bring on some physical sensations or even a full panic attack. It is important for exposures to be challenging and create anxious arousal, but they can also be fun—such as going to a concert, taking the subway to a fun place, going to the gym or spin class, going to the mall, riding in the car while sitting in the back seat with the heat on—any situation that will elicit panic-related feelings for the adolescent could be an appropriate situation to list on the hierarchy. A hierarchy is best when some activities are more difficult and some easier. If needed and/or appropriate, parents can be included in the process by helping to generate ideas for possible situations to include in the fear hierarchy. Patients are guided to assign an avoidance and a fear rating for every item on their fear hierarchy. This Fear Avoidance Hierarchy will be used throughout the exposure component of treatment.

Patients can be reminded about their success in completing interoceptive exposure exercises, and told that they can expect to see a similar symptom pattern during the situational exposure practice, just as if they were "riding a wave." That is, the symptoms initially rise, they crest, and then they recede. By engaging in exposures, the patient will learn to change their thoughts about the dangerousness of the situation, they will begin to weaken conditioned fear reactions and develop healthier associations, and importantly, they will learn to reduce their levels of avoidance and impairment. Patients are taught that while feared situations can trigger panic attacks, just *thinking* about doing an exposure (anticipatory anxiety) can often be much more difficult than actually doing an exposure. Furthermore, the patient must be taught that as soon as they learn not to fear the physical sensations, the sensations tend to dissipate quickly. Situational exposure practices can be done in session as well as outside of session as homework practice. Some exposure practices can be done with therapist accompaniment, whereas other exposures can be done with parents or done independently. It is critical, however, that the therapist or parent does not become a "safety person" who inadvertently facilitates avoidance of feelings. The particular format of exposure practice varies, based on factors such as the developmental level of the child, the magnitude of avoidance and fear, and the particular situations that the adolescent is avoiding. These can all be tailored flexibly to the particular needs of each patient. Having direct conversations about the patients' particular hesitations about exposure, the most common excuses for not completing exposures, any previous unsuccessful or successful attempts at exposure, as well as conversations reviewing the patients' goals for treatment, can maximize the chances that the patient's exposure practice will be successful.

Combinations of Interoceptive Exposures and Situational Exposures. To make exposure practices more challenging, patients can be encouraged to integrate interoceptive exposures with their situational exposure practices (e.g., running in place to elicit heart racing and then walking into a crowded shopping mall, or spinning around and then entering a movie theater and sitting in the middle seat where easy escape can be more difficult). Patients are encouraged to remind themselves that they are not "victims" of panic but rather are active observers or "scientists" who are tracking the ways in which their symptoms dissipate over time. These combinations of exposure practices can and should be tailored to each individual patient, with input from the patient on which interoceptive exercises are most similar to "naturally occurring panic."

Relapse Prevention

Before terminating treatment, it is often helpful to review the patient's progress and to assess any "costs" to getting better (e.g., having to attend school again due to panic improving). Given the nature of panic, it helps when patients are informed about the normal fluctuations of panic, and how panic sometimes re-emerges during periods of stress, and the differences between expected normal fluctuations, a "lapse" (which can be addressed with some booster sessions and/or a review of core concepts and further exposure practices) and a "relapse" (full and persistent return of symptoms or avoidance to pretreatment levels or higher). By encouraging appropriate expectations, patients will not become alarmed or catastrophize if and when a random panic attack occurs. Lastly, it is important for patients to develop a plan for continued exposure practice. It can be helpful for the patient to create a new Fear Avoidance Hierarchy to be used for continued future practice even once treatment has ended.

FLEXIBLE, PATIENT-FOCUSED IMPLEMENTATION

In addition to the critical core treatment components described thus far, some other components can be helpful to include in the treatment of panic, based on the particular needs of the patient and the family. The core treatment components also can be implemented in a variety of ways. For example, a therapist might add rewards for patients who need additional motivation, or include parents in treatment who need extra help reducing accommodations. A therapist might vary the format of therapy (e.g., weekly vs. intensive treatment) based on the patient's needs, vary the types of exposures delivered (e.g., interoceptive exposures, in-vivo exposures or both), or add therapy components (e.g., breathing retraining) as needed. Therapy setting variables and patient variables are also important to consider when deciding how to tailor panic treatment to a particular patient. We review each of these optional components and variations, and discuss existing literature that provides some guidance on which patients might benefit most from them. We review exemplary empirical evaluations on the treatment of adolescent panic, and discuss important considerations for the ways one could implement the panic treatment protocol with flexibility.

OPTIONAL TREATMENT COMPONENTS WHEN FLEXIBLY TAILORING TREATMENT

Use of Rewards

For some adolescents the most salient reward of treatment is the reduction of fear and panic, but others may benefit from small tangible rewards or special rewarding activities after treatment accomplishments. These rewards are best when tailored to the adolescent's preferences, and thus implemented flexibly. It is recommended that rewards are relationship enhancing (e.g., going out for a treat with a parent or good friend), and that they are relatively small and inexpensive. It can be helpful for the patient to brainstorm a list of rewards that they find motivating, and to include on the Fear Hierarchy which rewards will be earned after specific accomplishments. Examples of rewards could include small inexpensive items (e.g., an addition to a small collection), special time with family members (e.g., going out to a movie or favorite restaurant), making a favorite dinner with family members, and so on. For patients who are experiencing depression and need to engage in behavioral activation, an appropriate reward could be planning to go on an outing with a friend, or doing a special activity with a friend or family member. Generally speaking, the rewards list is organized so that smaller rewards are connected with easier exposures, and bigger rewards are connected with more difficult exposures. Given that adolescents each have particular types of activities, hobbies, or objects that they find rewarding, this component of treatment is implemented flexibly, tailored to the individual adolescent. Some adolescents might prefer not to incorporate rewards into their treatment, and instead might find it to be sufficiently rewarding to track their gradual progress and improvement. Rewards have been included in existing CBT for panic, but therapists are instructed to discuss with parents and patients the purpose of rewards, as well as the types of rewards that tend to be most effective (e.g., Angelosante et al., 2009; Pincus et al., 2010). To date, research on which subgroups of patients might benefit most from rewards, or how rewards or incentives can increase motivation, remains to be conducted. That said, there is a growing body of literature on individual sensitivity to incentives/rewards, the effects of different types of incentives on task performance, and on how anxiety can alter the influence of incentives (Dorfman et al., 2016; Hardin et al., 2007).

Parental Involvement in Treatment

Research shows that parenting plays a modest but significant role in the development and maintenance of childhood anxiety (McLeod et al., 2007; Möller et al., 2016). Given these findings, wisdom suggests that parent participation in youth therapy may enhance outcomes. The impact of parent participation in youth therapy has been the subject of several meta-analyses, with some evidence suggesting that parent participation contributes to greater treatment gains (Dowell & Ogles, 2010). Studies on youth CBT, however, have not shown a conclusive benefit of parent participation in treatment (Breinholst et al., 2012; Kendall et al, 2008; Manassis et al., 2014; Ollendick et al., 2015; Thulin et al., 2014).

To date, only a few studies have specifically investigated the influence of parent involvement in treatment for youth panic disorder. In the first randomized clinical trial (Pincus et al., 2010), youth aged 14 to 17 were randomized to either a self-monitoring control condition or to an 11-session weekly active treatment condition that included CBT skills focused specifically on panic (e.g., psychoeducation, cognitive work, breathing retraining, interoceptive exposures, in-vivo situational exposures [without therapist accompaniment], and a minimal parent component). For the parent component of treatment, parents were included in the last 10 minutes of four different sessions; they also were provided with educational reading material about adolescent panic disorder. Youth who received the CBT treatment showed significant reduction in severity of panic, self-reported anxiety, anxiety sensitivity, and depression, in comparison to the youth in the control condition. Youth maintained their gains at three- and six-month follow-up. Although the sample size was not large, this study provided initial support for the feasibility of using a developmentally tailored, CBT package with minimal parent involvement for adolescents with panic. The design of the trial, however, did not allow for testing the relative benefit of adding parents in treatment.

A larger randomized clinical trial was conducted to determine the efficacy of an intensive (eight-day) CBT program for adolescents ages 11 to 18 with panic disorder, with participants randomly assigned to either a treatment condition with a substantial parent component or treatment without a parent component (Angelosante et al., 2009; Pincus et al., 2014). Youth in both conditions participated in sessions that lasted two to six hours each day and covered the following core treatment components: psychoeducation about panic, development of the fear avoidance hierarchy, cognitive restructuring, interoceptive exposure exercises, situational exposures, and relapse prevention skills. Parents in the condition with parent involvement were provided with extensive reading material about adolescent panic, including parent-specific panic handouts (e.g., "Common Parent Reactions to Anxious Teens," or "Behavioral Principles for Parenting Anxious Youth"); they also were included in portions of all sessions and taught how to conduct exposure practices. In addition, they accompanied youth on some exposure practices. Those in the condition without a parent component were not provided with any of these materials or direct instruction. Overall, the results showed that the intensive treatment for panic disorder (both with and without parent involvement) reduced the rate and severity of panic disorder, decreased patients' fear and avoidance, reduced the number of comorbid clinical disorders in addition to panic, and eliminated adolescent's attentional bias toward panic-relevant and other threatening stimuli (Weiner et al., 2012). Of note, results showed relatively equivalent positive outcomes for participants with parent involvement or without parental involvement (Gallo et al., 2012, 2014; Pincus et al., 2014; Pincus, Elkins, & Hardway, 2014; Pincus & Hardway, 2019).

In a subsequent investigation of the impact of panic treatment on depressive symptoms using the same sample, Hardway and colleagues (2015) found no overall benefit or detriment to involving parents in treatment. The authors did find that younger adolescents showed greater reductions in depressive symptoms when their parents were minimally involved in the panic treatment (Hardway et al., 2015). These results suggest that age may be an important consideration when deciding whether to involve parents in panic treatment for youth with co-occurring depression.

Other work highlights both the potential benefits and downsides of including parents in treatment for youth panic disorder. For example, involved parents can reinforce homework compliance, serve as exposure coaches, and encourage the use of skills between sessions and after termination. In contrast, parents may diminish their child's sense of mastery and act as safety signals during exposures (Angelosante et al., 2009). Research is required to understand whether individual factors influence the utility of parent involvement in panic treatment. Factors may include the family's cultural values, the nature of the youth-parent relationship (e.g., amicable or contentious), and the youth's desire for autonomy. Overall, research to date has not shown a conclusive benefit to involving parents in adolescents' treatment for panic disorder.

Although it would seem important for parents to have knowledge about their adolescents' treatment so that they can reinforce therapy concepts, facilitate adolescents' approach behavior, and so on, it is also possible that being too involved in treatment can interfere with adolescents' growing sense of independence and become a source of conflict (e.g., nagging or arguing with the adolescent to complete therapy homework). An important goal of continued studies is to determine whether there are particular subgroups of adolescents who would benefit most from having parents in treatment, and what type of parental involvement would work best for which teens. It may very well be the case that families who show high levels of parental overprotection, family accommodation, and maladaptive parent-child interactions that can inadvertently reinforce child anxiety symptoms might benefit most from a family component that augments traditional exposure therapy (Kendall et al., 2008). Indeed, research has highlighted the importance of continued study of the optimal ways to involve parents in the treatment of anxious youth, particularly youth with panic disorder (Angelosante et al., 2009).

Breathing Awareness/Breathing Retraining

Learning how to become aware of one's breathing, and learning to slow one's breathing, has been an optional part of panic treatment (Hoffman & Mattis, 2000; Mattis & Pincus, 2004; Pincus et al., 2008). By guiding a patient through a brief hyperventilation exercise, the patient learns why "over breathing" is a common reaction in panic, and how it has the effect of lowering the carbon dioxide in one's cells. The patient is taught the similarity between the feelings experienced during the hyperventilation exercise and the symptoms that one might feel during panic. The therapist illustrates how engaging in frequent sighing, yawning, or rapid shallow breathing can inadvertently elicit dizziness or palpitations, which can bring on panic. This knowledge can help demystify the idea that panic comes from "out of the blue." It can help patients recognize the subtle triggers for panic that formerly might not have been in their awareness.

Research has not yet been conducted on which patients might benefit most from learning to become more aware of their breathing and learning to slow their breathing, but it has been suggested that this might be most helpful for adolescents who are very sensitive to breathing-related panic cues or those who have a tendency to hyperventilate during panic attacks (Pincus et al., 2008). Many patients initially report that panic feels out of their control, and understanding the many subtle triggers for panic can help them feel like panic is more controllable and more predictable. For patients who report that they tend to sigh a lot, or overbreathe by using their chest muscles rather than their abdominal muscles, it also can help for them to become more aware of these behaviors and to learn to exert voluntary control over their breathing. It can even be helpful for patients to learn how to change and slow down their breathing patterns; this could help decrease the frequency of physical sensations that could trigger panic. Teens are taught to place one hand on their chest and one hand on their diaphragm, making sure that their hand on their diaphragm is rising and falling with each breath. Patients are given instructions for home practice of slowing one's breathing by counting and breathing at a slower rate. Given that learning to gain control over one's breathing is a concrete skill that is relatively easy to learn, it is not surprising that it is often reported by adolescents as one of the most beneficial and helpful skills they learned during their treatment (Pincus et al., 2010).

OPTIONAL FORMAT VARIATIONS

Therapist-Assisted In-Vivo Exposures versus Independent In-Vivo Exposures

Exposure tasks are core, but actual exposures vary in their format. One study of an 11-session weekly treatment for panic disorder did not include therapist-assisted in-vivo exposures but relied solely on adolescents completing independent in-vivo exposures as homework (Pincus et al. 2010). Another trial of an intensive eight-day treatment for panic in adolescence incorporated both therapist-assisted and independent situational in-vivo exposures (Angelosante et al., 2009; Pincus et al., 2014). A nonrandomized comparison of these two studies showed that both resulted in significant improvements in adolescents' panic and general anxiety symptoms, with the majority of youth in both trials no longer showing clinical levels of panic disorder (Chase et al., 2012).

   Although no systematic research has been conducted on which patients might benefit from which formats of exposure, it is plausible that many variables might impact this choice. Variables such as the therapy setting (e.g., inpatient or outpatient), therapist and patient time availability, patient motivation, and patient age might impact whether it could be best for therapists to accompany patients on some of their situational exposure practices. For example, a therapist-assisted exposure component might be particularly helpful for adolescents who are having difficulties entering situations on their own, or for those who need additional support as they learn how to conduct an exposure practice effectively. For patients who are struggling or who have lower motivation, it could be helpful to have a therapist involved to provide positive reminders about how life might improve if panic were not interfering, and about how the short-term anxiety involved in an exposure could result in long-term gains. Alternatively, if the therapist is too involved in exposures, the therapist could soon be seen as a "safety person" who could inadvertently facilitate avoidance and interfere with the exposure eliciting sufficient levels of anxiety. In this case, it might be more effective for the therapist to phase out their presence during exposures and to provide praise and support only after the adolescent patient has completed the exposure. Thus, studies have varied in whether exposures have occurred in session or entirely out of the therapy session, but the existing literature indicates that as long as situational exposures are occurring, and as long as the patient has opportunities for independent exposure practice, patients typically show clinical improvement.

Excluding In-Vivo Exposures and Conducting Only Interoceptive Exposures

In-vivo exposures have been a prominent part of CBT for panic disorder both in youth and adults (e.g., Angelosante et al., 2009). When treating adults, however, some evidence suggests that the inclusion of in-vivo exposures does not necessarily increase the treatment effects. For example, in an attempt to make the treatment briefer, Otto and colleagues (2012) developed a five-session treatment consisting of psychoeducation, cognitive restructuring, and interoceptive exposures, and found effect sizes comparable to standard treatments. Similarly, Craske and colleagues (2003) compared the effects of Panic Control Treatment, with interoceptive exposures only, to Panic Control Treatment with both interoceptive and in-vivo exposures. In this study, both groups received psychoeducation, breathing retraining, cognitive restructuring, and interoceptive exposures. One group then was assigned to practice in-vivo exposures at home and the other group engaged in a discussion of in-vivo exposures and other skills. No difference was found between the two groups in terms of the treatment outcomes. Finally, in a meta-analysis that included 72 studies of CBT for panic disorder in adults, Pompoli and colleagues (2018) reported that interoceptive exposures along with face-to-face sessions yielded the highest efficacy. Although these findings have not been replicated in youth, the evidence from adult literature suggests that in-vivo exposures may be an optional component. It is important to mention, however, that the majority of the previous studies (i.e., Craske et al., 2003 and the ones included in the meta-analysis by Pompoli et al., 2018) incorporated in-vivo exposures as homework. It is possible that therapist-guided in-vivo exposures yield stronger effects than in-vivo exposures assigned as homework. Additional studies in youth are needed to determine which types of exposures (in vivo or interoceptive or both) are most indicated for particular patient subgroups who have panic disorder.

Intensive versus Weekly Treatment

There have been variations in the length and format of manual-based panic treatment for adolescents, with one randomized trial testing delivery of an 11-session treatment (one-hour-long weekly sessions) delivered over 12 weeks (Pincus et al., 2010), and another testing delivery of the same treatment delivered over the course of eight days with three to nine hours of treatment per day (Angelosante et al., 2009; Pincus et al., 2014). Chase and colleagues (2012) conducted a nonrandomized comparison of these two trials and found that both resulted in significant improvements in adolescents' panic and general anxiety symptoms, with the majority of youth in both trials no longer showing clinical levels of panic disorder. Those patients who received weekly treatment, however, showed greater decreases in depressive symptoms than those in the intensive program. Thus, for patients who show depressed mood in addition to panic disorder, it may be more effective to deliver treatment in a more traditional weekly format than an intensive format. Alternatively, those who receive intensive treatment might also benefit from an additional course of sessions to help with their depressed mood. Intensive approaches to treatment might offer other benefits, however, such as more expedient improvement in panic symptoms, as well as more rapid return to healthy developmental functioning and quicker resumption of everyday activities. Furthermore, patients who have more severe agoraphobia in addition to panic disorder might respond particularly well to an intensive approach because the extended sessions allow for therapists to accompany the patient in real-life situations to reduce agoraphobic avoidance (Chase et al., 2012). Some families might prefer the intensive format for logistical reasons (e.g., difficulty traveling to weekly sessions, living a long distance from the clinic) and to help a child more quickly re-enter school for those who are avoiding school situations. Follow-up research will inform us about which youth might respond best to an intensive or weekly format of treatment, but it is clear that both appear to be effective treatment formats.

Individual versus Group Treatment

Another aspect of flexible implementation of treatments is individual versus group delivery of CBT. Group CBT is likely more cost-effective than individual CBT and may allow for faster access to services, but no studies to date have compared the implementation of CBT specifically in youth with panic disorder in group versus in individual formats. Available data from trials of youth with anxiety disorders in general as well as adults with panic disorder are suggestive. For example, Manassis and colleagues (2002) found no difference in treatment gains following a course of individual versus group CBT in children 8 to 12 years of age (1.2% of the participants had panic disorder). Similarly, in a sample of 182 children ages 8 to 15 years diagnosed with an anxiety disorder (none of the participants had panic disorder), Wergeland and colleagues (2014) found no difference in recovery rates between the youth randomized to the group versus the individual format of CBT. In adults with panic disorder, similar findings were reported. Marchand and colleagues (2009) found no difference between individual, group, and brief CBT in adults with panic disorder. Overall, the findings suggest that group treatment may be as effective as individual treatment. Research is needed, however, to determine the optimal delivery mode for youth with panic disorder.

Online Delivery: Synchronous Videoconferencing-Based and Asynchronous Computer-Based Delivery

Several formats of computer-based delivery of evidence-based anxiety treatments have gained traction in recent years: synchronous, videoconferencing-based treatment, and asynchronous, computer-based treatment (or combinations of the two). Both of these technology-based delivery formats have the potential of increasing accessibility to evidence-based care, and both have the potential to reduce logistical barriers (such as travel time or transportation fees) that could contribute to missed sessions (Carpenter et al., 2018; Comer, 2016; Doss et al., 2017; Khanna & Kendall, 2010). Although few studies to date have specifically focused on testing online delivery of treatment for panic disorder in adolescents, one study is currently investigating the feasibility of delivering online panic treatment to youth in public school settings (Pincus, 2018). Youth who have participated to date have reported improvements in the frequency of their panic and decreases in avoidance and impairment.

Although no studies have examined online delivery of treatment for panic disorder specifically, studies have examined the effects of Internet-delivered CBT in youth with anxiety disorders more generally. Vigerland and colleagues (2016) randomized 93 children ages 8 to 12 to either Internet-delivered CBT (computer-based modules for children and parents combined with some therapist contact via messaging) or waitlist control (5% of the sample had a diagnosis of panic disorder). The results indicated that Internet-delivered CBT was more effective than the waitlist condition, based on both therapist and parent ratings. Khanna and Kendall (2010) randomized 49 children ages 7 to 12 to either face-to-face individual CBT, computer-based CBT with partial therapist involvement, or an attentional control condition. Two of the participants (4%) had a principal diagnosis of panic disorder. The children demonstrated significant improvement in both active treatment conditions. In a sample of 115 adolescents (ages 12 to 18), randomized to online, in-person or waitlist conditions, Spence and colleagues (2011) found no differences between online versus in-person delivery of CBT, demonstrating that both are beneficial. In this study, similar to most of the previously described studies, the therapist involvement in the online treatment was minimal and therapeutic contact was solely in the form of e-mail. Their sample, however, did not have any youth with panic disorder. More recently, Carpenter and colleagues (2018) reported a pilot examination of an entirely synchronous, videoconferencing-based family-based CBT for anxious youth delivered in their home setting. The treatment was found to be highly acceptable to families (e.g., high treatment retention, high client satisfaction, strong therapeutic alliance) and highly effective (90.9% of treatment completers were deemed treatment responders). Gains were maintained at the three-month follow-up assessment. Patients in this study had social anxiety, separation anxiety, or generalized anxiety disorder (no patients with panic disorder), but the authors suggest that videoconferencing formats hold tremendous promise for broadening the reach of quality care for youth with anxiety disorders in general—it is likely that patients with panic disorder also will respond well to this treatment format.

What can we learn from studies that compared online versus face-to-face delivery of treatment for panic disorder in adults? Bouchard and colleagues (2004) delivered CBT for panic disorder to 10 adults face-to-face and 11 adults remotely, via videoconferencing, and found that both formats were effective with no meaningful difference between the formats. Kiropoulos and colleagues (2008) compared Internet-based panic treatment with minimal therapist contact via e-mail to therapist-delivered panic treatment in 86 adults, and also found both to be effective and no difference between the conditions. Similar findings were reported in other studies (e.g., Klein et al., 2006). Accordingly, the literature on panic disorder in adults suggests that both online treatment and therapist-delivered telehealth treatment are as effective as face-to-face treatment. This is similar to the findings in child and adolescent literature on CBT for anxiety disorders in general. Although research is needed to establish the effectiveness of online or technology-based treatments for panic disorder in youth, the existing research findings suggest that various formats of online treatment for panic disorder may be feasible and practical solutions to facilitate treatment delivery and increase access to care.

PATIENT VARIABLES TO CONSIDER WHEN TAILORING TREATMENT TO PATIENTS

Age or Developmental Level

The empirically supported treatments for panic disorder in youth have been largely based on CBT approaches developed for adults, but with developmental tailoring to be appropriate for adolescents (e.g., Angelosante et al., 2009; Hoffman & Mattis, 2000; Pincus et al., 2008). These age-appropriate treatments for adolescents used simpler language, along with attractive, adolescent-friendly graphics, as well as examples and metaphors pertinent to adolescents to explain treatment-related concepts. These panic treatments are for adolescents aged 12 to 17 years, which is a wide age range. There are developmental considerations that might affect the implementation for youth of different ages within adolescence. For example, younger adolescents might find it more beneficial to have parents involved than older adolescents. Older adolescents may be able to engage in independent exposures more easily than younger adolescents. At present, there are few findings to guide whether there should be differential delivery of treatment by age for adolescents with panic disorder. One study suggests that younger adolescents who had panic disorder and comorbid depression showed greater reductions in depressive symptoms when their parents were minimally involved in the panic treatment (Hardway et al., 2015). Future studies might explore developmental variations, not just age, that could help tailor treatment to youth of different developmental levels. For example, some younger youth might need more illustrations and simpler language to understand the psychoeducation, while this might be less acceptable to older adolescents.

Mental Health Comorbidities

Panic disorder often occurs concurrently and sequentially with other mental health disorders. For example, in a large sample of youth presenting to a mood and anxiety disorder clinic, panic disorder was most highly comorbid with major depressive disorder, generalized anxiety disorder, separation anxiety disorder, and bipolar disorder (Diler et al., 2004). Other research shows that panic attacks in particular are associated with an elevated risk of later depression (e.g., Goodwin et al., 2004). With respect to depression, these findings are consistent with extant research showing high rates of comorbidity between anxiety and depressive disorders in youth (Seligman & Ollendick, 1998).

Co-occurring psychological disorders represent an important consideration in the flexible treatment of youth with panic disorder. Evidence from an intensive, eight-day CBT for youth panic disorder found that the intervention had a secondary benefit of reducing participants' depression as well as improving comorbid anxiety disorders (Gallo et al., 2012; Hardway et al., 2015). Findings from these studies suggest that although disorders other than panic disorder were not specific treatment targets, treatment for panic disorder also alleviated symptoms of specific phobia, generalized anxiety disorder, and social phobia. Thus, treatment gains appeared to generalize to alleviate symptoms of other disorders.

No known studies to date have examined whether having a comorbid anxiety disorder at pretreatment differentially impacts treatment outcomes for youth with panic disorder. Looking to the research on youth anxiety more broadly (e.g., Walkup et al., 2008), few studies have found a significant influence of comorbidities on treatment outcomes despite co-occurring psychological disorders being common among anxious youth (for review, see Ollendick et al., 2008). Effective anxiety interventions may target comorbid disorders directly via common treatment elements, or indirectly via reductions in anxiety and its sequelae. For example, CBT is a well-established psychosocial treatment for both adolescent anxiety (Higa-McMillan et al., 2016) and adolescent depression (Weersing et al., 2017). Future research may explore whether youth with particular comorbidities are more likely to respond to panic treatment, or whether there might be optimal sequencing of effective intervention components in youth with panic and multiple psychological disorders.

Medical Comorbidities

Some research suggests that at least half of children with anxiety disorders have a comorbid physical illness, with allergies and asthma being the most prevalent comorbid illnesses (Chavira et al., 2008). Those children with anxiety who have a comorbid physical illness have been shown to exhibit greater levels of emotional problems, more somatic complaints, more functional impairment and more care-giver strain than anxious children without a physical illness or with only physical illness and no anxiety (Chavira et al., 2008). Accordingly, clinicians are wise to assess for medical comorbidities, especially for patients with panic disorder. Panic disorder is frequently comorbid with respiratory illness (e.g., asthma), cardiovas-cular illness, diabetes, and irritable bowel syndrome (Meuret et al., 2017). Asthma, in particular, is associated with higher rates of panic among youth (Goodwin et al., 2003) and adults (Hasler et al., 2005). High rates of comorbidity between panic disorder and asthma may be exacerbated by substantial overlap in many of the physical (e.g., chest tightness), psychological (e.g., increased attention to so-matic symptoms), and behavioral (e.g., avoidance) effects of the two conditions. Further complicating matters, treatment of coexisting panic and asthma requires special consideration, because some treatment practices such as carrying out in-teroceptive exposure exercises can carry the risk of triggering asthma symptoms. It is possible with these patients to select interoceptive exposure exercises that trigger panic but not asthma; it can also be helpful to distinguish for the patient the difference between breathing-related changes that occur during asthma (e.g., wheezing) and the breathing-related changes that occur naturally with panic (e.g., more rapid heart rate).

Given the prevalence of co-occurring asthma and panic and the substan-tial overlap in symptoms, combined treatment for comorbid panic and asthma represents an important mental and medical health initiative. Current evi-dence from small trials in the adult literature suggest that combined CBT with asthma education improves both panic and asthma-related outcomes (Feldman et al., 2016; Lehrer et al., 2008; Ross et al., 2005). In addition to established CBT components such as psychoeducation, cognitive techniques, and exposure, combined treatments provide education about asthma, often including informa-tion about asthma physiology, management (e.g., proper medication use), and differentiating between asthma and panic symptoms. Clinicians may find that in-tegrating asthma education in treatment facilitates the appropriate application of CBT techniques, such as exposure. Other researchers suggest that, in addition to providing skills for differentiating between asthma and anxiety symptoms, standard CBT may need to be modified with alternate strategies, such as objective symptom monitoring and an Asthma Action Plan (Deshmukh et al., 2007).

Pretreatment Levels of Fear and Avoidance

Given that panic treatments have been shown to improve outcomes for many, but not all adolescents, it is important to explore the characteristics of the youth who are more (and less) likely to respond to various treatment formats, such as intensive or weekly, or telehealth-based treatments. Given that fear and avoidance are central targets for panic treatment, the heterogeneity in youth's baseline levels of fear and avoidance may be linked to the heterogeneity in youth's treatment response. One study explored whether baseline levels of fear and avoidance predicted treatment response for youth who received an intensive treatment for panic disorder (Elkins et al., 2016). Results showed that the treatment effects were predicted by the extent of pretreatment fear and avoidance, with greater improvements shown among adolescents with more moderate, relative to higher, levels of fear and avoidance. This finding suggests that intensive treatment may be an effective alternative to weekly care, particularly for those presenting with moderate levels of fear and avoidance. Given that the majority of cases of adolescent panic are more moderate in their severity, most youth with panic should be well served by an intensive treatment format as an alternative to a weekly treatment.

Cultural Considerations

Several studies have examined the rate of panic disorder symptomatology in various racial/ethnic groups (e.g., Barrera et al., 2010), and the findings suggest that the experience of panic symptoms may differ across groups (Asnaani et al., 2010). One study investigated a cultural adaptation of CBT for panic disorder (Carter et al., 2003) evaluating a culturally adapted Panic Control Treatment in African American women. The adaptations included delivering the treatment in a group format by an African American therapist, ensuring that the group was homogeneous, and including discussions of issues of race in treatment. The treatment group demonstrated significant improvement in comparison to the waitlist control.

In a review, Graham and colleagues (2013) discuss potential adaptations to adult CBT in general to make it more culturally sensitive. Some examples of suggested adaptations include educating therapists about the given cultural group, discussing the experience of being marginalized, and modifying exposures to consider cultural experiences. No studies to date have examined cultural adaptations of panic disorder treatments in youth specifically. Pina and colleagues (2003), however, compared the effects of exposure-based CBT for anxiety disorders among 162 Hispanic/Latino and European-American children and adolescents (ages 6 to 16), demonstrating that both groups responded favorably to treatment. Hinton and Patel (2017) offer a culturally informed, transdiagnostic model for how CBT can decrease anxiety in a culturally sensitive way. At present, research is needed to evaluate the merits of cultural adaptations.

Setting Variables

Evidence-based panic treatment for adolescents can be delivered in a variety of settings, such as outpatient clinics, inpatient hospital units, primary care, and school settings, making it versatile and transportable. Flexibility in treatment delivery might be needed depending on the setting of treatment. For example, in some clinical settings, it is not possible for a therapist to conduct massed in-vivo exposures for many hours with a patient; in these cases, it may be necessary for the adolescent to conduct in-vivo exposures as homework, or for the adolescent to conduct exposures along with a parent. Delivering treatment in pediatric care settings for youth with unexplained somatic symptoms may require special considerations. Given that there is a high prevalence of youth who report to pediatric medical offices with medically unexplained somatic symptoms who may actually have panic disorder, it may be important to tailor the panic treatment to focus more on the relationship between physical sensations and anxiety, and to help tailor the cognitive restructuring component of treatment so that the patient learns to restructure somatic cognitions and to de-catastrophize physical discomfort. The adolescent panic protocol already addresses some of the reasons for the most common somatic complaints such as stomachaches, palpitations, muscle tension, sweating, and trembling/shaking, so spending additional time on the causes of these symptoms might be helpful for youth presenting to a primary care setting with fear of them. It also might be helpful to provide parents of youth presenting in primary care with additional education not only about panic, but about the relationship between somatic and anxiety symptoms and how to help youth manage them. Although this can be accomplished by tailoring the standard adolescent panic protocol, some researchers also have adapted general anxiety treatments so that they more directly address both the anxiety and physical symptoms (e.g., Reigada et al., 2008).

Panic disorder treatment has not been formally evaluated for in school-settings, but there has been a proliferation of research on school-based psychosocial interventions for anxiety. In a meta-analysis of school-based CBT, Mychailyszyn and colleagues (2012) found that school-based CBT was moderately effective in reducing students' anxiety, though the reported results were not maintained after a 12-month follow-up. More recent work with anxious adolescents found that both a brief five-session and standard ten-session school-based CBT program reduced adolescents' anxiety symptoms, depression symptoms, and impairment, with outcomes sustained after one year (Haugland et al., 2020). Given similarities between CBT treatments for anxiety and CBT treatments for panic disorder specifically, these results suggest that implementing CBT in school-settings is promising.

SUMMARY AND FUTURE DIRECTIONS

Research on panic disorder in adolescence has burgeoned, resulting in manual-based and evidence-based treatments that help youth return to healthier developmental trajectories. There are essential components of panic treatment that are required to maintain fidelity, but optimal care requires that therapists deliver the core treatment components flexibly, tailoring the treatment to their particular teen. Existing empirical findings provide guidance on *when* a treatment is best tailored to a patient, *for whom* it should be tailored, and *how* it should be tailored. When guided by existing research, we begin to cultivate patient-focused implementation of treatment for youth with panic disorder. As suggested by Kendall and colleagues, a manual-based treatment is a guide, but having *flexibility* in one's delivery of the treatment is part of best practices (Kendall et al., 2008). Treatment protocols should not be implemented rigidly, or adhered to without careful consideration of individual patient needs.

Although patient-centered approaches to care can result in rapid patient improvement, there is still work to be done, given that data show that 30% to 40% of patients do not respond sufficiently to our evidence-based approaches (Silverman et al., 2008). Testing of variations in panic treatment format, novel methods of treatment delivery, and adjunctive treatment components might help the subset of youth who do not currently show sufficient treatment response. Future studies might investigate further how to best include parents in panic treatment, whether peers could be incorporated into exposure practices to boost youth's motivation to engage in exposures, whether a motivational enhancement component could be helpful for particular subpopulations of youth, and whether there are effective ways to implement treatment for panic so that it is widely available to youth into school settings.

Continued investigations are needed to answer the general Kiesler (1966) question, "What works for whom under which conditions?" For example, continued examination is needed to understand the ways that cultural and socioeconomic variables might influence outcome. Furthermore, it is possible that certain subsamples of patients would respond better to particular formats of treatment, or particular variations of treatment. Given the fact that large numbers of youth with psychological disorders such as panic disorder never receive services (Merikangas et al., 2010), and given the fact that most youth who do receive services never receive evidence-based care (Comer & Barlow, 2014; McHugh & Barlow, 2010), it is a priority for the field to determine methods for increasing youth's access to all evidence-based care, including panic treatment. As suggested by Kendall and Beidas (2007), delivering evidence-based care with flexibility and fidelity will help to facilitate the dissemination of empirically supported practices more widely. By combining knowledge from future empirical studies on panic disorder with clinician feedback and insight about their flexible use of panic treatment manuals, we will facilitate continued progress toward making panic treatments more effective for youth of diverse backgrounds in a variety of settings.

REFERENCES

American Psychiatric Association. (2013). *Diagnostic and statistical manual of mental disorders* (5th ed.). Author. https://doi.org/10.1176/appi.books.9780890425596

Angelosante, A. G., Pincus, D. B., Whitton, S. W., Cheron, D., & Pian, J. (2009). Implementation of an intensive treatment protocol for adolescents with panic disorder and agoraphobia. *Cognitive and Behavioral Practice, 16*(3), 345–357. https://doi.org/10.1016/j.cbpra.2009.03.002

Asnaani, A., Richey, J. A., Dimaite, R., Hinton, D. E., & Hofmann, S. G. (2010). A cross-ethnic comparison of lifetime prevalence rates of anxiety disorders. *The Journal of Nervous and Mental Disease, 198*(8), 551–555. https://doi.org/10.1097/NMD.0b013e3181ea169f

Barrera, T. L., Wilson, K. P., & Norton, P. J. (2010). The experience of panic symptoms across racial groups in a student sample. *Journal of Anxiety Disorders, 24*(8), 873–878. https://doi.org/10.1016/j.janxdis.2010.06.010

Beidas, R. S., Benjamin, C. L., Puleo, C. M., Edmunds, J. M., & Kendall, P. C. (2010). Flexible applications of the Coping Cat Program for anxious youth. *Cognitive and Behavioral Practice, 17*(2), 142–153. https://doi.org/10.1016/j.cbpra.2009.11.002

Bouchard, S., Paquin, B., Payeur, R., Allard, M., Rivard, V., Fournier, T., Renaud, P., & Lapierre, J. (2004). Delivering cognitive-behavior therapy for panic disorder with agoraphobia in videoconference. *Telemedicine Journal and E-Health, 10*(1),13-25. https://doi.org/10.1089/153056204773644535

Bouton, M. E., Mineka, S., & Barlow, D. H. (2001). A modern learning theory perspective on the etiology of panic disorder. *Psychological Review, 108* (1), 4–32. https://doi.org/10.1037/0033-295X.108.1.4

Breinholst, S., Esbjørn, B. H., Reinholdt-Dunne, M. L., & Stallard, P. (2012). CBT for the treatment of child anxiety disorders: A review of why parental involvement has not enhanced outcomes. *Journal of Anxiety Disorders, 26*(3), 416–424. https://doi.org/10.1016/j.janxdis.2011.12.014

Carpenter, A. L., Pincus, D. B., Furr, J. M., & Comer, J. S. (2018). Working from home: An initial pilot examination of videoconferencing-based cognitive behavioral therapy for anxious youth delivered to the home setting. *Behavior Therapy, 49*(6), 917–930. https://doi.org/10.1016/j.beth.2018.01.007

Carter, M. M., Sbrocco, T., Gore, K. L., Marin, N. W., & Lewis, E. L. (2003). Cognitive-behavioral group therapy versus a wait-list control in the treatment of African American women with panic disorder. *Cognitive Therapy and Research, 27*(5), 505–518. https://doi.org/10.1023/A:1026350903639

Chase, R. M., Whitton, S. W. & Pincus, D. B. (2012). Treatment of adolescent panic disorder: A non-randomized comparison of intensive versus weekly CBT. *Child and Family Behavior Therapy, 34,* 305–323. https://doi.org/10.1080/07317107.2012.732873

Chavira, D. A., Garland, A. F., Daley, S., & Hough, R. (2008). The impact of medical comorbidity on mental health and functional health outcomes among children with anxiety disorders. *Journal of Developmental and Behavioral Pediatrics: JDBP, 29*(5), 394–402. https://doi.org/10.1097/DBP.0b013e3181836a5b

Chorpita, B. F., Becker, K. D., & Daleiden, E. L. (2002). Understanding the common elements of evidence-based practice: Misconceptions and clinical examples. *Journal of the American Academy of Child and Adolescent Psychiatry, 46*(5), 647–652. https://doi.org/10.1097/chi.0b013e318033ff71

Comer, J. S. (2016). Introduction to the special series: Applying new technologies to extend the scope and accessibility of mental health care. *Cognitive and Behavioral Practice, 22*(3), 253–257. https://doi.org/10.1016/j.cbpra.2015.04.002

Comer, J. S., & Barlow, D. H. (2014). The occasional case against broad dissemination and implementation: Retaining a role for specialty care in the delivery of psychological treatments. *American Psychologist, 69*, 1–18. https://doi.org/10.1037/a0033582

Craske, M. G., DeCola, J. P., Sachs, A. D., & Pontillo, D. C. (2003). Panic control treatment for agoraphobia. *Journal of Anxiety Disorders, 17*(3), 321–333. https://doi.org/10.1016/S0887-6185(02)00203-7

Craske, M. G., Treanor, M., Conway, C. C., Zbozinek, T., & Vervliet, B. (2014). Maximizing exposure therapy: An inhibitory learning approach. *Behaviour Research and Therapy, 58*, 10–23. https://doi.org/10.1016/j.brat.2014.04.006

Deshmukh, V. M., Toelle, B. G., Usherwood, T., O'Grady, B., & Jenkins, C. R. (2007). Anxiety, panic and adult asthma: A cognitive-behavioral perspective. *Respiratory Medicine, 101*(2), 194–202. https://doi.org/10.1016/j.rmed.2006.05.005

Diler, R. S., Birmaher, B., Brent, D. A., Axelson, D. A., Firinciogullari, S., Chiapetta, L., & Bridge, J. (2004). Phenomenology of panic disorder in youth. *Depression and Anxiety, 20*(1), 39–43. https://doi.org/10.1002/da.20018

Dorfman, J., Rosen, D., Pine, D., & Ernst, M. (2016). Anxiety and gender influence reward-related processes in children and adolescents. *Journal of Child and Adolescent Psychopharmacology, 26*(4), 380–390. https://dx.doi.org/10.1089%2Fcap.2015.0008

Doss, B. D., Feinberg, L. K., Rothman, K., Roddy, M. K., & Comer, J. S. (2017). Using technology to enhance and expand interventions for couples and families: Conceptual and methodological considerations. *Journal of Family Psychology, 31*(8), 983–993. https://psycnet.apa.org/doi/10.1037/fam0000349

Dowell, K. A., & Ogles, B. M. (2010). The effects of parent participation on child psychotherapy outcome: A meta-analytic review. *Journal of Clinical Child & Adolescent Psychology, 39*(2), 151–162. https://doi.org/10.1080/15374410903532585

Elkins, R. M., Gallo, K. P., Pincus, D. B., & Comer, J. S. (2016). Moderators of intensive CBT for adolescent panic disorder: The roles of fear and avoidance. *Child and Adolescent Mental Health, 21*(1), 30–36. PMCID: PMC4768300 https://dx.doi.org/10.1111%2Fcamh.12122

Feldman, J. M., Matte, L., Interian, A., Lehrer, P. M., Lu, S. E., Scheckner, B., Steinberg, D. M., Oken, T., Kotay, A., Sinha, S., & Shim, C. (2016). Psychological treatment of comorbid asthma and panic disorder in Latino adults: Results from a randomized controlled trial. *Behaviour Research and Therapy, 87*, 142–154. https://doi.org/10.1016/j.brat.2016.09.007

Gallo, K., Buzzella, B., Chan, P., Whitton, S. W., & Pincus, D. B. (2012). The impact of an eight-day intensive treatment for adolescent panic disorder and agoraphobia on comorbid diagnoses. *Behavior Therapy, 42*, 153–159. https://doi.org/10.1016/j.beth.2011.05.002

Gallo, K. P., Cooper-Vince, C. E., Hardway, C., Pincus, D. B., & Comer, J. S. (2014). Trajectories of change across outcomes in intensive treatment for adolescent panic disorder and agoraphobia. *Journal of Clinical Child and Adolescent Psychology, 43*(5), 742–750. https://doi.org/10.1080/15374416.2013.794701

Goodwin, R. D., Fergusson, D. M., & Horwood, L. J. (2004). Panic attacks and the risk of depression among young adults in the community. *Psychotherapy and Psychosomatics, 73*(3), 158–165. https://doi.org/10.1159/000076453

Goodwin, R. D., Pine, D. S., & Hoven, C. W. (2003). Asthma and panic attacks among youth in the community. *Journal of Asthma, 40*(2), 139–145. https://doi.org/10.1081/JAS-120017984

Graham, J. R., Sorenson, S., & Hayes-Skelton, S. A. (2013). Enhancing the cultural sensitivity of cognitive behavioral interventions for anxiety in diverse populations. *The Behavior Therapist, 36*(5), 101–108. https://www.ncbi.nlm.nih.gov/pubmed/25392598

Hardin, M. G., Schroth, E., Pine, D. S., & Ernst, M. (2007). Incentive-related modulation of cognitive control in healthy, anxious and depressed adolescents: Development and psychopathology related differences. *Journal of Child Psychology and Psychiatry, 48*(5), 446–454. https://dx.doi.org/10.1111%2Fj.1469-7610.2006.01722.x

Hardway, C. L., Pincus, D. B., Gallo, K. P., & Comer, J. S. (2015). Parental involvement in intensive treatment for adolescent panic disorder and its impact on depression. *Journal of Child and Family Studies, 24*(11), 3306–3317. https://doi.org/10.1007/s10826-015-0133-7

Hasler, G., Gergen, P. J., Kleinbaum, D. G., Ajdacic, V., Gamma, A., Eich, D., Rössler, W., & Angst, J. (2005). Asthma and panic in young adults. *American Journal of Respiratory and Critical Care Medicine, 171*(11), 1224–1230. https://doi.org/10.1164/rccm.200412-1669OC

Haugland, B. S. M., Haaland, Å. T., Baste, V., Bjaastad, J. F., Hoffart, A., Rapee, R. M., Raknes, S., Himle, J. A., Husabø, E., & Wergeland, G. J. (2020). Effectiveness of brief and standard school-based cognitive-behavioral interventions for adolescents with anxiety: A randomized non-inferiority study. *Journal of the American Academy of Child & Adolescent Psychiatry, 59*(4), 552–564.e2. https://doi.org/10.1016/j.jaac.2019.12.003

Higa-McMillan, C. K., Francis, S. E., Rith-Najarian, L., & Chorpita, B. F. (2016). Evidence base update: 50 years of research on treatment for child and adolescent anxiety. *Journal of Clinical Child & Adolescent Psychology, 45*(2), 91–113. https://doi.org/10.1080/15374416.2015.1046177

Hinton, D., & Patel, A. (2017). Cultural adaptations of cognitive behavioral therapy. *Psychiatric Clinics of North America, 40*(4), 701–714. https://doi.org/10.1016/j.psc.2017.08.006

Hoffman, E. C., & Mattis, S. G. (2000). A developmental adaptation of Panic Control Treatment for panic disorder in adolescence. *Cognitive and Behavioral Practice, 7*(3), 253–261. https://doi.org/10.1016/s1077-7229(00)80081-4

Kendall, P. C., & Beidas, R. (2007). Smoothing the trail for dissemination of evidence-based practices for youth: Flexibility within fidelity. *Professional Psychology: Research and Practice, 38*, 13–20. https://psycnet.apa.org/doi/10.1037/0735-7028.38.1.13

Kendall, P. C., Chu, B., Gifford, A., Hayes, C., & Nauta, M. (1998). Breathing life into a manual. *Cognitive and Behavioral Practice, 5*(2), 177–198. https://psycnet.apa.org/doi/10.1016/S1077-7229(98)80004-7

Kendall, P. C., & Frank, H. (2018). Implementing evidence-based treatment protocols: Flexibility within fidelity. *Clinical Psychology: Science and Practice, 25*, 1–12. https://doi.org/10.1111/cpsp.12271

Kendall, P. C., Gosch, E., Furr, J., & Sood, E. (2008). Flexibility within fidelity. *Journal of the American Academy of Child and Adolescent Psychiatry, 47*, 987–993. https://psycnet.apa.org/doi/10.1097/CHI.0b013e31817eed2f

Kendall P. C., & Hedtke, K. (2006a). *Cognitive-behavioral therapy for anxious children: Therapist manual.* 3. Ardmore, PA: Workbook Publishing.

Kendall, P. C., & Hedtke, K. (2006b). *The Coping Cat workbook.* Ardmore, PA: Workbook Publishing.

Kendall, P. C., Hudson, J. L., Gosch, E., Flannery-Schroeder, E., & Suveg, C. (2008). Cognitive behavioral therapy for anxiety disordered youth: A randomized clinical trial evaluating child and family modalities. *Journal of Consulting and Clinical Psychology, 76*(2), 282–297. https://doi.org/10.1037/0022-006x.76.2.282

Khanna, M. S., & Kendall, P. C. (2010). Computer-assisted cognitive behavioral therapy for child anxiety: Results of a randomized clinical trial. *Journal of Consulting and Clinical Psychology. 78*(5), 737–745. https://doi.org/10.1037/a0019739

Kiesler, D. J. (1966). Some myths of psychotherapy research and the search for a paradigm. *Psychological Bulletin, 65*(2), 110–136. https://doi.org/10.1037/h0022911

Kiropoulos, L. A., Klein, B., Austin, D. W., Gilson, K., Pier, C., Mitchell, J., & Ciechomski, L. (2008). Is internet-based CBT for panic disorder and agoraphobia as effective as face-to-face CBT? *Journal of Anxiety Disorders, 22*(8), 1273–1284. https://doi.org/10.1016/j.janxdis.2008.01.008

Klein, B., Richards, J. C., & Austin, D. W. (2006). Efficacy of internet therapy for panic disorder. *Journal of Behavior Therapy and Experimental Psychiatry, 37*(3), 213–238. https://doi.org/10.1016/j.jbtep.2005.07.001

Lehrer, P. M., Karavidas, M. K., Lu, S. E., Feldman, J., Kranitz, L., Abraham, S., Sanderson, W., & Reynolds, R. (2008). Psychological treatment of comorbid asthma and panic disorder: A pilot study. *Journal of Anxiety Disorders, 22*(4), 671–683. https://doi.org/10.1016/j.janxdis.2007.07.001

Manassis, K., Lee, T. C., Bennett, K., Zhao, X. Y., Mendlowitz, S., Duda, S., Saini, M., Wilansky, P., Baer, S., Barrett, P., Bodden, D., Cobham, V. E., Dadds, M. R., Flannery-Schroeder, E., Ginsburg, G., Heyne, D., Hudson, J. L., Kendall, P. C., Liber, J., . . . Wood, J. J. (2014). Types of parental involvement in CBT with anxious youth: A preliminary meta-analysis. *Journal of Consulting and Clinical Psychology, 82*(6), 1163–1172. https://doi.org/10.1037/a0036969

Manassis, K., Mendlowitz, S. L., Scapillato, D., Avery, D., Fiksenbaum, L., Freire, M., Monga, A., & Owens, M. (2002). Group and individual cognitive-behavioral therapy for childhood anxiety disorders: A randomized trial. *Journal of the American Academy of Child and Adolescent Psychiatry. 41*(12), 1423–1430. https://doi.org/10.1097/00004583-200212000-00013

Marchand, A., Roberge, P., Primiano, S., & Germain, V. (2009). A randomized, controlled clinical trial of standard, group and brief cognitive-behavioral therapy for panic disorder with agoraphobia: A two-year follow-up. *Journal of Anxiety Disorders, 23*(8), 1139–1147. https://doi.org/10.1016/j.janxdis.2009.07.019

Mattis, S. G., & Pincus, D. B. (2004). Treatment of SAD and panic disorder in children and adolescents. In P. M. Barrett & T. H. Ollendick (Eds.), *Handbook of interventions that work with children and adolescents: Prevention and treatment* (pp. 145–169). Wiley. doi:10.1002/9780470753385

McHugh, R. K., & Barlow, D. H. (2010). The dissemination and implementation of evidence-based psychological treatments: A review of current efforts. *American Psychologist, 65*, 73–84. https://doi.org/10.1037/a0018121

McLeod, B. D., Wood, J. J., & Weisz, J. R. (2007). Examining the association between parenting and childhood anxiety: A meta-analysis. *Clinical Psychology Review, 27*(2), 155–172. https://doi.org/10.1016/j.cpr.2006.09.002

Merikangas, K. R., He, J., Burstein, M., Swanson, S. A., Avenevoli, S., Cui, L., Benjet, C., Georgiades, K., Swendsen, J. (2010). Lifetime prevalence of mental disorders in U.S. adolescents: Results from the National Comorbidity Survey Replication-Adolescent Supplement (NCS-A). *Journal of the American Academy of Child and Adolescent Psychiatry, 49*(10), 980–989. https://doi.org/10.1016/j.jaac.2010.05.017

Meuret, A. E., Kroll, J., & Ritz, T. (2017). Panic disorder comorbidity with medical conditions and treatment implications. *Annual Review of Clinical Psychology, 13*, 209–240. https://doi.org/10.1146/annurev-clinpsy-021815-093044

Möller, E. L., Nikolić, M., Majdandžić, M., & Bögels, S. M. (2016). Associations between maternal and paternal parenting behaviors, anxiety and its precursors in early childhood: A meta-analysis. *Clinical Psychology Review, 45*, 17–33. https://doi.org/10.1016/j.cpr.2016.03.002

Mychailyszyn, M. P., Brodman, D. M., Read, K. L., & Kendall, P. C. (2012). Cognitive-Behavioral school-based interventions for anxious and depressed youth: A meta-analysis of outcomes. *Clinical Psychology: Science and Practice, 19*(2), 129–153. https://doi.org/10.1111/j.1468-2850.2012.01279.x

Ollendick, T. H. (1995). Cognitive behavioral treatment of panic disorder with agoraphobia in adolescents: A multiple baseline design analysis. *Behavior Therapy, 26*(3), 517–531. https://psycnet.apa.org/doi/10.1016/S0005-7894(05)80098-X

Ollendick, T. H., Halldorsdottir, T., Fraire, M. G., Austin, K. E., Noguchi, R. J., Lewis, K. M., Jarrett, M. A., Cunningham, N. R., Canavera, K., Allen, K. B., & Whitmore, M. J. (2015). Specific phobias in youth: a randomized controlled trial comparing one-session treatment to a parent-augmented one-session treatment. *Behavior Therapy, 46*(2), 141–155. https://doi.org/10.1016/j.beth.2014.09.004

Ollendick, T., Jarrett, M., Grills-Taquechel, A. E., Hovey, L. D., & Wolff, J. C. (2008). Comorbidity as a predictor and moderator of treatment outcome in youth with anxiety, affective, attention deficit/hyperactivity disorder, and oppositional/conduct disorders. *Clinical Psychology Review, 28*(8), 1447–1471. https://doi.org/10.1016/j.cpr.2008.09.003

Ollendick, T., & Pincus, D. B. (2008). Panic disorder in adolescents. In R. Steele & M. Roberts (Eds.), *Handbook of evidence based therapies for children and adolescents.* (pp. 83–102). Springer. https://doi.org/10.1007/978-0-387-73691-4_6

Otto, M. W., Tolin, D. F., Nations, K. R., Utschig, A. C., Rothbaum, B. O., Hofmann, S. G., & Smits, J. A. J. (2012). Five sessions and counting: Considering ultra-brief treatment for panic disorder. *Depression and Anxiety, 29*(6), 465–470. https://doi.org/10.1002/da.21910

Pina, A. A., Silverman, W. K., Fuentes, R. M., Kurtines, W. M., & Weems, C. F. (2003). Exposure-based cognitive-behavioral treatment for phobic and anxiety disorders: Treatment effects and maintenance for Hispanic/Latino relative to European-American youths. *Journal of the American Academy of Child and Adolescent Psychiatry, 42*(10), 1179–1187. https://doi.org/10.1097/00004583-200310000-00008

Pincus, D. B. (2018, February 22). *Recent advances in the development of psychological treatments for adolescents with panic disorder* [Keynote presentation]. Miami International Child and Adolescent Mental Health Conference, Miami, FL, United States.

Pincus, D. B., Ehrenreich, J. T., & Mattis, S. G. (2008). *Mastery of anxiety and panic for adolescents: Riding the wave. Therapist Guide.* Oxford University Press.

Pincus, D. B., Ehrenreich, J. T., Whitton, S. A., Mattis, S. M., & Barlow, D. H. (2010). Cognitive behavioral treatment of panic disorder in adolescence. *Journal of*

Clinical Child and Adolescent Psychology, 39(5), 638–649. https://doi.org/10.1080/15374416.2010.501288

Pincus, D. B., Elkins, R. M., & Hardway, C. (2014). Intensive treatments for adolescent panic disorder and agoraphobia: Helping youth move beyond avoidance. *Psychopathology Review, 1*(1), 189–194. https://doi.org/10.5127%2Fpr.033313

Pincus, D. B., & Hardway, C. (2019). Brief intensive treatments. In L. Farrell, P. Muris, & T. Ollendick (Eds.), *Innovations in CBT for childhood anxiety, OCD, and PTSD: Improving access and outcomes* (pp. 130–159). Cambridge University Press. https://doi.org/10.1017/9781108235655

Pincus, D. B., Korn, A., & Difonte, M. (2017). Panic disorder. In C. A. Flessner & J. Piacentini (Eds.), *Clinical handbook of psychological disorders in children and adolescents: A step-by-step treatment manual.* Guilford Press.

Pincus, D. B., Leyfer, O., Hardway, C., Elkins, R., & Comer, J. (2014, November). *Recent advances in the development of psychological treatments for adolescents with panic disorder* [Paper presentation]. Association for Behavioral and Cognitive Therapies, 48th annual meeting, Philadelphia, PA, United States.

Pompoli, A., Furukawa, T. A., Efthimiou, O., Imai, H., Tajika, A., & Salanti, G. (2018). Dismantling cognitive-behaviour therapy for panic disorder: A systematic review and component network meta-analysis. *Psychological Medicine, 48*(12), 1945–1953. https://doi.org/10.1017/S0033291717003919

Rapee, R. M., Craske, M. G., & Barlow, D. H. (1995). Assessment instrument for panic disorder that includes fear of sensation-producing activities: The Albany Panic and Phobia Questionnaire, *Anxiety, 1*, 114–122. https://doi.org/10.1002/anxi.3070010303

Rapee, R., Lyneham, H., Schniering, C., Wuthrich, V., Abbott, M., Hudson, J., & Wignall, A. (2006a). *Cool Kids therapist manual: For the Cool Kids child and adolescent anxiety programs.* Centre for Emotional Health, Macquarie University: Sydney, Australia.

Reigada, L. C., Fisher, P. H., Cutler, C., & Masia Warner, C. (2008). An innovative treatment approach for children with anxiety disorders and medically unexplained somatic complaints. *Cognitive and Behavioral Practice, 15*(2), 140–147. https://doi.org/10.1016/j.cbpra.2007.08.003

Ross, C. J. M., Davis, T. M. A., & Macdonald, G. F. (2005). Cognitive-behavioral treatment combined with asthma education for adults with asthma and coexisting panic disorder. *Clinical Nursing Research, 14*(2), 131–157. https://doi.org/10.1177/1054773804273863

Schmidt, N. B., & Trakowski, J. (2004). Interoceptive assessment and exposure in panic disorder: A descriptive study. *Cognitive and Behavioral Practice, 11*(1), 81–92. https://psycnet.apa.org/doi/10.1016/S1077-7229(04)80010-5

Seligman, L. D., & Ollendick, T. H. (1998). Comorbidity of anxiety and depression in children and adolescents: An integrative review. *Clinical Child and Family Psychology Review, 1*(2), 125–144. https://doi.org/10.1023/A:1021887712873

Seligman, L. D., & Ollendick, T. H. (2011). Cognitive behavioral therapy for anxiety disorders in youth. *Child and Adolescent Psychiatry Clinics of North America, 20*(2), 217–238.https://doi.org/10.1016/j.chc.2011.01.003

Silverman, W. K., Pina, A. A., & Viswesvaran, C. (2008). Evidence-based psychosocial treatments for phobic and anxiety disorders in children and adolescents. *Journal of*

Clinical Child and Adolescent Psychology, 37(1), 105–130. https://doi.org/10.1080/15374410701817907

Spence, S. H., Donovan, D. L., March, S., Gamble, A., . . . Kenardy, J. (2011). A randomized controlled trial of online versus clinic-based CBT for adolescent anxiety. *Journal of Consulting and Clinical Psychology, 79*(5), 629–642. https://doi.org/10.1037/a0024512

Thulin, U., Svirsky, L., Serlachius, E., Andersson, G., & Öst, L.-G. (2014). The effect of parent involvement in the treatment of anxiety disorders in children: A meta-analysis. *Cognitive Behaviour Therapy, 43*(3), 185–200. https://doi.org/10.1080/16506073.2014.923928

Vigerland, S., Ljótsson, B., Thulin, U., Öst, L. G., Andersson, G., & Serlachius, E. (2016). Internet-delivered cognitive behavioural therapy for children with anxiety disorders: A randomised controlled trial. *Behaviour Research and Therapy, 76*, 47–56. https://doi.org/10.1016/j.brat.2015.11.006

Walkup, J., Albano, A. M., Piacentini, J., Birmaher, B., Compton, S., Sherrill, J., Ginsburg, G., Rynn, M., McCracken, J., Waslick, B., Iyengar, S., March, J., & Kendall, P. C. (2008). Cognitive behavioral therapy, sertraline, or a combination in childhood anxiety. *New England Journal of Medicine, 359*, 2753–2766. https://doi.org/10.1056/nejmoa0804633

Weersing, V. R., Jeffreys, M., Do, M.-C. T., Schwartz, K. T. G., & Bolano, C. (2017). Evidence base update of psychosocial treatments for child and adolescent depression. *Journal of Clinical Child & Adolescent Psychology, 46*(1), 11–43. https://doi.org/10.1080/15374416.2016.1220310

Weiner, C., Perloe, A., Whitton, S., & Pincus, D. B. (2012). Attentional bias in adolescents with panic disorder: Changes over an 8-day intensive treatment program. *Behavioural and Cognitive Psychotherapy, 40*, 193–204. https://doi.org/10.1017/s1352465811000580

Wergeland, G. J. H., Fjermestad, K. W., Marin, C. E., Haugland, B. S. M., Bjaastad, J. F., Oeding, K., Bjelland, I., Silverman, W. K., Öst, L.-G., Havik, O. E., & Heiervang, E. R. (2014). An effectiveness study of individual vs. group cognitive behavioral therapy for anxiety disorders in youth. *Behaviour Research and Therapy, 57*, 1–12. https://doi.org/10.1016/j.brat.2014.03.007

13

Tourette and Trichotillomania

Adapting Treatment While Maintaining Fidelity

JENNIFER R. ALEXANDER, JORDAN T. STIEDE,
AND DOUGLAS W. WOODS ■

INTRODUCTION

Trichotillomania (TTM; also referred to as hair pulling disorder) and Tourette disorder (TD) exist in separate diagnostic categories (American Psychiatric Association [APA], 2013) but exhibit functional similarities and respond to similar treatments (Himle et al., 2004; Lamothe et al., 2020). After reviewing the characteristics of each disorder, we describe habit reversal training (HRT) and function-based interventions, which serve as core therapeutic elements in the treatment of both TTM and TD. Additional treatment strategies that occur as part of standard protocols for both disorders are discussed and followed by a review of the treatment efficacy research. Consistent with the call for "flexibility within fidelity" (Kendall & Beidas, 2007; Kendall & Frank, 2018), we close with an example of a flexible implementation of these treatments in a case example.

Trichotillomania Characteristics

Trichotillomania is an obsessive-compulsive related disorder characterized by recurrent hair pulling that leads to hair loss and impairment and continues despite attempts to stop (APA, 2013). Whereas nonpathological (i.e., nonimpairing) hair pulling often emerges in infancy/early childhood and subsides on its own (Santhanam et al., 2008; Stein et al., 2010; Swedo et al., 1992), pathological hair pulling typically emerges in late childhood/early adolescence (Ricketts et al., 2019). The severity of TTM tends to wax and wane over time (Tolin et al., 2007) but is typically chronic when left untreated (Grant & Chamberlain, 2016).

The prevalence of TTM among children and adolescents is not well understood due to an absence of large epidemiological studies (Duke et al., 2010). However, the lifetime prevalence of TTM is believed to be greater than 1% (Franklin et al., 2010; King et al., 1995). Children with TTM are more likely to experience a negative impact in academics (e.g., missing classes), social life (e.g., avoiding social events due to embarrassment around hair loss), and self-esteem (Franklin et al., 2008; Walther et al., 2014). TTM also can be associated with physical impairment such as scarring, gastrointestinal difficulties when hair is ingested after pulling, and muscle strain due to the recurring motions associated with hair pulling (e.g., Labouliere & Storch, 2012).

Children and adolescents with TTM often meet criteria for other mental health disorders, and comorbidity often impacts TTM expression and treatment. The most commonly occurring comorbid disorders are anxiety disorders (McGuire et al., 2012; Walther et al., 2014), attention-deficit/hyperactivity disorder (ADHD), and oppositional defiant disorder (McGuire et al., 2012). Youth with TTM also commonly engage in other body-focused repetitive behaviors (BFRBs), such as skin picking and nail biting (Walther et al., 2014).

Tourette Disorder Characteristics

Tourette disorder is a childhood-onset condition that involves the performance of multiple motor and one or more vocal tics for at least one year (APA, 2013). Tics are sudden, repetitive, nonrhythmic movements/vocalizations that can be categorized as simple or complex. Simple tics are subtle, purposeless movements or sounds, while complex tics involve coordinated actions of multiple muscle groups and may consist of combinations of simple tics. TD occurs in about .6% to .8% of youth and is more prevalent in boys (Robertson, 2015; Scahill et al., 2014; Scharf et al., 2015). Most individuals with TD experience premonitory urges, which are uncomfortable physical sensations relieved by the performance of tics (Brandt et al., 2016; Capriotti et al., 2014; Himle et al., 2007; Leckman et al., 1993). Contextual factors, such as certain places, people, and feelings can impact tic expression (Conelea & Woods, 2008).

Treatment seeking youth with tic disorders generally have mild-to-moderate tic severity and related impairment linked to academic, psychosocial, and familial difficulties and reduced quality of life (Conelea et al., 2014; Scahill et al., 2009; Specht et al., 2011; Storch et al., 2007). Tics typically begin around age 6, peak in severity around age 10, and steadily decline into adolescence and young adulthood (Bloch et al., 2006: Espil et al., 2020; Leckman et al., 1998; Rizzo et al., 2012). The majority of children with TD experience another mental health condition (Hirschtritt et al., 2015; Lebowitz et al., 2012; Sambrani et al., 2016). ADHD and obsessive-compulsive disorder (OCD) are the most common, and emerging research suggests anxiety disorders are also common (Specht et al., 2011). Individuals with tics plus comorbidities tend to have poorer quality of life compared to those who present with tics alone (Eapen et al., 2016; Eddy et al., 2011).

TREATMENT FOR TRICHOTILLOMANIA AND TOURETTE DISORDER

Various psychopharmacological and psychological treatments have been investigated for these conditions. Treatments studied for TTM include n-acetylcysteine (Bloch et al., 2013), milk thistle (Grant et al., 2019), naltrexone (De Sousa, 2008), behavior therapy (e.g., Franklin et al., 2010; Rahman et al., 2017; Tolin et al., 2007), acceptance and commitment therapy (E. B. Lee et al., 2020), and a computerized cognitive retraining program designed to increase response inhibition (H. J. Lee et al., 2018). Examples of treatments for TD include alpha-2 adrenergic agonists (Weisman et al., 2013), typical and atypical neuroleptics (Quezada & Coffman, 2018; Shapiro et al., 1989), and some forms of behavior therapy, including Habit Reversal Training (HRT; Bate et al., 2011), comprehensive behavioral intervention for tics (CBIT; Piacentini et al., 2010), and exposure and response prevention (ERP; Verdellen et al., 2004). Behavior therapy consisting primarily of HRT and function-based intervention has proven to be particularly effective for both disorders. These elements are described in further detail later.

Traditional Habit Reversal Training Elements

Azrin and Nunn (1973) developed HRT, a multicomponent intervention demonstrated to significantly reduce repetitive behaviors, such as tics, hair pulling, nail biting, and thumb sucking. Over the last 50 years, researchers have suggested the awareness training (AT), competing response (CR) training, and social support (SS) components of HRT are the primary components responsible for the intervention's effectiveness in treating youth with TTM and TD (Miltenberger et al., 1985; Woods & Miltenberger, 1996; Woods et al., 1996).

Awareness Training (AT). The purpose of AT is to increase children's awareness of their target behavior. In TTM, the target behavior is hair pulling, and in TD, the target behaviors are tics, with one tic being targeted at a time. In AT, children are first taught to develop a thorough description of their target behavior (*response description*). In developing a *good* description, the therapist and child work together to detail the ways in which various muscle groups (e.g., fingers, hands, arms, shoulders) are involved in producing the target behavior, the typical body posture they hold while performing the behavior, *and* the internal sensations they feel prior to the behavior. After developing this *detailed* description, children are guided through a *response detection* exercise in which they are tasked with notifying their clinician (e.g., by raising their hand) whenever they engage in the target behavior or notice any warning signs indicating the target behavior is about to occur (e.g., premonitory urges, itching, holding various body postures). While doing this "detection" exercise, children are simultaneously asked to complete a seemingly unrelated task (e.g., playing a game or conversing about another topic) to enhance generalization of awareness. When children correctly acknowledge the behavior or warning sign by raising their finger, the therapist praises them. If they engage in the target behavior, but forget to acknowledge its occurrence, the therapist stops the session and points out the occurrence to them. By the end of AT, the goal is for children to be aware of at least 80% of their target behaviors.

Competing Response (CR) Training. CR training is completed after AT. In CR training, children are taught to do a behavior that is incompatible with the target habit. They are instructed to do this "competing" behavior every time they begin to do the target behavior (i.e., pulling or tic), or if they notice any warning signs for these behaviors. Children are encouraged to hold their CR for a minute or until the urge to perform the target behavior goes away, whichever is longer. When developing CRs, it can be helpful to keep four rules in mind. First, a CR should make the target behavior impossible or significantly harder to do. Second, children should be able to hold their CRs for one minute or longer. Third, CRs should be relatively subtle, meaning they should not draw much attention from others. Finally, CRs should be portable in the sense that children should be able to do their CRs anywhere at any time. Examples of commonly used CRs are included in Table 13.1.

Social Support (SS) Component. Social support is designed to reinforce children's use of CRs. In SS, identified support persons (e.g., parents, guardians) are taught to support children's efforts in managing the target behavior by offering gentle praise and reminders around the appropriate implementation of their CRs. For example, parents might gently remind their teen to use her CR upon noticing the teen tic while watching TV. In another setting, parents may offer praise when noticing the teen practicing her CR without being prompted.

Table 13.1. Examples of Competing Responses (CRs)

TTM		TD	
Target Behavior	CR	*Target Behavior*	CR
Hair pulling	Form fists with hands and simultaneously pull shoulders down away from ears	Eye darting tic	Focus eyes on one spot in the room and engage in slow, controlled blinking every 1–3 seconds
	Hold hands to thighs	Neck rolling tic	Gently tense neck muscles with chin down slightly
	Clasp hands together and place them on lap or behind the back	Coughing tic	Purse lips, relaxed breathing in and out through nose

Function-Based Interventions

Function-based interventions are designed to reduce the likelihood of target behaviors by eliminating or modifying variables that appear to trigger, facilitate, or reinforce the target behaviors. To develop effective functional interventions, the clinician, youth, and family must first complete a functional analysis of the youth's behavior. This analysis should identify: (1) the situations/settings/activities wherein the youth pulls/tics most (e.g., the bathroom, classroom) and least frequently (e.g., while others are around, while playing a musical instrument); (2) tools used to complete the behavior (e.g., tweezers in the case of hair pulling); (3) internal experiences that typically precede and follow pulling/ticcing; and (4) external events that typically happen after the pulling/ticcing (e.g., performance of rituals with pulled hair; others' responses to the target behavior such as teasing or being told to stop; being excluded or excused from an activity or situation because of the target behavior).

In conducting the functional analysis, it may be helpful for clinicians to have youth and their parents monitor the target behavior at home prior to completing the functional analysis. After identifying contextual variables surrounding the target behavior, treating clinicians will need to work with the family to determine whether and how to modify each variable in a manner that will make the target behavior less likely. Examples of commonly used function-based procedures are included in Table 13.2.

Table 13.2. EXAMPLES OF FUNCTION-BASED INTERVENTIONS TO MANAGE HABITS
GIVEN PARTICULAR CONTEXTUAL TRIGGERS

Hair Pulling Contextual Variables	Functional Interventions/Procedures
Greater tendency to pull hair in bathroom	• Limiting time in bathroom (e.g., via time-limits) • Covering mirrors in the bathroom • Dimming the lights over the bathroom mirror
Tendency to use tweezers to pull hair	• Having children throw out tweezers or give to trusted person to store for them
Tendency to pull hair while "zoning" out (e.g., watching TV)	• Wearing a hat and gloves • Keeping hands occupied at all times (e.g., holding onto fidget toys) • Maintaining a body posture that does not facilitate hair pulling (e.g., sitting in the center of the couch)
Tendency to put hair on lips/in mouth after pulling hair with fingers	• Wearing gloves, bandaids, or finger covers • Applying bitter nail polish to fingers or another safe, mild, relatively unpleasant tasting substance or device on fingers/hands • Providing an alternative toy/device for children to play with

Table 13.2. CONTINUED

Tic Contextual Variables	Functional Interventions/Procedures
Tendency to tic while watching TV	• Limiting daily television time • Having a social support person watch television with the child • Having social support persons/other visual reminders to remind the child that this is a good time to practice CR exercises
Tendency to tic while in class	• Discussing the child's tics with the teacher and providing guidelines on how they can support her • Seating the child in a location that will decrease the noticeability of tics • Allowing the child to take short breaks during class
Tendency to tic in the car	• Seating the child in a location that will not interfere with the driver • Taking short breaks during long car rides • Scheduling car rides during times that tics may be less severe • Having social support persons/other visual reminders to remind the child that this is a good place to practice CRs
Tendency to not complete homework assignments when tics are present	• Having the child work on homework until assignments are completed • Allowing the child to have short breaks, not contingent on bouts of tics • Having social support persons/other visual reminders to remind the child to practice CR exercises

Additional Treatment Components beyond Habit Reversal Training and Function-Based Interventions

Although HRT and function-based interventions are the two primary/essential therapeutic approaches used to treat both tics and hair pulling, standard treatment protocols for both disorders include additional treatment strategies, described here.

Supplemental Interventions for TTM. When treating children with TTM, HRT and functional interventions are supplemented with additional strategies. Reward programs are used to reinforce the completion of various treatment-related behaviors, including participating in therapy sessions, completing therapy homework, and implementing function-based procedures and CRs (Snorrason et al., 2016). A flexible and creative rewards program may be particularly helpful when working with younger children.

In addition to implementing an appropriate and feasible rewards program, taking a "bossing back" approach (similar to "bossing back OCD") also may be helpful in treating children with TTM. Ultimately, this approach teaches youth to (1) externalize TTM as a bully or monster that gets its strength from the child's hair pulling and (2) view blocking hair pulling via function-based procedures and CRs as a means to defeat the TTM "bully/monster."

For older children and adolescents, it may be beneficial to supplement traditional HRT with strategies that target various psychological factors that have been hypothesized to maintain TTM hair pulling. Perhaps the most common adjunctive therapy components include cognitive-behavior therapy (CBT), acceptance and commitment therapy (ACT), and dialectical behavior therapy (DBT). CBT-enhanced HRT protocols for children and adolescents with TTM (e.g., Rahman et al., 2017; Tolin et al., 2007) call for supplementing HRT with CBT to reduce stress/distress and promote appropriate use of HRT skills. This includes progressive muscle relaxation, cognitive restructuring (e.g., targeting beliefs around stressful situations), problem-solving around issues secondary to TTM (e.g., school issues), and relapse prevention. ACT-enhanced HRT protocols (e.g., AEBT-TTM; Woods & Twohig, 2008) call for supplementing HRT with ACT-based exercises (e.g., mindfulness, cognitive defusion, behavioral commitment) that help individuals understand that pulling is part of a broad strategy they employ to help control undesirable internal experiences and commit to letting go of that behavioral tendency in favor of acting in ways that are more consistent with their life values. Similarly, DBT-enhanced HRT protocols (Keuthen et al., 2012; Keuthen & Sprich, 2012) call for supplementing HRT with modified DBT modules on mindfulness, emotion regulation skills, and distress tolerance to both promote behavioral management of hair pulling via HRT skills and enable the development and use of more adaptive self-regulation practices. Limited evidence from various studies provides support for the efficacy of CBT-enhanced HRT protocols in children (Rahman et al., 2017; Tolin et al., 2007) and CBT-enhanced, ACT-enhanced, and DBT-enhanced HRT in adolescents (Fine et al., 2012; Rahman et al., 2017; Tolin et al., 2007; Welch & Kim, 2012).

Supplemental Interventions for TD. Building on HRT and functional intervention strategies, Woods and colleagues (2008) developed CBIT, which includes components of relaxation training and a motivational reward program. These additional procedures target other factors that may impact tic severity. For instance, relaxation techniques (e.g., diaphragmatic breathing and progressive muscle relaxation) target internal phenomena, such as stress and anxiety, that may worsen tic severity. Using these skills may reduce the likelihood of tics during stressful situations (Woods et al., 2008). Likewise, a motivational reward program is implemented to reinforce attending sessions, participating in session activities, and completing homework assignments. As part of this program, children are rewarded for tic management efforts, not tic reduction, which helps increase treatment compliance of unmotivated individuals.

Standard Organization and Course of Treatment for Trichotillomania

In implementing behavior therapy for TTM, a clinician typically spends the first session providing children and their families with general psychoeducation about TTM and the rationale for behavior therapy. Next, clinicians spend at least one to two sessions gathering information about the contextual variables surrounding children's hair pulling and working with children and their families to develop functional interventions based on this information. Generally, clinicians will continue to dedicate a portion of each remaining session to checking in with children about their use of functional interventions and modify the procedures if/ when necessary. The focus of treatment next transitions to HRT. When applied to hair pulling, AT, CR training, and SS components often can be introduced and completed in one to two sessions. In some instances, however, clinicians may find it is necessary to spend more time implementing specific components (e.g., children who have trouble becoming aware of their pulling may require extra time in AT). After focusing on functional interventions and HRT, clinicians can shift the primary focus of sessions onto supplemental therapeutic techniques (e.g., CBT, ACT, and DBT) as needed, although they will continue to check on accurate implementation of the HRT and functional intervention.

Standard Organization and Course of Treatment for Tourette Disorder

Standard CBIT is a manual-based, eight-session program delivered over 10 weeks for individuals 9 years and older (Woods et al., 2008). The first two sessions are 90 minutes in duration, while the remaining sessions are 60 minutes. Clinicians meet with individuals weekly for the first six sessions, followed by two-week intervals between the remaining sessions. For children, sessions are conducted with caregivers present, but older adolescents may choose to meet individually, with caregivers being debriefed at the end of the session. The first session consists of an explanation of treatment rationale, psychoeducation about tic disorders, and an introduction to functional interventions. Clinicians also create a hierarchy of tics to be addressed in treatment, and a motivational reward program is implemented for child patients. Subsequent sessions consist of functional interventions and HRT for each tic on the hierarchy. Training in diaphragmatic breathing and progressive muscle relaxation are added to Sessions Four and Five, respectively. Further, relapse prevention is introduced in Session Seven, and treatment procedures and relapse prevention are reviewed in the last session. Homework is assigned throughout treatment and consists of monitoring the tics, practicing CR exercises and relaxation techniques, and implementing functional interventions.

Efficacy of Behavior Therapy for Trichotillomania

The most efficacious treatment currently available for pediatric TTM is behavior therapy, specifically HRT plus function-based interventions. Experts view HRT as the first-line treatment for TTM across the lifespan (Flessner et al., 2010). Supporting this conclusion, two randomized controlled trials (RCTs) in children with TTM have found behavior therapy to be efficacious. Franklin and colleagues (2010) found that HRT was more efficacious than a minimal attention control condition, although findings from that study raised some questions regarding maintenance of HRT treatment gains. In another study, Rahman and colleagues (2017) found that HRT was more effective at reducing hair pulling severity than "treatment as usual," which included other forms of psychotherapy, medication, school-based interventions, and no treatment. Although some (~25%) participants lost their responder status following the conclusion of treatment, hair pulling reductions were largely maintained one- and three-months posttreatment (Rahman et al., 2017). Echoing what has been found in studies examining HRT efficacy in children, meta-analyses also have highlighted behavior therapy as the most efficacious treatment for TTM in adults (Bloch et al., 2007; Farhat et al., 2020; McGuire et al., 2014; Slikboer et al., 2017).

Efficacy of Behavior Therapy for Tourette Disorder

The most efficacious nonpharmacological treatment for TD is behavior therapy, with CBIT being the most well-supported treatment in children (Murphy et al., 2013; Pringsheim et al., 2019; Steeves et al., 2012; Verdellen et al., 2011). Recently, a multidisciplinary panel of tic experts indicated that CBIT should be considered a first-line treatment option for children with tics (Pringsheim et al., 2019). Anchoring both recommendations were data from a RCT of 126 children with TD, which demonstrated that CBIT was more effective than psychoeducation and supportive therapy (PST) at reducing tic severity and related impairment (Piacentini et al., 2010). In the study, 53% of children who received CBIT significantly responded to treatment, with 87% of responders showing continued benefits at six-months post treatment. An 11-year follow-up of this trial found that children who had originally responded to CBIT maintained their gains at long-term follow-up, while nonresponders still showed tic severity improvements but gains were not as meaningful (Espil et al., 2020). Tic-related impairment was similar at follow-up among all participants, but effective CBIT and PST treatment reduced impairment more rapidly (Espil et al., 2020). Finally, CBIT delivered via different modalities, such as videoconference (Himle et al., 2012) and a Voice over Internet Protocol (VoIP; Ricketts, Goetz, et al., 2016), also have demonstrated significant improvements in tic severity and related impairment.

FLEXIBLE IMPLEMENTATION OF THE PROTOCOLS

Fidelity with standard behavior therapy protocols for TTM and TD requires flexible implementation by the therapist. By their very nature, the functional assessments that lead to functional interventions for TTM and TD will yield different triggers and reinforcers for the target behavior, depending on the child's history. Such diversity in function will lead a good therapist to recommend different functional interventions to fit the unique needs of the child and his or her family. Similarly, in HRT, the competing responses chosen for each child will differ depending on the individual's specific tics. Beyond the inherent flexibility in the existing protocols, research on factors associated with treatment outcome suggest other areas in which flexible treatment implementation may be warranted.

Flexible Implementation of Behavior Therapy for Trichotillomania

To date, few studies have investigated predictors or moderators of TTM treatment, partially due to the small number of TTM RCTs that have been conducted (Slikboer et al., 2017). Studies that have investigated predictors and moderators of outcome have largely done so using adult samples. One such study found that more therapeutic contact hours led to better outcomes (McGuire et al., 2014) and that the addition of ACT and/or DBT components led to better treatment outcomes than traditional HRT + function-based interventions (McGuire et al., 2014). Nevertheless, a more recent meta-analysis failed to offer support for these findings (Farhat et al., 2020). Notably, neither McGuire and colleagues (2014) or Farhat and colleagues (2020) found any evidence to suggest that factors, such as age or comorbidity status, are associated with TTM treatment outcome.

Flexibility in Functional Interventions. Although research has not yet consistently identified differential predictors of TTM treatment outcomes, factors such as hair pulling characteristics, pulling style, and pulling function, do influence treatment implementation. Indeed, there is substantial variation in children's specific hair pulling phenomenology, and understanding this variation within a functional assessment framework is essential in developing flexible, yet effective interventions. For example, some affected individuals report multiple hair pulling binges or episodes in any given day (Tolin et al., 2007), and each of these episodes can last anywhere from seconds to hours (Mansueto et al., 1997). Children and adolescents with TTM pull their hair from various body sites, though the most commonly reported are the scalp, eyebrows, and eyelashes (Franklin et al., 2008; Walther et al., 2014). There is also heterogeneity in how affected children pull their hair. Most often, children use their fingers, but some report using tweezers, mirrors, or other tools to aid in their pulling at least some of the time (Walsh & McDougle, 2012).

Based on an individual's specific pulling action, different treatment procedures may be necessary. For instance, youth who use their fingers to engage in hours-long pulling binges from their scalp may particularly benefit from procedures that physically block ready access to hair pulling (e.g., wearing gloves on their hands, wearing bandages on their fingers, wearing a hat). Similarly, someone pulling from their lashes or eyebrows may be asked to wear nonprescription reading glasses to diminish access to pulling areas, and any individual who pulls may be asked to put petroleum jelly on their fingertips in high-risk situations to make pulling more difficult.

In addition to the diverse expression of the pulling behavior, there is diversity in the settings and stimuli that trigger pulling, each of which requires its own flexible intervention. Reports indicate that affected children most commonly pull in the bathroom, a private bedroom, the living room, and the car and that affected children rarely pull while others are around (Labouliere & Storch, 2012). Youth who have a tendency to pull their hair while in the bathrooms or private bedrooms, as well as those who tend to refrain from pulling while others are around, may benefit from having time limits placed around alone time. For instance, limits may be placed around how long they are to be in the bathroom (e.g., 10 to 15 minutes to shower and get ready for bed), and timers may be used to help them adhere to these time restrictions. Likewise, to naturally limit time in their bedrooms, children may be asked to only use their rooms for sleeping, changing clothes, or quickly performing other tasks.

In addition to setting time limits in preferred pulling settings, functional interventions can involve changing the evocative aspects of these settings. For instance, if children tend to pull in the bathroom while looking in a mirror, clinicians may consider having their family cover the bathroom mirror and remove some or all of the lights over the bathroom mirror to dim the lighting available to them. Similarly, for children who tend to pull their hair while sitting on their bed in their bedroom or sitting on the couch in the living room, clinicians may consider changing how and/or where they sit in these rooms. For instance, they may be asked to consider sitting in a straight back chair without armrests in instances when such chairs are available. Alternatively, they may be asked to sit in the middle of the couch as opposed to on the sides of the couch so their hand is no longer propped on an armrest and therefore closer to the hair. In addition, children may be asked to keep their hands occupied when they are in settings in which they typically pull their hair.

Finally, pulling can lead to a diverse set of consequences that may serve to strengthen or maintain the behavior. For example, more than half of children with TTM engage in at least one post-pulling ritual (Labouliere & Storch, 2012). Such rituals can include playing with pulled hair, closely examining pulled hair, placing pulled hair on lips, and ingesting pulled hair (Labouliere & Storch, 2012). These rituals are thought to reinforce hair pulling by providing pleasurable sensory stimulation (Morris et al., 2013). In cases where tactile stimulation may reinforce the behavior, gloves can be used to dampen the pleasurable tactile stimulation youth receive from playing with their hair. In addition, encouraging the child to find an alternative, more acceptable method of deriving similar tactile stimulation also may be helpful. Such methods may include having the child rub loose threads on their lips and giving the child fidget toys or other stimuli that provide similar sensations as that of hair.

Experience of unpleasant emotions secondary to hair pulling is also commonly reported in therapy (e.g., feeling embarrassed about TTM hair loss). In instances when emotional reactions to pulling tend to trigger more hair pulling, it will be beneficial for clinicians to ensure that children learn adaptive ways of responding to such negative emotions other than hair pulling or manipulation. Implementing CBT, DBT, and ACT techniques may prove particularly helpful for meeting this goal.

Flexibility within HRT for TTM. Although HRT is a relatively fixed treatment procedure, some degree of flexibility and creativity is required within the core HRT components of AT, CR, and SS. With AT, affected children often shy away from pulling in front of others, which can complicate response detection activities. Clinicians who encounter a child who does not pull her hair during session may simply have her simulate hair pulling. Likewise, the therapist may have children focus primarily on their body posture during HRT response detection and signify whenever they notice they are assuming any of their posture-related hair pulling warning signs (e.g., leaning their head to the side, moving their hand toward their head). To the extent that is possible and reasonable, it may also be beneficial for clinicians to have children do an in-session activity that frequently co-occurs with hair pulling (e.g., watching a YouTube video on their phone, scrolling through their social media page of choice, reading through a magazine or book the clinician provides). This step may trigger the behavior and offer them an opportunity to practice detecting when they are engaging in any hair pulling or hair pulling warning signs.

For children who experience difficulties accurately detecting their hair pulling, it will be particularly important for clinicians to assign self-monitoring homework assignments to assist in improving their awareness. These assignments may entail having children and their support persons keep detailed records of their hair pulling episodes during prescribed times (e.g., during family TV time). Clinicians also may consider asking them to wear various stimuli that will provide auditory or olfactory feedback whenever they engage in various posture-related hair pulling warning signs (e.g., bracelets that make noise or vibrate when the arms move, hand lotions with strong scents; HabitAware, 2020; Morris et al., 2013).

Flexibility is required during CR training. After initially agreeing to use a specific CR, some children will report having not used it regularly. In such cases, it will be important for clinicians to work with them to determine barriers to implementation. If noncompliance occurred because the child frequently forgot to use the CR, she can be encouraged to place reminder notes in high-risk areas. In contrast, if it becomes clear that inconsistent CR use was due to the youth's dislike of their CR, clinicians may work with them to identify an alternative CR that is more agreeable and likely to be more consistently used by the child. Finally, it may be that CR noncompliance is due to a lack of motivation. In such cases, clinicians may consider working to boost the child's motivation to use the CR (e.g., via motivational interviewing or other appropriate therapeutic strategies, such as cognitive restructuring around using the CR in question) or to determine whether it is the child or parent who is more motivated for behavior change.

Flexibility based on Emotion Regulation Function. Effective implementation of behavior therapy for TTM requires an understanding of children's hair pulling style, because it has been hypothesized that different styles of TTM may benefit from different treatments (Alexander et al., 2016; Flessner, Conelea, et al., 2008). The two pulling styles most frequently discussed in the literature are "automatic" and "focused." Automatic pulling refers to hair pulling that occurs outside of one's awareness (Flessner, Woods, et al., 2008). Such pulling may occur while affected persons are completing a sedentary activity in which it is possible to "zone out," such as watching television. In contrast, focused pulling refers to pulling that occurs within affected persons' awareness and in response to an internal event (e.g., sensory/emotional experiences and thoughts about the way certain hairs appear or feel; Flessner et al., 2010). Generally, it is thought that automatic pulling may be more responsive to traditional HRT and functional interventions, whereas focused pulling may benefit from HRT and function-based interventions supplemented with CBT, ACT, or DBT, because such approaches may be useful for providing them with alternative methods for regulating and/or responding to the emotional experiences that can trigger hair pulling (Flessner, Conelea, et al., 2008).

Flexible Implementation of Standard Comprehensive Behavioral Intervention for Tics for Tourette Disorder

Few studies have examined factors associated with differential outcomes from behavior therapy for children with tic disorders. Nevertheless, combined data from the child (Piacentini et al., 2010) and adult (Wilhelm et al., 2012) CBIT outcome trials showed that CBIT had a greater effect for those not on tic medication at baseline (Sukhodolsky et al., 2017). Other variables such as tic phenomenology, age, sex, family functioning, treatment expectancy, and co-occurring ADHD, OCD, and anxiety disorders were not associated with outcome. Further, McGuire and colleagues (2013) found that specific types of tics did not predict greater reductions, suggesting that CBIT is effective across all types of tics. Interestingly, tics with premonitory urges were more likely to attenuate following CBIT relative to PST (McGuire et al., 2015), indicating that tics without an urge may be more transient and can diminish without treatment, while tics with urges should be prioritized in CBIT.

Sukhodolsky and colleagues (2017) showed that several variables predicted treatment outcome, and each of these provide opportunities for flexible implementation of the standard treatment protocol. For instance, greater baseline premonitory urge severity was associated with poorer outcomes, suggesting that children with stronger urges have more difficulty learning to manage tics (Sukhodolsky et al., 2017) and thus may need additional sessions to practice competing response exercises. Mindfulness-based strategies also could be used when premonitory urge severity is impacting treatment. Reese and colleagues (2015) demonstrated that an eight-week trial of mindfulness-based stress reduction led to significant improvements in tic severity and related impairment for 18 individuals with tic disorders. Participants in this study were instructed to mindfully notice the urge to tic and use breathing exercises until the urge subsided, while not trying to tic or eliminate the urge in any way. Gev and colleagues (2016) also demonstrated that urge acceptance reduced tic severity and urge intensity. Clinicians may use these approaches in CBIT if children struggle with competing response exercises due to greater urge intensity.

Döpfner and Rothenberger (2007) suggested that more impairing conditions such as ADHD should be treated before beginning CBIT treatment because severe comorbid symptoms can negatively impact behavior therapy outcomes. Even after ADHD treatment, children with comorbid ADHD often struggle with adherence to HRT procedures. Therefore, the standard CBIT reward program can be enhanced to increase focus on therapeutic activities. For instance, clinicians could help parents create a token economy system for children to receive rewards for using CRs at home, and they could add extra rewards for the correct use of CR exercises in session. Clinicians also may need to examine the structure of sessions and implement short breaks if the child is less focused.

Other research suggests anxiety may negatively impact response to treatment. Sukhodolsky and colleagues (2017) demonstrated less tic reduction following CBIT (Sukhodolsky et al., 2017), and Nissen and colleagues (2019) found that high anxiety led to less improvement in functional impairment. Further, Conelea and colleagues (2011) showed that acute stress disrupted tic suppression ability. Although studies have demonstrated that relaxation techniques may not be a necessary component for all children who receive CBIT (Dreison & Lagges, 2017), additional therapeutic focus on reducing anxiety may be beneficial.

For individuals with co-occurring OCD, it can be difficult to differentiate complex motor tics from compulsions; therefore, clinicians should assess youth's experiences before performing the behavior. Tics are usually associated with decreases in uncomfortable sensory phenomena, whereas compulsions are related to decreases in anxiety or the prevention of catastrophic consequences (Mansueto & Keuler, 2005). Nevertheless, CBIT can be slightly modified by treating both "not just right" compulsions and complex tics with ERP plus CR training. For instance, if an individual feels compelled to touch an object, clinicians can expose the child to the object and instruct him/her to perform a CR, such as crossing their arms, during response prevention.

Flexibility within Functional Interventions. For each child, clinicians recommend functional interventions associated with environmental factors that impact tic expression. Depending on the child, clinicians focus on various settings (e.g., home, school), activities (e.g., sports, clubs), and emotional states (e.g., excitement, anxiety) that exacerbate tics (Woods et al., 2008). For instance, for children whose tics worsen in school, clinicians should communicate with teachers to explain the uncontrollability of tics and provide guidelines on how the teachers can support the child. The child may benefit from short breaks from classroom activities, not contingent on bouts of tics, or from sitting in a location of the classroom that reduces the noticeability of tics. For children who tic more before bedtime, clinicians should help structure a consistent bedtime routine each night. Potential tic exacerbating activities, such as watching television and completing homework, should be completed at least 30 minutes before bedtime, and children may practice relaxation techniques in bed. For youth who report tic exacerbation during anxiety-provoking situations, clinicians should implement strategies to reduce anxious responses that worsen tics. For example, the child could engage in relaxation techniques, such as deep breathing, and clinicians could introduce cognitive restructuring of anxious thoughts (see also Rifkin et al., this book). Finally, before entering any situation that exacerbates tics, a support person should remind children to engage in CRs if they feel the urge to tic.

Reactions to tics can strengthen or maintain the behavior, and reducing such consequences requires the clinician to be flexible. For instance, children may report receiving social attention after tics, such as teasing, laughter, or someone telling the child to stop ticcing. In such cases, parents and teachers should provide those around the child with specific instructions to ignore tics. If parents tend to comfort children during bouts of tics, clinicians should explain how these reactions also may reinforce tic expression and work with parents to develop methods of providing the child comfort in a fashion not contingent on tics. If classmates contingently react to tics, the clinician or child could present tic psychoeducation to help them understand the importance of a tic neutral environment. Although parents are generally encouraged to ignore tics, exceptions may occur for painful/dangerous tics. For example, if children exhibit self-abusive tics, such as hitting themselves, parents can interrupt these behaviors while providing minimal attention. In some cases, children's tics result in them being removed from aversive settings or situations. For example, a child may be asked to leave a classroom or stop doing homework because of tics. Should this occur, strategies designed to keep the child in the situation should be developed. For example, if classroom tics occur, but become distracting to others, the child can be moved to a less noticeable place within the classroom while still participating in the class. Similarly, children should not be allowed to skip homework assignments due to tics, but short homework breaks can be implemented not contingent on bouts of tics.

Flexibility within HRT. In standard HRT for TD, awareness training is usually completed in 20 to 25 minutes. However, if children have poor awareness of a tic, therapists can dedicate full sessions to awareness training and use additional techniques to increase awareness. For instance, youth with difficulties describing tics may benefit from using mirrors or video recordings of themselves ticcing, which could help them more accurately describe the behaviors. The response detection exercise also could initially be completed in front of a mirror, or children could notify the clinician when the target tic is seen in a video of themselves. If youth continue to struggle with tic detection, clinicians can perform the children's target tic and ask them to point out when the therapist engages in the target behavior. After reliably acknowledging target tics demonstrated by the therapist, the children can transition to standard response detection in which they detect their own tics. If response detection is impacted because children rarely tic in session, clinicians can use the results of the functional assessment to trigger tics. In doing so, the clinician, with parental consent and child assent, exposes the child to tic-exacerbating stimuli in session with the hope of triggering tics. For example, if discussing the premonitory urge exacerbates tics for a child, the therapist may start talking about the urge. Likewise, for children who tic more while watching television, the therapist and child may watch television during the session as a way of evoking tics. If these strategies do not work, clinicians could also ask children to intentionally perform the target tic and acknowledge those occurrences.

Competing response training also can be flexibly implemented in a number of ways. First, if children dislike the CR, clinicians can adjust the exercise to make it more comfortable. This is possible because for most tics, multiple CRs could be used to physically prevent the completion of the behavior. Further, children with certain vocal tics may dislike that the CR (e.g., pursed lips while breathing through the nose) prevents them from talking. In situations where talking is necessary, they can stop the CR to briefly respond, but immediately return to the exercise after talking. Additionally, with close friends and family members, children could have a signal that indicates they will respond once the premonitory urge diminishes.

When a CR is ineffective, clinicians should assess why children are not improving. For example, poor awareness may lead to children not using the CR, so clinicians could spend more time on awareness training. If clinicians notice poor CR compliance, they can implement additional reward programs in which youth receive rewards for correct CR use at home and in session. Support individuals also could remind children to use CRs before entering situations in which tics are usually more severe (e.g., in the car, at dinner, during homework). Finally, intense premonitory urges may lead to ineffective CRs. When children experience premonitory urges that last well past one minute, clinicians can ask them to rate the urge intensity on a 0 to 10 scale. Then, clinicians can record an urge rating every 30 seconds and show them that the urge gradually decreases with time. Instead of waiting until the urge completely diminishes, children also could stop the CR when it reaches a manageable level, such as a rating of one or two (Woods et al., 2008). If the child continues to struggle with urge intensity, clinicians could implement mindfulness-based strategies, such as tic-specific meditation (Reese et al., 2015).

With respect to implementing SS, a number of issues arise that require flexibility on the part of the clinician. Children typically benefit from receiving praise and reminders from SS persons, but some may find SS to be more punishing than rewarding. In these situations, clinicians can discontinue SS but implement other strategies to remind children to use CRs. For instance, youth who tend to tic while playing video games may benefit from a reminder note on the video game console. Additionally, instead of using a support person, children could set reminders on their phones for times when tics are more likely, such as right after school or during bedtime routines.

Social support persons sometimes find it difficult to notice the child's covert tics and/or extremely discreet CRs. In these situations, youth can tell the support person or have a signal (e.g., raise finger) when they perform these behaviors. Such notification can allow the support person to praise the use of the exercise. In addition, clinicians can assign homework in which support persons play games with children during the week while focusing on CR practice. Finally, parents are typically the support persons; but when parents have fewer interactions with the child or the parent/child relationship is difficult, an older sibling, babysitter, or other family member could step into this role. Important to note is the finding from Flessner and colleagues (2005) who showed that HRT may be equally effective with or without SS.

In addition, behavior therapy for tics has been flexibly implemented with respect to the age of the child, the overall protocol structure, and flexibility within the use of standard therapy techniques. These variations are described here.

Flexibility Based on Age. The original CBIT protocol was developed for children ages 9 and older. Nevertheless, the protocol may be flexibly implemented with younger children. For example, Bennett and colleagues (2020) demonstrated several ways in which standard CBIT (Woods et al., 2008) can be restructured for children under age 9 years. In this modified protocol, the first session only included parents, and the focus was on psychoeducation about tic disorders and emphasizing the importance of creating a tic neutral environment. Next, instead of immediately starting HRT, therapists played "The Opposite Game" (TOG) with the children to teach concepts underlying HRT. TOG is designed to assess their readiness for HRT by increasing tic awareness and teaching the opposite action concept of a CR through a call-and-response style similar to the childhood game "Simon Says." Once children understood TOG concepts, they began to use CRs contingent upon urges or the actual occurrence of tics. Throughout this process, TOG and HRT were administered with a developmentally sensitive play approach. The use of this approach with 15 young children with tic disorders led to significant decreases in clinician-rated and parent-reported tic severity at posttreatment, with a 50% response rate. Improvements were maintained at three-month follow-up, and parents reported high acceptability (Bennett et al., 2020).

Flexibility in Protocol Structure. In some circumstances, the traditional eight-session format over 10 weeks is not possible. In such cases, different treatment courses may be necessary. In one randomized controlled trial, Chen and colleagues (2019) compared modified CBIT to a control condition in 46 children with TD. Modified CBIT consisted of standard CBIT (Woods et al., 2008) abbreviated into four 30- to 45-minute sessions over three months. Participants who received modified CBIT experienced significantly greater reductions in tic severity compared to those in the control group, with improvements maintained at three months posttreatment. Blount and Raj (2018) also implemented a modified version of CBIT that compressed standard CBIT into eight sessions over four days.

Four of five participants showed clinically significant decreases in tic severity at posttreatment, and two of three participants who completed the one-month follow-up demonstrated continued benefit.

Access to treatment may be limited for some families, sometimes due to a lack of fully trained CBIT therapists. To address this issue, Ricketts, Gilbert, and colleagues (2016) examined the efficacy of CBIT with 14 children in child neurology and developmental pediatric clinics (CBIT-NP). Treatment consisted of six, 20- to 25-minute sessions delivered over six to eight weeks by a nurse or practicing physician with little behavior therapy experience. Prior to the first session, participants were asked to review information about tic disorders and environmental influences on tics from a clinic-provided workbook and supplemental DVD. The first session consisted of brief psychoeducation and simplified functional intervention procedures, while subsequent sessions included HRT for one tic per week. Results demonstrated significant decreases in tic severity and related impairment, with 56% of study completers exhibiting treatment response at posttreatment. These studies suggest that CBIT can still be effective if administered with fewer treatment sessions or delivered by nonpsychologist tic experts; however, future studies with larger sample sizes are needed.

Flexibility in Techniques. The aforementioned studies showed that CBIT can be delivered in various courses, in different formats, and by novice CBIT therapists. Another recent study also demonstrated how specific techniques can be delivered flexibly and still yield positive effects. In a pediatric psychiatry clinic, Dreison and Lagges (2017) conducted a retrospective chart review to assess the effectiveness of clinic-based CBIT in comparison to standard CBIT. Results showed that flexible use of the CBIT manual in a standard clinic led to significant reductions in tic severity in 10 children and adolescents with TD; 70% demonstrated positive treatment response. Compared to the CBIT manual, the motivational rewards program and progressive muscle relaxation techniques were implemented with significantly fewer youth, suggesting that these techniques may not be as important to treatment outcome. Additionally, clinicians only completed HRT for an average of three tics, which is three fewer than standard CBIT. This suggests that children can learn HRT techniques and generalize them to tics outside of session. HRT was the most utilized CBIT component of clinic-based treatment but was only integrated into 64.5% of sessions, and function-based interventions were only present in 37.4%. Both percentages are significantly lower than standard CBIT treatment (90.9% and 100%, respectively). Overall, Dreison and Lagges (2017) found significant reductions in tic severity with flexible use of the CBIT manual.

CASE EXAMPLE

To illustrate how therapists flexibly implement HRT and functional interventions, consider the case example of a clinician working with Jessica, a 15-year-old female diagnosed with TTM and generalized anxiety disorder (GAD).

The Initial Assessment

Clinician: Jessica, why don't we talk about your hair pulling in more detail? I hear you've been pulling your hair for about two years. It sounds like you don't feel you have any control over your pulling and that your main goal in working with me is to learn how to better manage it. Is that correct?

Jessica: Yes, I hate that I pull my hair. It's really embarrassing, especially now that my eyebrows and eyelashes are just gone. No one's outright made fun of me, but I'm worried people will, and when I start worrying about all of that, I usually pull more. I don't know. I want to stop pulling my hair, but when I'm really upset, all I want to do is feel better, and pulling helps. But after I stop and realize what I've done, I usually wind up feeling really angry at myself and even more worried, which can sometimes make me start pulling even more

Clinician: First, thank you for sharing all of that. It's helpful to hear how you feel about your hair pulling and to get a sense for what hair pulling can sometimes look like for you. From what you've told me so far, it sounds like your anxiety and hair pulling often go hand in hand.

Jessica: Yeah, seems like whenever I'm really anxious or really stressed about something, I start feeling like I "want" to pull my hair. Unfortunately for me, I worry about pretty much everything, which means I often feel tempted to pull my hair.

Just the other night, I got stressed out because I couldn't figure out how to do a math problem I was working on. And then, I started thinking about how I would probably never figure that problem out, which would mean I'd end up failing that assignment, and then I might end up not graduating high school, which would mean my parents would disown me. Before I knew it, I was crying in my room while pulling my hair and continuing to freak out about my future.

Clinician: I see, so it sounds like we can confidently count anxiety, and perhaps strong emotions in general, as a hair pulling trigger for you. This is helpful to know, and we will use this knowledge to help guide what we do in here. May I ask, do you only pull your hair when you're anxious or feeling a strong emotion?

Jessica: Well, I have also noticed that sometimes I pull my hair when I'm zoning out, like when I'm watching TV or something.

Clinician: OK, got it. Based on what you've shared so far, it sounds like HRT, along with functional interventions, will be very useful for you. We will use HRT to help give you the behavioral tools you will need to manage your hair pulling, and we will use functional interventions to change small aspects of your environment in a way that will make your hair pulling less likely. In addition to these treatments, it also sounds like we will want to work on developing some tools to help you with managing your anxiety. How does that sound?

Based on the information gleaned from the above conversation, the treating clinician may now be considering structuring treatment as follows: (1) completing a more extensive functional assessment of Jessica's hair pulling; (2) developing functional strategies to make Jessica's hair pulling less likely; (3) implementing HRT components—with special attention on AT given Jessica's occasional proclivity to pull her hair while zoning out; and (4) implementing supplemental therapeutic techniques to help Jessica better manage the worry that triggers the pulling. Given Jessica's age, the treating clinician could consider supplementing HRT with either CBT, ACT, or DBT. To decide on which of these supplemental approaches to use, the clinician will need to consider Jessica's presentation of worry and her current developmental level.

Creating Functional Interventions

In the following example, the clinician asks Jessica and her mother, Kerry, a series of questions to better understand the contextual variables associated with Jessica's hair pulling. Upon gleaning this information, the clinician notes potential functional strategies that may be beneficial for Jessica.

> *Clinician:* Today, we will be coming up with plans for how we will go about changing some of the things in your everyday life that make hair pulling seem so irresistible for you at times. To create these plans, we're going to spend some time uncovering your hair pulling patterns. Let's start with one type of pattern that is often relatively easy to identify. Where are you typically when you pull your hair? Do you tend to pull your hair mostly when you're at home? Do you ever pull while you're at school?
>
> *Jessica:* I've pulled while at school a couple of times, but that hasn't happened in about a year now. I mostly just pull my hair when I'm at home.
>
> *Kerry:* I've never seen her pull her hair. The only way I can tell she's been pulling her hair is if I notice she has new bald spots, or if I happen to find a clump of hair in the trash or on the ground.
>
> *Jessica:* Yea, I don't think I've ever pulled my hair when I knew other people were around. A lot of the time, I pull my hair when I'm doing homework or listening to music in my room with my door closed. I also tend to pull my hair when I'm on the couch in the den and I'm super absorbed in what I'm watching on TV. Sometimes, I'll pull my hair in the bathroom when I'm getting ready for bed at night and mentally going over everything that happened that day.
>
> *Clinician:* Got it. Well, it sounds like there are already a couple of strategies we can think about for you. Perhaps we could have you wear a hat and gloves while you are at home as a way of blocking your ability to engage in hair pulling easily. Another strategy we might consider is trying to limit the amount of time you spend alone with your door shut. When

you are in your room, we could also have you try focusing primarily on completing more cognitively engaging activities as opposed to spending chunks of time primarily listening to music.

Jessica: Well, I'm not going to wear a hat or gloves while I'm at home all the time. That's weird. But I think limiting my alone time might work. Maybe that will help with worry spirals too—seems like I'm less likely to start feeling intense worry when I'm not alone.

Clinician: OK, thank you for your honesty about your willingness versus unwillingness to engage in the strategies I mentioned. I also appreciate your point about your tendency to get into a worry spiral when you're alone; I think that is something we will want to come back to talk about some more. When you are doing homework or listening to music in your room and when you are watching TV in the den, what are you typically doing with your hands? Are they usually free?

Jessica: Actually, I usually end up kind of zoning out when I'm doing those things, so I'm not 100% sure what I'm usually doing with my hands at those times. I'm guessing my hands are usually free, though.

Kerry: Almost every time I see you sitting on the couch, your hands are resting on your head. I can picture it now—you usually sit on the right side of the couch, with your elbow on the arm rest and your head laying in your hand.

Clinician: Based on what you both are saying, I think we should add a couple other strategies to the list for consideration. One might entail having you keep your hands busy at all times, perhaps by keeping both of your hands on your laptop while doing homework or holding the remote while you watch TV. Another might entail having you sit in the center of the couch when you watch TV so your arms aren't up by your head.

Jessica: Yeah, that might work! What about when I'm in the bathroom, though?

Clinician: Great question. To create a strategy for your bathroom hair pulling, let's see if you can walk me through what it looks like when you're pulling your hair while in the bathroom. Are you typically looking in the mirror? Using tweezers? Playing with your hair?

Kerry: Who knows what she is doing in there? She can spend hours in the bathroom when she is getting ready for bed at night.

Jessica: Usually, if I'm pulling my hair in the bathroom, it's because I'm worrying or it's because I've found some weird-looking hair I saw while looking in the mirror. For some reason, when I see weird-looking hair, it's pretty easy to convince myself that I need to pull that hair out before anyone else sees it, and I'll promise myself I'll only pull one hair. Then, I'll usually get my tweezers and go at my hair.

Clinician: Perhaps we can consider having your mom hold on to your tweezers from now on. We can also consider a couple additional strategies for your bathroom hair pulling: we could potentially set a time limit for getting ready for bed each evening (perhaps 20 minutes) and we could potentially dim the lights over the bathroom mirror.

Jessica: That could work!

Clinician: I'm glad you're willing to consider those suggestions.

The clinician in this instance chose to simultaneously complete a functional analysis of Jessica's hair pulling and brainstorm potential functional strategies for Jessica. However, the clinician may have just as easily decided to refrain from brainstorming potential function-based procedures for Jessica until they completed a thorough functional analysis of Jessica's hair pulling. In either case, it will be important for clinicians to work with the adolescent and their family to consider the feasibility of each of the strategies, including their willingness and ability to implement them. In this example, Jessica explicitly indicated her unwillingness to implement one of the potential function-based procedures the clinician proposed. Although the clinician may have chosen to spend more time exploring Jessica's unwillingness and/or targeting the thoughts and beliefs driving Jessica's unwillingness, it will ultimately be important for clinicians to refrain from assigning strategies that are unlikely to be utilized.

Awareness Training (AT)

The following is an example of implementing AT. In this example, the clinician primarily focuses on developing Jessica's awareness of her eyebrow pulling.

Clinician: Now, we're going to start using HRT principles to target your hair pulling more directly. We're going to start by doing something called AT. We're going to help you become more aware of what you're doing when you pull your hair, the signals that warn you that you're about to start pulling your hair, and your hair pulling in general. Let's start by coming up with a really detailed description of your pulling. I'm going to ask you to walk me through what usually happens when you pull your hair. If it helps, just pretend like you're pulling your hair now.

Jessica: OK. [Jessica proceeds to pretend like she is pulling her hair.]

Clinician: Great! Now, I want you to really try to concentrate on what your body is doing while you complete this exercise, because I'm going to ask you to describe it to me as if I can't see you right now. The first thing I'm going to ask you to describe is what hand and which fingers do you notice yourself using to pull your hair?

Jessica: I'm using my thumb and index finger on my right hand. Really, I only pull with my right hand.

Clinician: Got it. Now, tell me, what do you notice about your body posture right now? Are you sitting straight, or are you slouched to the side?

Jessica: I'm slouched over to the right.

Clinician: You are indeed. Now, let's see if we can describe what you mean by that in even greater detail. What is your neck doing right now? Is it straight or bent? Do you notice anything else about the positioning of the rest of your body? What about your head? Your right arm and hand? Your torso?

Jessica: Well, my head is resting on my right hand, and I can feel my fingers on my hair. So, my neck is bent to the right side, which means my head is tilted to my right side. I can also feel that my stomach is sort of bent to the right side.

Clinician: Way to be so detailed! I think we can consider your current posture a warning signal—that is, sitting in this manner is probably a warning sign for you that you could start pulling your hair at any moment. In this way, it seems similar to the anxiety or urge you sometimes feel right before you pull your hair.

Jessica: Yes, I think you're right.

Clinician: As such, it will be really important for us to have you increase your ability to recognize when you are sitting in this manner. We also want to increase your ability to recognize your other hair pulling warning signals. With that goal in mind, let's play a quick game where we spend five minutes talking about something unrelated to hair pulling. While we're talking, I want you to raise your left index finger whenever you notice yourself (1) shifting into the body position that you usually hold while pulling your hair, (2) feeling an urge to pull, or (3) engaging in hair pulling. I will be sure to also raise my index finger whenever I notice your posture-related pulling warning signal or I notice you pulling, and I will interrupt you to let you know if I think you should have raised your index finger but didn't. Any questions about how to play this game?

Jessica: Nope, I think I understand. [Jessica and the clinician proceed to play this response detection game. Despite multiple points of feedback from the clinician, however, Jessica exhibits difficulty catching when she is engaging in hair pulling/manipulation behaviors. After 20 minutes and four instances in which Jessica began manipulating her hair without her awareness, the clinician decides to end the game.]

Clinician: Jessica, that was a really good effort. I can tell that you are taking therapy seriously because you want to get better control over your pulling. I can also tell that, despite your understanding of the awareness game we're playing and the effort I see you exerting to try to be aware of your hair pulling, it's proving difficult for you to notice in real time when your hand moves up to your scalp. For that reason, I'm thinking we might want to take awareness training to another level. Let's talk about having you and your parents look into securing a HabitAware Keen bracelet so that you can get some out-of-session practice with awareness. This is a device we can buy online and it can be programmed to vibrate every time you start doing the pulling action. It will help with your awareness.

As part of AT, it is important for clinicians to spend ample time supporting adolescents' development of detailed descriptions of their hair pulling and their hair pulling warning signals (i.e., typical hair pulling body posture, urges, itchiness, anxiety). Note that practicing recognizing hair pulling and hair pulling warning signals is considered a critical component of AT. Therefore, clinicians need to ensure adolescents have ample time to practice recognizing these phenomena in session.

Competing Response (CR) Training

After Jessica shows marked improvement in her ability to be aware in real time of her hair pulling and hair pulling warning signals, the clinician goes on to implement CR training. The following is an example of how CR training may be implemented.

> *Clinician:* Now, we're going to do something called CR training. As part of this, we're going to come up with a CR. Or, said differently, we're going to come up with a way for you to physically block your hair pulling. We will want to do our best to find a single CR that will work to block pulling hair both from your scalp and your eyebrows. This blocker will need to follow four rules.
> [Clinician goes on to describe the four rules for CRs.]
> Based on these rules, do you have any ideas for what we could have you do to block your hair pulling?
> *Jessica:* Maybe I can ball my hand into fists like this or sit on my hands like this.
> [Jessica proceeds to demonstrate what both of these behaviors would look like.]
> *Clinician:* Great ideas! Let's see how they hold up to the rules. Would balling your hand into a fist or sitting on your hands make hair pulling impossible or harder to do?
> *Jessica:* Yes! And I know I can do both of those things for a minute or longer.
> *Clinician:* That's true. I also think it's fair to say that those behaviors wouldn't draw too much attention. What do you think?
> *Jessica:* I agree.
> *Clinician:* Great! Starting right now, let's have you do these behaviors every time you notice your hair pulling warning signals—like your pulling urges or the body posture you hold when you pull your hair. Let's also have you do these behaviors whenever you notice yourself pulling your hair. Do you remember how long we want you to hold these blocking behaviors?
> *Jessica:* Yeah, for a minute or until my warning signals go away.

After deciding on CRs, it is wise for clinicians to dedicate some session time to having their patients practice their CRs. In addition, it will be ideal for clinicians to implement an expectation that, going forward, their patients will use their CRs as appropriate when they are in sessions. Clinicians also may consider having them complete dedicated CR practice for homework. Such practice may entail having patients set aside three to four 20-minute periods wherein they focus on utilizing their CRs anytime they pull their hair or notice a pulling warning signal.

Social Support (SS)

The following is an example of how the SS HRT component may be implemented.

> *Clinician:* OK, Kerry. Let's spend some time talking about how you and Dad can support Jessica's use of her HRT skills.
>
> *Kerry:* That would be great, because I feel like I have no idea how to support Jessica with this. I know her father, Michael, feels the same way.
>
> *Jessica:* Yeah, I remember there was one time a long time ago when Dad somehow caught me pulling my hair in the den and he just told me to stop. He didn't really yell or anything, but I was really embarrassed, and I immediately went to my room, closed the door, and just pulled some more.
>
> *Clinician:* Kerry, let's think through what Jessica needs from you and Michael as it relates to her efforts to manage her pulling. Jessica has already indicated she finds her TTM very distressing. Because of this, she wants to work toward reducing her pulling. Based on that, we can conclude that Jessica is already motivated to use her newly acquired HRT skills; she is also likely to feel upset whenever she engages in hair pulling. As such, we can guess that it will be important for you and Michael to understand that Jessica is already very self-motivated for change, which means you will not need to exert any efforts to increase her motivation. It seems likely that what she will need from the both of you is considerate support and validation. From that perspective, if you ever notice (1) she is pulling her hair, (2) she is exhibiting her hair pulling sitting posture, or (3) she is not using her function-based interventions, let's have you neutrally remind her to practice her HRT skills. Let's try not to go overboard with reminders, however. One reminder per setting or every one to two hours is enough. On the flip side, every time you notice her using her hair pulling management skills, I'm going to ask that you and Michael offer her praise. Feel free to be very enthusiastic with this praise— let's acknowledge that, oftentimes, using her hair pulling management skills requires effort.
>
> How does that sound to you all?
>
> *Kerry & Jessica:* That sounds great!

Keep in mind that it is important for clinicians to first check in with their patients and support persons before implementing the SS component to gauge whether it will be beneficial for them to have their identified support persons perform the described HRT SS behaviors. In instances when it is decided that implementing the SS component would be helpful, some creativity in terms of how support is delivered by support persons may be necessary. For instance, in instances when youth express concern about having their support persons give verbal reminders about hair pulling management skills, clinicians may suggest the adoption of an alternative reminder system wherein a code word or a physical signal is used to convey to them that they need to implement their hair pulling management skills.

In the above case example, if Jessica returned to therapy the following week and reported that she has been experiencing increased worry since her parents started implementing SS as discussed in therapy primarily because she feels like her parents are constantly watching her and waiting for to make mistakes, the treating clinician would do well to reconsider having her parents provide SS.

CONCLUSION

Trichotillomania and Tourette Disorder are highly heterogeneous and impairing disorders that impact individuals of all ages. Based on the evidence that is currently available, HRT in conjunction with functional interventions is an effective treatment for TTM and TD. We describe the key features of the manual-based treatments (behavior therapy protocols), as well as ways these protocols can be flexibly implemented for those with TTM and TD.

Clinicians interested in getting more detailed descriptions of HRT for TTM and TD are referred to Azrin and Nunn (1973). Clinicians interested in learning more about protocols for enhanced behavior treatments for TTM are referred to: (1) Franklin and Tolin (2007) for CBT-enhanced HRT; (2) Woods and Twohig (2008) for ACT-enhanced HRT; and (3) Keuthen and Sprich (2012) for DBT-enhanced HRT. Clinicians interested in learning more about protocols for enhanced behavior treatments for TD are referred to Woods and colleagues (2008).

REFERENCES

Alexander, J. R., Houghton, D. C., Twohig, M. P., Franklin, M. E., Saunders, S. M., Neal-Barnett, A. M., Compton, S. N., & Woods, D. W. (2016). Factor analysis of the Milwaukee Inventory for Subtypes of Trichotillomania-Adult Version. *Journal of Obsessive-Compulsive and Related Disorders, 11*, 31–38. https://doi.org/10.1016/j.jocrd.2016.08.001

American Psychiatric Association. (2013). *Diagnostic and statistical manual of mental disorders* (5th ed.). Author.

Azrin, N. H., & Nunn, R. G. (1973). Habit-reversal: A method of eliminating nervous habits and tics. *Behaviour Research and Therapy, 11*(4), 619–628. https://doi.org/10.1016/0005-7967(73)90119-8

Bate, K. S., Malouff, J. M., Thorsteinsson, E. T., & Bhullar, N. (2011). The efficacy of habit reversal therapy for tics, habit disorders, and stuttering: A meta-analytic review. *Clinical Psychology Review, 31*, 865–871. https://doi.org/10.1016/j.cpr.2011.03.013

Bennett, S. M., Capriotti, M., Bauer, C., Chang, S., Keller, A. E., & Walkup J. (2020). Development and open trial of a psychosocial intervention for young children with chronic tics: The CBIT-JR study. *Behavior Therapy, 51*, 659–669. https://doi.org/10.1016/j.beth.2019.10.004

Bloch, M. H., Landeros-Weisenberger, A., Dombrowski, P., Kelmendi, B., Wegner, R., Nudel, J., Pittenger, C., Leckman, J. F., & Coric, V. (2007). Systematic review: Pharmacological and behavioral treatment for trichotillomania. *Biological Psychiatry, 62*, 839–846. https://doi.org/10.1016/j.biopsych.2007.05.019

Bloch, M. H., Panza, K. E., Grant, J. E., Pittenger, C., & Leckman, J. F. (2013). N-acetylcysteine in the treatment of pediatric trichotillomania: A randomized, double-blind, placebo-controlled add-on trial. *Journal of the American Academy of Child and Adolescent Psychiatry, 52*(3), 231–240. https://doi.org/10.1016/j.jaac.2012.12.020

Bloch, M. H., Peterson, B. S., Scahill, L., Otka, J., Katsovich, L., Zhang, H., & Leckman, J. F. (2006). Adulthood outcome of tic and obsessive-compulsive symptom severity in children with Tourette syndrome. *Archives of Pediatrics and Adolescent Medicine, 160*, 65–69. https://doi.org/10.1001/archpedi.160.1.65

Blount, T. H., & Raj, J. J. (2018). Intensive outpatient comprehensive behavioral intervention for tics: A clinical replication series. *Cognitive and Behavioral Practice, 25*, 156–167.

Brandt, V. C., Beck, C., Sajin, V., Baaske, M. K., Bäumer, T., Beste, C., Anders, S., &Münchau, A. (2016). Temporal relationship between premonitory urges and tics in Gilles de la Tourette syndrome. *Cortex, 77*, 24–37. https://doi.org/10.1016/j.cortex.2016.01.008

Capriotti, M. R., Brandt, B. C., Turkel, J. E., Lee, H. J., & Woods, D. W. (2014). Negative reinforcement and premonitory urges in youth with Tourette syndrome: An experimental evaluation. *Behavior Modification, 38*(2), 276–296. https://doi.org/10.1177/0145445514531015

Chen, C. W., Wang, H. S., Chang H., & Hsuech, C. (2019). Effectiveness of a modified comprehensive behavioral intervention for tics for children and adolescents with Tourette's syndrome: A randomized controlled trial. *Journal of Advanced Nursing, 76*, 903–915. https://doi.org/10.1111/jan.14279

Conelea, C. A., Ramanujam, K., Walther, M. R., Freeman, J. B., & Garcia, A. M. (2014). Is there a relationship between tic frequency and physiological arousal? Examination in a sample of children with co-occurring tic and anxiety disorders. *Behavior Modification, 38*(2), 217–234. https://doi.org/10.1177/0145445514528239

Conelea, C. A., & Woods, D. W. (2008). The influence of contextual factors on tic expression in Tourette's syndrome: A review. *Journal of Psychosomatic Research, 65*, 487–496. https://doi.org/10.1016/j.jpsychores.2008.04.010

Conelea, C. A., Woods, D. W., & Brandt, B. C. (2011). The impact of a stress induction task on tic frequencies in youth with Tourette Syndrome. *Behaviour Research and Therapy, 49*, 492–497. https://doi.org/10.1016/j.brat.2011.05.006

De Sousa, A. (2008). An open-label pilot study of naltrexone in childhood-onset trichotillomania. *Journal of Child and Adolescent Psychopharmacology, 18*(1), 30–33. https://doi.org/10.1089/cap.2006.0111

Döpfner, M., & Rothenberger, A. (2007). Behavior therapy in tic-disorders with co-existing ADHD. *European Child and Adolescent Psychiatry, 16,* 89–99. https://doi.org/10.1007/s00787-007-1011-7

Dreison, K. C., & Lagges, A. A. (2017). Effectiveness of the Comprehensive Behavioral Intervention for Tics (CBIT) in a pediatric psychiatry clinic: A retrospective chart review. *Clinical Practice in Pediatric Psychology, 5*(2), 180–185. https://doi.org/10.1037/cpp0000189

Duke, D. C., Keeley, M. L., Geffken, G. R., & Storch, E. A. (2010). Trichotillomania: A current review. *Clinical Psychology Review, 30*(2), 181–193. https://doi.org/10.1016/j.cpr.2009.10.008

Eapen, V., Cavanna, A. E., & Robertson, M. M. (2016). Comorbidities, social impact, and quality of life in Tourette syndrome. *Frontiers in Psychiatry, 7,* 97. https://doi.org/10.3389/fpsyt.2016.00097

Eddy, C., Rizzo, R., Gulisano, M., Agodi, A., Barchitta, M., Calì, P., Robertson, M. M., & Cavanna, A. E. (2011). Quality of life in young people with Tourette syndrome: A controlled study. *Journal of Neurology, 258,* 291–301. https://doi.org/10.1007/s00415-010-5754-6

Espil, F., Woods, D. W., Specht, M., Bennett, S. M., Walkup, J. T., Ricketts, E. J., McGuire, J. F., Stiede, J. T., Schild, J. S., Chang, S. W., Peterson, A. L., Scahill, L., Wilhelm, S., &Piacentini, J. (2021). Long-term outcomes of behavior therapy for youth with Tourette disorder.[Manuscript submitted for publication].

Farhat, L. C., Olfson, E., Nasir, M., Levine, J. L., Li, F., Miguel, E. C., & Bloch, M. H. (2020). Pharmacological and behavioral treatment for trichotillomania: An updated systematic review with meta-analysis. *Depression and Anxiety, 37,* 715–727. https://doi.org/10.1002/da.23028

Fine, K. M., Walther, M. R., Joseph, J. M., Robinson, J., Ricketts, E. J., Bowe, W. E., & Woods, D. W. (2012). Acceptance-Enhanced Behavior Therapy for Trichotillomania in adolescents. *Cognitive and Behavioral Practice, 19*(3), 463–471. https://doi.org/10.1016/j.cbpra.2011.10.002

Flessner, C. A., Conelea, C. A., Woods, D. W., Franklin, M. E., Keuthen, N. J., & Cashin, S. E. (2008). Styles of pulling in trichotillomania: Exploring differences in symptom severity, phenomenology, and functional impact. *Behaviour Research and Therapy, 46*(3), 345–357. https://doi.org/10.1016/j.brat.2007.12.009

Flessner, C. A., Miltenberger, R. G., Egemo, K., Kelso, P., Jostad, C., Johnson, B., Gatheridge, B. J., & Neighbors, C. (2005). An evaluation of the social support component of simplified habit reversal. *Behavior Therapy, 36,* 35–42. https://doi.org/10.1016/S0005-7894(05)80052-8

Flessner, C. A., Penzel, F., & Keuthen, N. J. (2010). Current treatment practices for children and adults with trichotillomania: Consensus among experts. *Cognitive and Behavioral Practice, 17*(3), 290–300. https://doi.org/10.1016/j.cbpra.2009.10.006

Flessner, C. A., Woods, D. W., Franklin, M. E., Cashin, S. E., Keuthen, N. J., Mansueto, C. S., Lerner, E., Penzel, F., Golomb, R., Mouton-Odum, S., Novak, C., O'Sullivan, R. L., Pauls, D., Piacentini, J., Stein, D., Thienemann, M., Walkup, J. T., & Wright, H. H. (2008). The Milwaukee Inventory for Subtypes of Trichotillomania-Adult Version

(MIST-A): Development of an instrument for the assessment of "focused" and "automatic" hair pulling. *Journal of Psychopathology and Behavioral Assessment, 30*(1), 20–30. https://doi.org/10.1007/s10862-007-9073-x

Franklin, M. E., Edson, A. L., & Freeman, J. B. (2010). Behavior therapy for pediatric trichotillomania: Exploring the effects of age on treatment outcome. *Child and Adolescent Psychiatry and Mental Health, 4,* 18. https://doi.org/10.1186/1753-2000-4-18

Franklin, M. E., Flessner, C. A., Woods, D. W., Keuthen, N. J., Piacentini, J. C., Moore, P., Stein, D. J., Cohen, S. B., & Wilson, M. A. (2008). The child and adolescent trichotillomania impact project: Descriptive psychopathology, comorbidity, functional impairment, and treatment utilization. *Journal of Developmental and Behavioral Pediatrics, 29*(6), 493–500. https://doi.org/10.1097/DBP.0b013e31818d4328

Franklin, M. E., & Tolin, D. F. (2007). Treating trichotillomania: Cognitive-behavioral therapy for hair pulling and related problems. In *Treating trichotillomania: Cognitive-behavioral therapy for hair pulling and related problems.* Springer Science + Business Media.

Gev, E., Pilowsky-Peleg, T., Fennig, S., Benaroya-Milshtein, N., Woods, D. W., Piacentini, J., Apter, A., & Steinberg, T. (2016). Acceptance of premonitory urges and tics. *Journal of Obsessive-Compulsive and Related Disorders, 10,* 78–83. https://doi.org/10.1016/j.jocrd.2016.06.001

Grant, J. E., & Chamberlain, S. R. (2016). Trichotillomania. *American Journal of Psychiatry, 173*(9), 868–874. https://doi.org/10.1176/appi.ajp.2016.15111432

Grant, J. E., Redden, S. A., & Chamberlain, S. R. (2019). Milk thistle treatment for children and adults with trichotillomania: A double-blind, placebo-controlled, crossover negative study. *Journal of Clinical Psychopharmacology, 39*(2), 129–134. https://doi.org/10.1097/JCP.0000000000001005

HabitAware. (2020). *How Keen works.* HabitAware. https://habitaware.com/pages/how-it-works

Himle, M. B., Flessner, C. A., & Woods, D. W. (2004). Advances in the behavior analytic treatment of trichotillomania and Tourette's Syndrome. *Journal of Early and Intensive Behavior Intervention, 1,* 57–64. https://doi.org/10.1037/h0100282

Himle, M. B., Freitag, M., Walther, M., Franklin, S. A., Laura, E., & Woods, D. W. (2012). A randomized pilot trial comparing videoconferences versus face-to-face delivery of behavioral therapy for childhood tic disorders. *Behavior Research and Therapy, 50,* 565–570. https://doi.org/10.1016/j.brat.2012.05.009

Himle, M. B., Woods, D. W., Conelea, C. A., Bauer, C. C., & Rice, K. A. (2007). Investigating the effects of tic suppression on premonitory urge ratings in children and adolescents with Tourette's syndrome. *Behaviour Research and Therapy, 45,* 2964–2976. https://doi.org/10.1016/j.brat.2007.08.007

Hirschtritt, M. E., Lee, P. C., Pauls, D. L., Dion, Y., Grados, M. A., Illmann, C., King, R. A., Sandor, P., McMahon, W. M., Lyon, G. J., Cath, D. C., Kurlan, R., Robertson, M. M., Osiecki, L., Scharf, J. M., & Mathews, C. A. (2015). Lifetime prevalence, age of risk, and genetic relationships of comorbid psychiatric disorders in Tourette syndrome. *JAMA Psychiatry, 72*(4), 325–333. https://doi.org/10.1001/jamapsychiatry.2014.2650

Kendall, P. C., & Frank, H. (2018). Implementing evidence-based treatment protocols: Flexibility within fidelity. *Clinical Psychology: Science and Practice, 25,* 1–12. doi: 10.1111/cpsp.12271.

Kendall, P. C., & Beidas, R. (2007). Smoothing the trail for dissemination of evidence-based practices for youth: Flexibility within fidelity. *Professional Psychology: Research and Practice, 38*, 13–20.

Keuthen, N. J., Rothbaum, B. O., Fama, J., Altenburger, E., Falkenstein, M. J., Sprich, S. E., Kearns, M., Meunier, S., Jenike, M. A., & Welch, S. S. (2012). DBT-enhanced cognitive-behavioral treatment for trichotillomania: A randomized controlled trial. *Journal of Behavioral Addictions, 1*(3), 106–114. https://doi.org/10.1556/JBA.1.2012.003

Keuthen, N. J., & Sprich, S. E. (2012). Utilizing DBT skills to augment traditional CBT for trichotillomania: An adult case study. *Cognitive and Behavioral Practice, 19*(2), 372–380. https://doi.org/10.1016/j.cbpra.2011.02.004

King, R. A., Zohar, A. H., Ratzoni, G., Binder, M., Kron, S., Dycian, A., Cohen, D. J., Pauls, D. L., & Apter, A. (1995). An epidemiological study of trichotillomania in Israeli adolescents. *Journal of the American Academy of Child and Adolescent Psychiatry, 34*(9), 1212–1215. https://doi.org/10.1097/00004583-199509000-00019

Labouliere, C. D., & Storch, E. A. (2012). Pediatric trichotillomania: Clinical presentation, treatment, and implications for nursing professionals. *Journal of Pediatric Nursing, 27*(3), 225–232. https://doi.org/10.1016/j.pedn.2011.01.028

Lamothe, H., Baleyte, J. M., Mallet, L., & Pelissolo, A. (2020). Trichotillomania is more related to Tourette disorder than to obsessive-compulsive disorder. *Brazilian Journal of Psychiatry, 42*, 87–104. https://doi.org/10.1590/1516-4446-2019-0471

Lebowitz, E. R., Motlagh, M. G., Katsovich, L., King, R. A., Lombroso, P. J., Grantz, H., Lin, H., Bentley, M. J., Gilbert, D. L., Singer, H. S., Coffey, B. J., Kurlan, R. M., &Leckman, J. F. (2012). Tourette syndrome in youth with and without obsessive compulsive disorder and attention deficit hyperactivity disorder. *European Child and Adolescent Psychiatry, 21*, 451–457. https://doi.org/10.1007/s00787-012-0278-5

Leckman, J. F., Walker, D. E., & Cohen, D. J. (1993). Premonitory urges in Tourette's syndrome. *American Journal of Psychiatry, 150*, 98–102. https://doi.org/10.1176/ajp.150.1.98

Leckman, J. F., Zhang, H., Vitale, A., Lahnin, F., Lynch, K., Bondi, C., Kim, Y. S., &Peterson, B. S. (1998). Course of tic severity in Tourette syndrome: The first two decades. *Pediatrics, 102*, 14–19. https://doi.org/10.1542/peds.102.1.14

Lee, E. B., Homan, K. J., Morrison, K. L., Ong, C. W., Levin, M. E., & Twohig, M. P. (2020). Acceptance and Commitment Therapy for trichotillomania: A randomized controlled trial of adults and adolescents. *Behavior Modification, 44*(1), 70–91. https://doi.org/10.1177/0145445518794366

Lee, H. J., Espil, F. M., Bauer, C. C., Siwiec, S. G., & Woods, D. W. (2018). Computerized response inhibition training for children with trichotillomania. *Psychiatry Research, 262*, 20–27. https://doi.org/10.1016/j.psychres.2017.12.070

Mansueto, C. S., & Keuler, D. J. (2005). Tic or compulsion? It's Tourettic OCD. *Behavior Modification, 29*, 784–799. https://doi.org/10.1177/0145445505279261

Mansueto, C. S., Stemberger, R. M. T., Thomas, A. M., & Golomb, R. G. (1997). Trichotillomania: A comprehensive behavioral model. *Clinical Psychology Review, 17*(5), 567–577. https://doi.org/10.1016/S0272-7358(97)00028-7

McGuire, J. F., Kugler, B. B., Park, J. M., Horng, B., Lewin, A. B., Murphy, T. K., & Storch, E. A. (2012). Evidence-based assessment of compulsive skin picking, chronic tic disorders and trichotillomania in children. *Child Psychiatry and Human Development, 43*(6), pp. 855–883. https://doi.org/10.1007/s10578-012-0300-7

McGuire, J. F., Nyirabahizi, E., Kircanski, K., Piacentini, J., Peterson, A. L., Woods, D. W., Wilhelm, S., Walkup, J. T., & Scahill, L. (2013). A cluster analysis of tic symptoms in children and adults with Tourette syndrome: Clinical correlates and treatment outcome. *Psychiatry Research, 210,* 1198–1204. https://doi.org/10.1016/j.psychres.2013.09.021

McGuire, J. F., Piacentini, J., Scahill, L., Woods, D. W., Villarreal, R., Wilhelm, S., Walkup, J. T., &Peterson, A. L. (2015). Bothersome tics in patients with chronic tic disorders: Characteristics and individualized treatment response to behavior therapy. *Behaviour Research and Therapy, 70,* 56–63. https://doi.org/10.1016/j.brat.2015.05.006

Miltenberger, R. G., Fuqua, R. W., & McKinley, T. (1985). Habit reversal with muscle tics: Replication and component analysis. *Behavior Therapy, 16,* 39–50. https://doi.org/10.1016/S0005-7894(85)80054-X

Morris, S. H., Zickgraf, H. F., Dingfelder, H. E., & Franklin, M. E. (2013). Habit reversal training in trichotillomania: Guide for the clinician. *Expert Review of Neurotherapeutics,13*(9),1069–1077.https://doi.org/10.1586/14737175.2013.827477

Murphy, T. K., Lewin, A. B., Storch, E. A., & Stock, S. (2013). Practice parameter for the assessment and treatment of children and adolescents with tic disorders: Committee on Quality Issues (CQI). *Journal of the American Academy of Child & Adolescent Psychiatry, 52,* 1341–1349. https://doi.org/10.1016/j.jaac.2013.09.015

Nissen, J. B., Partner, E. T., & Thomsen, P. H. (2019). Predictors of therapeutic treatment outcome in adolescent chronic tic disorders. *BJPsych Open, 5,* 1–6. https://doi.org/10.1192/bjo.2019.56

Piacentini, J., Woods, D. W., Scahill, L., Wilhelm, S., Peterson, A. L., Chang, S., Ginsburg, G. S., Deckersbach, T., Dziura, J., Levi-Pearl, S., & Walkup, J. T. (2010). Behavior therapy for children with Tourette disorder: A randomized controlled trial. *JAMA: The Journal of the American Medical Association, 303*(19), 1929–1937. https://doi.org/10.1001/jama.2010.607

Pringsheim, T., Holler-Managan, Y., Koun, M. S., Jankovic, J., Piacentini, J., Cavanna, A. E., Martino, D., Muller-Vahl, K., Woods, D. W., Robinson, M., Jarvie, E., Roessner, V., &Oskoui, M. (2019). Comprehensive systematic review summary: Treatment of tics in people with Tourette syndrome and chronic tic disorders. *American Academy of Neurology, 92,* 907–915. https://doi.org/10.1212/WNL.0000000000007467

Quezada, J., & Coffman, K. A. (2018). Current approaches and new developments in the pharmacological management of Tourette syndrome. *CNS Drugs, 32,* 33–45. https://doi.org/10.1007/s40263-017-0486-0

Rahman, O., McGuire, J., Storch, E. A., & Lewin, A. B. (2017). Preliminary randomized controlled trial of habit reversal training for treatment of hair pulling in youth. *Journal of Child and Adolescent Psychopharmacology, 27*(2), 132–139. https://doi.org/10.1089/cap.2016.0085

Reese, H. E., Vallejo, Z., Rasmussen, J., Crowe, K., Rosenfield, E., & Wilhelm, S. (2015). Mindfulness-based stress reduction for Tourette syndrome and chronic tic disorder: A pilot study. *Journal of Psychosomatic Research, 78,* 293–298. https://doi.org/10.1016/j.jpsychores.2014.08.001

Ricketts, E. J., Gilbert, D. L., Zinner, S. H., Mink, J. W., Lipps, T. D., Wiegand, G. A., Vierhile, A. E., Ely, L. J., Piacentini, J., Walkup, J. T., Woods, D. W. (2016). Pilot testing behavior therapy for chronic tic disorders in neurology and developmental pediatrics clinics. *Journal of Child Neurology, 31*(4), 444–450. https://doi.org/10.1177/0883073815599257

Ricketts, E. J., Goetz, A. R., Capriotti, M. R., Bauer, C. C., Brei, N. G., Himle, M. B., Espil, F. M., Snorrason, I., Ran, D., Woods, D. W. (2016). A randomized waitlist-controlled pilot trial of voice over Internet protocol-delivered behavior therapy for youth with chronic tic disorders. *Journal of Telemedicine and Telecare, 22*, 153–162. https://doi.org/10.1177/1357633X15593192

Ricketts, E. J., Snorrason, I., Kircanski, K., Alexander, J. R., Stiede, J. T., Thamrin, H., Flessner, C. A., Franklin, M. E., Keuthen, N. J., Walther, M. R., Piacentini, J., Stein, D. J., & Woods, D. W. (2019). A latent profile analysis of age of onset in trichotillomania. *Annals of Clinical Psychiatry: Official Journal of the American Academy of Clinical Psychiatrists, 31*(3), 169–178.

Rizzo, R., Gulisano, M., Cali, P. V., & Curatolo, P. (2012). Long term clinical course of Tourette syndrome. *Brain & Development, 34*, 667–673. https://doi.org/10.1016/j.braindev.2011.11.006

Robertson, M. M. (2015). A personal 35 year perspective on Gilles de la Tourette syndrome: Prevalence, phenomenology, comorbidities, and coexistent psychopathologies. *The Lancet Psychiatry, 2*, 68–87. https://doi.org/10.1016/S2215-0366(14)00132-1

Sambrani, T., Jakubovski, E., & Muller-Vahl, K. R. (2016). New insights into clinical characteristics of Gilles de la Tourette syndrome: Findings in 1032 patients from a single German center. *Frontiers in Neuroscience, 10*, 415. https://doi.org/10.3389/fnins.2016.00415

Santhanam, R., Fairley, M., & Rogers, M. (2008). Is it trichotillomania? Hair pulling in childhood: A developmental perspective. *Clinical Child Psychology and Psychiatry, 13*(3), 409–418. https://doi.org/10.1177/1359104508090604

Scahill, L., Aman, M. G., McDougle, C. J., Arnold, L. E., McCracken, J. T., Handen, B., Johnson, C., Dziura, J., Butter, E., Sukhodolsky, D., Swiezy, N., Mulick, J., Stigler, K., Bearss, K., Ritz, L., Wagner, A., & Vitiello, B. (2009). Trial design challenges when combining medication and parent training in children with pervasive developmental disorders. *Journal of Autism and Developmental Disorders, 39*, 720–729. https://doi.org/10.1007/s10803-008-0675-2

Scahill, L., Specht, M., & Page, C. (2014). The prevalence of tic disorders and clinical characteristics in children. *Journal of Obsessive-Compulsive and Related Disorders, 3*, 394–400. https://doi.org/10.1016/j.jocrd.2014.06.002

Scharf, J. M., Miller, L. L., Gauvin, C. A., Alabiso, J., Mathews C. A., & Ben-Shlomo, Y. (2015). Population prevalence of Tourette syndrome: A systematic review and meta-analysis. *Movement Disorders, 30*, 221–228. https://doi.org/10.1002/mds.26089

Shapiro, E., Shapiro, A. K., Fulop, G., Hubbard, M., Mandeli, J., Nordlie, J., & Phillips, R. A. (1989). Controlled study of haloperidol, pimozide, and placebo for the treatment of Gilles de la Tourette's syndrome. *Archives of General Psychiatry, 46*, 722–730.

Slikboer, R., Nedeljkovic, M., Bowe, S. J., & Moulding, R. (2017). A systematic review and meta-analysis of behaviourally based psychological interventions and pharmacological interventions for trichotillomania. *Clinical Psychologist, 21*(1), 20–32. https://doi.org/10.1111/cp.12074

Snorrason, I., Walther, M. R., Elkin, T. D., & Woods, D. W. (2016). Treating trichotillomania (hair-pulling disorder) in a child. *Journal of Clinical Psychology, 72*(11), 1200–1208. https://doi.org/10.1002/jclp.22399

Specht, M. W., Woods, D. W., Piacentini, J., Scahill, L., Wilhelm, S., Peterson, A. L., Chang, S., Kepley, H., Deckersbach, T., Flessner, C., Buzzella, B. A., McGuire, J. F., Levi-Pearl, S., & Walkup, J. T. (2011). Clinical characteristics of children and adolescents with a primary tic disorder. *Journal of Developmental and Physical Disabilities, 23*, 15–31. https://doi.org/10.1007/s10882-010-9223-z

Steeves, T., McKinlay, B. D., Gorman, D., Billinguist, L. Day, L., Carroll, A., Dion, Y., Doja, A., Luscombe, S., Sandor, P., & Pringsheim, T. (2012). Canadian guidelines for the evidence-based treatment of tic disorders: Behavioural therapy, deep brain simulation, and transcranial magnetic stimulation. *The Canadian Journal of Psychiatry, 57*, 144–151. https://doi.org/10.1177/070674371205700303

Stein, D. J., Grant, J. E., Franklin, M. E., Keuthen, N., Lochner, C., Singer, H. S., & Woods, D. W. (2010). Trichotillomania (hair pulling disorder), skin picking disorder, and stereotypic movement disorder: Toward DSM-V. *Depression and Anxiety, 27*(6), 611–626. https://doi.org/10.1002/da.20700

Storch, E. A., Merlo, L. J., Lack, C., Milsom, V. A., Geffken, G. R., Goodman, W. K., & Murphy, T. K. (2007). Quality of life in youth with Tourette's syndrome and chronic tic disorder. *Journal of Clinical and Child Adolescent Psychology, 36*, 217–227. https://doi.org/10.1080/15374410701279545

Sukhodolsky, D. G., Woods, D. W., Piacentini, J. Wilhelm, S. Peterson, A. L., Katsovich, L., Dziura, J., Walkup, J. T., &Scahill, L. (2017). Moderators and predictors of response to behavior therapy for tics in Tourette syndrome. *American Academy of Neurology, 88*, 1029–1036. https://doi.org/10.1212/WNL.0000000000003710

Swedo, S. E., Leonard, H. L., Lenane, M. C., & Rettew, D. C. (1992). Trichotillomania: A profile of the disorder from infancy through adulthood. *International Pediatrics, 7*(2), 144–150.

Tolin, D. F., Franklin, M. E., Diefenbach, G. J., Anderson, E., & Meunier, S. A. (2007). Pediatric trichotillomania: Descriptive psychopathology and an open trial of cognitive behavioral therapy. *Cognitive Behaviour Therapy, 36*(3), 129–144. https://doi.org/10.1080/16506070701223230

Verdellen, C. W. J., Keijsers, G. P. J., Cath, D. C., & Hoogduin, C. A. L. (2004). Exposure with response prevention versus habit reversal in Tourette's syndrome: A controlled study. *Behaviour Research and Therapy, 42*, 501–511. https://doi.org/10.1016/S0005-7967(03)00154-2

Verdellen, C., Van de Griendt, J., Hartmann, A., Murphy, T., Androutsos, C., Aschauer, H., Baird, G., Bos-Veneman, N., Brambilla, A., Cardona, F., Cath, D. C., Cavanna, A. E., Czernecki, V., Dehning, S., Eapter, A., Farkas, L., Gadaros, J., Hauser, E., Heyman, I., Hedderly, T., et al. (2011). European clinical guidelines for Tourette syndrome and other tic disorders. Part III: Behavioural and psychosocial interventions. *European Child and Adolescent Psychiatry, 20*, 197–207. https://doi.org/10.1007/s00787-011-0167-3

Walsh, K. H., & McDougle, C. J. (2012). Trichotillomania: Presentation, etiology, diagnosis and therapy. *American Journal of Clinical Dermatology, 2,* 327–333. https://doi.org/10.2165/00128071-200102050-00007

Walther, M. R., Snorrason, I., Flessner, C. A., Franklin, M. E., Burkel, R., & Woods, D. W. (2014). The trichotillomania impact project in young children (TIP-YC): Clinical characteristics, comorbidity, functional impairment and treatment utilization. *Child Psychiatry and Human Development, 45*(1), 24–31. https://doi.org/10.1007/s10578-013-0373-y

Weisman, H., Qureshi, I. A., Leckman, J. F., Scahill, L., & Bloch, M. H. (2013). Systematic review: Pharmacological treatment of tic disorders—Efficacy of antipsychotic and alpha-2 adrenergic agonist agents. *Neuroscience and Biobehavioral Reviews, 37,* 1162–1171. https://doi.org/10.1016/j.neubiorev.2012.09.008

Welch, S. S., & Kim, J. (2012). DBT-enhanced cognitive behavioral therapy for adolescent trichotillomania: An adolescent case study. *Cognitive and Behavioral Practice, 19*(3), 483–493. https://doi.org/10.1016/j.cbpra.2011.11.002

Wilhelm, S., Peterson, A. L., Piacentini, J., Woods, D. W., Deckersbach, T., Sukhodolsky, D. G., Chang, S., Liu, H., Dziura, J., Walkup, J. T., & Scahill, L. (2012). Randomized trial of behavior therapy for adults with Tourette syndrome. *Archives of General Psychiatry, 69*(8), 795–803. https://doi.org/10.1001/archgenpsychiatry.2011.1528

Woods, D. W., & Miltenberger, R. G. (1996). A review of habit reversal with childhood habit disorders. *Education and Treatment of Children, 19*(2), 197–214.

Woods, D. W., Miltenberger, R. G., & Lumley, V. A. (1996). Sequential application of major habit-reversal components to treat motor tics in children. *Journal of Applied Behavior Analysis, 29*(4), 483–493. https://doi.org/10.1901/jaba.1996.29-483

Woods, D. W., Piacentini, J. C., Chang, S. W., Deckersbach, T., Ginsburg, G. S., Peterson, A. L., Scahill, L. D., Walkup, J. T., Wilhelm, S. (2008). *Managing Tourette syndrome: A behavioral intervention for children and adults.* Oxford University Press.

Woods, D. W., & Twohig, M. P. (2008). *Trichotillomania: An ACT-enhanced behavior therapy approach therapist guide.* Oxford University Press.

For the benefit of digital users, indexed terms that span two pages (e.g., 52–53) may, on occasion, appear on only one of those pages.

References to tables, figures, and boxes have an italic *t*, *f*, or *b* following the page number.